T0293389

Materials Design and Clinical Perspectives in Drug Delivery

Materials Design and Clinical Perspectives in Drug Delivery

Editor: Michael Mason

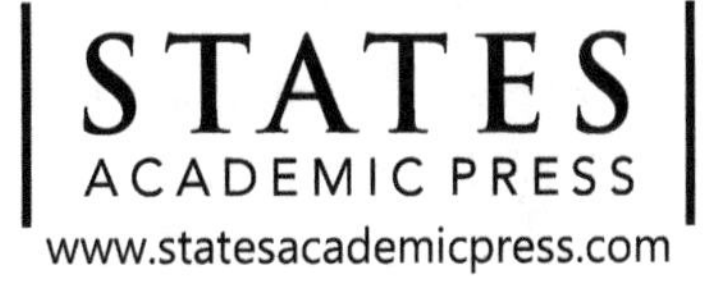

www.statesacademicpress.com

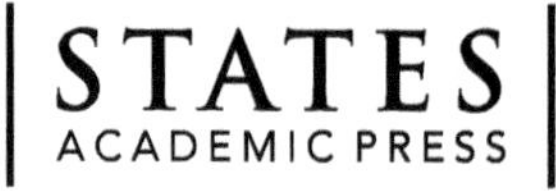

Cataloging-in-Publication Data

Materials design and clinical perspectives in drug delivery / edited by Michael Mason.
p. cm.
Includes bibliographical references and index.
ISBN 978-1-63989-798-8
1. Drug delivery systems. 2. Biomedical materials. 3. Drug delivery devices. 4. Drug targeting.
5. Clinical pharmacology. 6. Pharmaceutical technology. I. Mason, Michael.
RS199.5 .M38 2023
615.6--dc23

States Academic Press,
109 South 5th Street,
Brooklyn, NY 11249, USA

ISBN 978-1-63989-798-8 (Hardback)

Contents

Preface

Drug delivery refers to the formulations, storage systems, methods, production processes and technologies used to transport a pharmaceutical compound to its target site for achieving intended therapeutic effect. It aims to change the specificity and pharmacokinetics of the drug by combining it with various drug carriers, excipients and medical devices. The synthesis and design of effective drug delivery systems (DDS) is critical for healthcare and medicine. Nanotechnology and materials innovation are utilized together for making improvements in drug delivery. Liposomes, hydrogels, micelles and thin films with distinct biological and mechanical properties are used as carriers in novel drug delivery systems. Poly glycol acid (PGA) and their copolymers, poly lactide-co-glycolide (PLGA) as well as poly lactic acid (PLA) are some of the materials most frequently utilized in DDS development due to their properties of biocompatibility, biodegradability and ease of processing. This book provides comprehensive insights into materials design and clinical perspectives in drug delivery. Its extensive content provides the readers with a thorough understanding of the subject.

After months of intensive research and writing, this book is the end result of all who devoted their time and efforts in the initiation and progress of this book. It will surely be a source of reference in enhancing the required knowledge of the new developments in the area. During the course of developing this book, certain measures such as accuracy, authenticity and research focused analytical studies were given preference in order to produce a comprehensive book in the area of study.

This book would not have been possible without the efforts of the authors and the publisher. I extend my sincere thanks to them. Secondly, I express my gratitude to my family and well-wishers. And most importantly, I thank my students for constantly expressing their willingness and curiosity in enhancing their knowledge in the field, which encourages me to take up further research projects for the advancement of the area.

Editor

1

Design of Paracetamol Delivery Systems Based on Functionalized Ordered Mesoporous Carbons

Joanna Goscianska [1,*], Aleksander Ejsmont [1], Anna Olejnik [1], Dominika Ludowicz [2], Anna Stasiłowicz [2] and Judyta Cielecka-Piontek [2,*]

[1] Department of Chemical Technology, Faculty of Chemistry, Adam Mickiewicz University in Poznań, Uniwersytetu Poznańskiego 8, 61-614 Poznań, Poland; aleejs@amu.edu.pl (A.E.); annamar@amu.edu.pl (A.O.)

[2] Department of Pharmacognosy, Faculty of Pharmacy, Poznań University of Medical Sciences, Święcickiego 4, 61-781 Poznań, Poland; dominika.siakowska@interia.eu (D.L.); astasilowicz@ump.edu.pl (A.S.)

* Correspondence: asiagosc@amu.edu.pl (J.G.); jpiontek@ump.edu.pl (J.C.-P.)

Abstract: The oxidized ordered mesoporous carbons of cubic and hexagonal structure obtained by two templating methods (soft and hard) were applied for the first time as delivery systems for paracetamol—the most common antipyretic and analgesic drug in the world. The process of carbon oxidation was performed using an acidic ammonium persulfate solution at 60 °C for 6 h. The functionalization was found to reduce the specific surface area and pore volume of carbon materials, but it also led to an increasing number of acidic oxygen-containing functional groups. The most important element and the novelty of the presented study was the evaluation of adsorption and release ability of carbon carriers towards paracetamol. It was revealed that the sorption capacity and the drug release rate were mainly affected by the materials' textural parameters and the total amount of surface functional groups, notably different in pristine and oxidized samples. The adsorption of paracetamol on the surface of ordered mesoporous carbons occurred according to different mechanisms: donor–acceptor complexes and hydrogen bond formation. The adsorption kinetics was assessed using pseudo-first- and pseudo-second-order models. The regression results indicated that the adsorption kinetics was more accurately represented by the pseudo-second-order model. Paracetamol was adsorbed onto the carbon materials studied following the Langmuir type isotherm. The presence of oxygen-containing functional groups on the surface of ordered mesoporous carbons enhanced the amount of paracetamol adsorbed and its release rate. The optimal drug loading capacity and expected release pattern exhibited oxidized ordered mesoporous carbon with a hexagonal structure obtained by the hard template method.

Keywords: carbon carriers; active pharmaceutical ingredients; adsorption of paracetamol; kinetic modelling; permeability study

---

1. Introduction

The ever-increasing cost of the development of new therapeutic drugs, the long time it takes for their introduction onto the market, and the high risk of failure in clinical trials have stimulated efforts directed to the design of delivery systems of already known active pharmaceutical ingredients (APIs) with well-defined safety profiles and physicochemical properties [1]. Therefore, a lot of attention in the latest years has been given to develop and produce stable and selective API carriers. The use of an appropriate carrier and suitable method of active pharmaceutical ingredient incorporation into its structure can bring an improvement in the API bioavailability, prevent its recrystallization, limit the side effects, and lengthen the activity time in the human body [1–3]. Miscellaneous drug carriers have been developed and investigated, each of which has distinctive advantages. The most popular types of pharmaceutical vehicles include liposomes, lipid and metal nanoparticles, carbon nanotubes, mesoporous carbons, metal–organic frameworks (MOFs), and mesoporous silica of different structures such as MCM-41, MCM-48, SBA-15, and SBA-16 [1–10]. Amidst them, especially highly biocompatible ordered mesoporous carbons (OMCs) containing pores with a size ranging from 2 to 50 nm, which form a two- or three-dimensional network, can precisely tune the drug release rate and thus prolong its therapeutic effect [7,8]. Their peculiar features can be achieved in two main synthetic procedures, including hard template [11–13] (also called nanocasting) or soft template methods [14]. In the nanocasting, the ordered mesoporous silica (OMS) or zeolites are used as scaffolds. They are initially impregnated with precursors rich in carbon (e.g., sugars, furfuryl alcohol) and then carbonized at high temperature. In the last step, the matrices are removed by strong base or hydrofluoric acid [11–13]. Contrarily, in the soft template procedure, the OMCs are synthesized by co-assembly of carbon precursors (phenolic resins) and triblock copolymers (organic surfactants), which are subjected to carbonization [14]. After carbonization, the ordered mesoporous carbons are obtained that, depending on the selected method, are different not only in structure, but also in pores' ordering, morphology, and uniformity. Such materials are featured by well-developed specific surface area, large pore volume, and very good mechanical, thermal, and chemical stability. It allows for a wide range of post-synthetic modifications/functionalizations to proceed, for example, via grafting [15], impregnation [16], and sulfonation [17], but mostly through diverse oxidation [18–20]. Different oxidizing agents at varied temperatures enrich OMCs' surface in additional functional groups [21]. During such processes, it is important to preserve the material ordered structure and enhance their sorption capabilities towards the required adsorbate. Active pharmaceutical ingredients are especially challenging adsorbate because their bioavailability depends on many aspects that the drug carrier is supposed to maintain. Pharmaceutics usually exhibit low solubility, chemical lability, or poor permeability through biological membranes [22]. Therefore, the carriers applied have to be stable in aqueous media, harmless in biological systems, and should have a good affinity towards API. Moreover, the drug should also have the ability to release from the vehicle in required environment in the controlled manner [23–26]. In this study, paracetamol (also known as acetaminophen) was used as a model drug. This medicine is commonly applied to treat fever, cold and flu symptoms (when combined with decongestants and antihistamines), and mild and moderate pain [27]. Paracetamol is also recommended to control the fever symptoms of patients with coronavirus disease 2019 (COVID-19), who require conservative management and palliative care [28,29]. The overdosage of paracetamol may be responsible for liver damage, resulting in hepatic necroses. Acetaminophen is available in different forms, including capsules, tablets, liquids, soluble powders, and suppositories [27]. Furthermore, paracetamol can be delivered into the systemic blood from modified or immediate-release formulations. In order to control its dissolution over a certain time, it is essential to develop an appropriate vehicle that will improve drug efficiency. Therefore, the aim of the presented research was to synthesize pristine and oxidized ordered mesoporous carbons (ox-OMCs) of a different structure by the hard and soft template method and apply them as a novel platform for paracetamol. It is worth noting that, by tuning the type of carbon structure and introducing oxygen functionalities, it is possible to modulate the course of the drug release processes. Paracetamol has a relatively short half-life (4 h) and low solubility; therefore, the development of a carrier that will increase drug solubility and prolong its half-life was the target of this study. The effort was devoted to developing new nanomaterial-based therapeutics that will provide better drug release control.

2. Materials and Methods

2.1. Preparation of Mesoporous Carbon Carriers via Hard Template Method

The hard template method was used to synthesize ordered mesoporous carbons $C_{KIT\text{-}6}$ (cubic structure) and $C_{SBA\text{-}15}$ (hexagonal structure). In the first stage, OMS matrices KIT-6 and SBA-15 were prepared according to the reported procedures [5,6].

In the hydrothermal synthesis of KIT-6, the triblock copolymer Pluronic P123 (4 g, $EO_{20}PO_{70}EO_{20}$, Aldrich, St. Louis, MO, USA) was dissolved in the acidic solution (144 g of distilled water and 7.9 g of hydrochloric acid, Avantor Performance Materials Poland S.A.) at 35 °C. Subsequently, butan-1-ol (4 g, POCh) and tetraethyl orthosilicate (8.6 g, 98% wt, Aldrich) were added. The prepared solution was intensively mixed for 24 h at 35 °C and subjected to hydrothermal treatment for 24 h at 100 °C. The received precipitate was filtered, washed three times with distilled water, and dried in the oven at 100 °C overnight. The removal of triblock copolymer proceeded through calcination at 550 °C for 8 h.

The substrates for SBA-15 preparation were triblock copolymer Pluronic P123 (0.5 g, Aldrich), hydrochloric acid (19 mL, 1.6 mol/L, Avantor Performance Materials Poland S.A.), and TEOS (1.1 mL, tetraethyl orthosilicate, 98% wt., Aldrich). To an aqueous hydrochloric acid solution of Pluronic P123 maintained at 35 °C, TEOS was added dropwise upon stirring continuously for 6 h. Then, the as-prepared mixture was subjected to hydrothermal treatment in tightly closed polypropylene bottles in an oven for 24 h at 35 °C as a first stage, and for 6 h at 100 °C as a second stage. Then, the material obtained was filtered, washed three times, and dried at 100 °C for 12 h. Lastly, to remove the template, it was calcined for 8 h at 550 °C.

KIT-6 and SBA-15 silica materials were subjected to twice repeated impregnation with a sucrose solution. An exactly weighted portion of sucrose (1.25 g, Aldrich) was dissolved in sulfuric(VI) acid (0.14 mL, Avantor Performance Materials Poland S.A., Gleiwitz, Poland) and distilled water (5 mL). Next, as-prepared solution was added slowly to the flask containing OMS. The contents were heated in the oven firstly for 6 h at 100 °C, and then for 6 h at 160 °C. Afterwards, the obtained silica–carbon composites were treated again with a solution containing sucrose (0.8 g), sulfuric(VI) acid (0.09 mL), and distilled water (5 mL). The materials were heated in the oven for 6 h at 100 °C and then for the next 6 h at 160 °C. The composites obtained were carbonized for 3 h at 900 °C, at the temperature increase rate of 2.5 °C/min, and the remaining silica was washed out twice with 200 mL 5% of hydrofluoric acid solution (Avantor Performance Materials Poland S.A.). The materials were collected by filtration, washed with ethanol three times, and dried for 12 h at 100 °C. The carbon materials were labelled as $C_{KIT\text{-}6}$ and $C_{SBA\text{-}15}$, respectively.

2.2. Preparation of Mesoporous Carbon Carriers via Soft Template Method

Mesoporous carbon C_{ST} was obtained via the soft template method based on the co-assembly triblock copolymer Pluronic F127 (Sigma-Aldrich) and carbon precursor—resorcinol (Sigma-Aldrich). In the initial stage, Pluronic F127 (1.875 g) and resorcinol (1.88 g) were dissolved in the solution of ethanol (POCh, 96%) and distilled water (15.38 g, weight ratio C_2H_5OH/H_2O = 10:7) at room temperature and the as-prepared mixture was stirred vigorously. Subsequently, hydrochloric acid (0.14 mL, POCh, 36%) and formaldehyde solution (1.93 mL, Chempur, 37%) were added. The solution was stirred intensively until it became turbid. Two hours later, the two-phased mixture was separated; one (aqueous layer) was removed, while the other (organic layer) was stirred by a magnetic mixer for 72 h. The dark brown monolith received at this stage was subsequently heated up to 100 °C and kept for 24 h in a propylene bottle. Finally, it was carbonized in a tube furnace under nitrogen atmosphere at three stages: 5 h—180 °C, 4 h—400 °C, and 2 h—800 °C.

2.3. Functionalization of Mesoporous Carbon Carriers

OMC carriers were subjected to oxidation using acidic ammonium persulfate solution (APS, Sigma-Aldrich) with a concentration of 1 mol/L as a gentle oxidant. This procedure was applied to generate oxygen functionalities on the carbon surface. In a round-bottomed flask, the carbon materials (0.5 g) were flooded with APS solution (30 mL). The process of oxidation was performed under reflux upon vigorous stirring at 60 °C. After 6 h, the solids were filtered off, washed with ethanol and distilled water, followed by drying at 100 °C overnight. The oxidized carbon samples were denoted as $C_{SBA\text{-}15}$-APS, $C_{KIT\text{-}6}$-APS, and C_{ST}-APS.

2.4. Characterization of Materials

2.4.1. Low-Temperature Nitrogen Sorption

The pore structure of the synthesized carbon carriers was characterized by low-temperature nitrogen adsorption/desorption isotherms measured at −196 °C with the use of a Quantachrome Autosorb IQ apparatus. Before adsorption measurements, the pristine carbon samples were degassed in vacuum at 300 °C for 3 h, while oxidized carbon materials were degassed in vacuum at 150 °C for 3 h. The Brunauer–Emmett–Teller (BET) method was utilized for the determination of the surface areas (S_{BET}) of carbon carriers. The average pore size was estimated from the adsorption branch of isotherm using the Barret–Joyner–Halenda (BJH) method.

2.4.2. Powder X-ray Diffraction

The type and ordering of the mesoporous structure of the carbon carriers were identified by powder X-ray diffraction (XRD). XRD patterns were made at room temperature with a step size 0.02° in the small-angle range using a D8 Advance Diffractometer (Bruker) with the copper $K\alpha 1$ radiation (λ = 1.5406 Å).

2.4.3. Surface Oxygen Functional Groups

The number of surface oxygen functional groups of acidic and basic nature was determined by the Boehm method [30]. In the case of acidic groups, mesoporous material (0.2 g) was suspended in sodium hydroxide solution (25 mL, 0.1 mol/L, Chempur, Karlsruhe, Germany) and agitated at room temperature for 24 h. Afterwards, the liquid was separated from the solid sample by centrifugation for 10 min and titrated with a hydrochloric acid solution (0.1 mol/L, Chempur) in the presence of methyl orange as an indicator. In order to establish the total content of basic oxygen groups, the converse procedure was applied.

2.4.4. Infrared Spectroscopy

FT-IR (Fourier-transform infrared) spectra of the carbon materials before and after paracetamol adsorption were registered with the use of a Varian 640-IR spectrometer. The samples were studied in the form of tablets, obtained by pressing a mixture of anhydrous KBr (ca. 0.25 g) and the carbon material (0.3 mg) in a special steel ring, under a pressure of 10 MPa. The analysis was carried out in a wavenumber range of 4000–400 cm^{-1} (at a resolution of 0.5 cm^{-1}; number of scans: 64).

2.5. Paracetamol Adsorption Studies

In order to evaluate the adsorption abilities of the carbon materials towards paracetamol (PAR), a series of its solution was prepared, the concentration of which varied from 5 to 150 mg/L. The samples (0.025 g) were placed in flasks and flooded with 50 mL of a paracetamol solution of a certain concentration, and the contents were shaken in the temperature-controlled orbital shaker (KS 4000i control, IKA, Staufen im Breisgau, Germany) at a fixed shaking rate of 250 rpm over 24 h. After that, the drug solutions were separated from the adsorbents by centrifugation for 10 min and their absorbance was studied with the use of Agilent Cary 60 UV/vis spectrophotometer at the wavelength of 243 nm.

The amount of the paracetamol adsorbed per unit weight of OMCs, q_e (mg/g), was calculated according to the following equation:

$$q_e = \frac{(C_0 - C_e) \cdot V}{m} \tag{1}$$

where C_0 is the initial concentration of paracetamol (mg/L), C_e is the residual concentration of paracetamol (mg/L), V is the volume of the paracetamol solution (L), and m is the mass of the carrier (g).

Analysis of the adsorption data was carried out using Freundlich and Langmuir models [31,32]. The criterion of best fitting is the correlation coefficient R^2. The Langmuir isotherm is described by the following linear equation [31]:

$$\frac{C_e}{q_e} = \frac{1}{q_m K_L} + \frac{C_e}{q_m} \tag{2}$$

where C_e is the equilibrium concentration of paracetamol (mg/L), q_e is the quantity of drug adsorbed onto the adsorbent at equilibrium (mg/g), q_m is the maximum monolayer adsorption capacity of adsorbent (mg/g), and K_L is the Langmuir constant denoting the energy of adsorption and affinity of the binding sites (L/mg).

The linear form of the Freundlich equation is as follows [32]:

$$\ln q_e = \ln K_F + \frac{1}{n} \ln C_e \tag{3}$$

where q_e is the amount of paracetamol adsorbed at equilibrium (mg/g) and C_e is the equilibrium concentration of the drug (mg/L). K_F and n are the Freundlich constants; n gives an indication of how favorable the adsorption process is and K_F (mg/g $(\mathrm{L/mg})^{1/n}$) is related to the adsorption capacity of the adsorbents.

The kinetic studies of paracetamol adsorption were carried out to understand the adsorption rate and mechanism at the solid–liquid interface of mesoporous carbon carriers and drug molecules. In this context, linear forms of the pseudo-first- and pseudo-second-order models were applied to estimate the adsorption process by fitting the experimental data obtained. These models are given in Equations (4) and (5), in the same order [33,34]:

$$\ln(q_e - q_t) = \ln q_e - \frac{k_1 t}{2.303} \tag{4}$$

$$\frac{t}{q_t} = \frac{1}{k_2 q_e^2} + \frac{t}{q_e} \tag{5}$$

where q_e is the amount of the paracetamol adsorbed at equilibrium state (mg/g), q_t is the amount of the paracetamol adsorbed in time (mg/g), k_1 is the rate constant of adsorption in the pseudo-first-order model (min^{-1}), and k_2 is the rate constant of adsorption in the pseudo-second-order model (g/mg min).

2.6. Paracetamol Release Studies

Pure paracetamol and ordered mesoporous carbons with the adsorbed paracetamol were weighed to gelatin capsules placed in the springs in order to sink and prevent flotation on the surface of the medium. The analyses were performed using USP (United States Pharmacopoeia) dissolution paddle apparatus (Agilent 708-DS) in the gastric juice medium (pH 1.2) maintained at 37 °C and stirred at 50 rpm. At the defined time intervals, 5.0 mL of dissolution samples was withdrawn and replaced with an equal volume of temperature-equilibrated medium, and then filtered through a 0.45 µm membrane filter. The changes in concentration of paracetamol were measured using high-performance liquid chromatography (HPLC) with a DAD (Diode Array Detector) detector. The separations were performed using a stationary phase based on a Kinetex-C18 column (100 mm × 2.1 mm; 5 µm) at 37 °C. The mobile phase consisted of 0.1% formic acid and acetonitrile (90:10, *v/v*) with the flow rate of 0.5 mL/min. The injection volume was 5 µL and the detection wavelength was set at 243 nm.

The paracetamol release data were fitted to kinetic models including zero-order (percentage of acetaminophen release versus time), first-order (log of the percentage of acetaminophen remaining versus time), Higuchi's model (percentage of acetaminophen release versus square root of time), the Korsmeyer–Peppas model (log of the percentage of acetaminophen release versus log time), and the Hixson–Crowell model (cube root of the percentage of acetaminophen remaining versus time) [35,36]. Additionally, R^2 was calculated to determine which model follows the selected release profile.

The two-factor values f_1 and f_2 introduced by Moore and Flanner were used to compare dissolution profiles. The f_1 and f_2 values are defined by the following equations:

$$f_1 = \frac{\sum_{j=1}^{n} |R_j - T_j|}{\sum_{j=1}^{n} R_j} \times 100 \tag{6}$$

$$f_2 = 50 \times \log\left(\left(1 + \left(\frac{1}{n}\right)\sum_{j=1}^{n} |R_j - T_j|^2\right)^{-\frac{1}{2}} \times 100\right) \tag{7}$$

where n is the number of time points, R_j is the percentage of the reference dissolved product in the medium, T_j is the percentage of the dissolved tested product, and t is the time point. Dissolution profiles are similar when the f_1 value is close to 0 and f_2 is close to 100 (between 50 and 100); Table 1 [37].

Table 1. Interpretation of f_1 and f_2 factors.

	f_1 (Difference Factor)	f_2 (Similarity Factor)
Identical profiles	0	100
Similar profiles	0–15	50–100
Different profiles	>15	<50

2.7. Permeability Study

In vitro gastrointestinal (GIT) permeability test was performed using PAMPA (parallel artificial membrane permeability assay). The kit consists of a 96-well microfilter plate divided into two chambers, donor and acceptor, separated by a 120 μm thick microfilter disc coated with a 20% (*w*/*v*) dodecane solution of a lecithin mixture (Pion, Inc., Billerica, MA, USA). The samples solutions were added to the donor compartments. After adding the acceptor solution to the acceptor wells, both parts—donor and acceptor—were placed together, and the sandwich was incubated for 3 h at the temperature of 37 °C in a humidity-saturated atmosphere. Afterwards, both chambers were split, and the concentrations of donor and acceptor solutions were measured using UV spectroscopy at 243 nm. The apparent permeability coefficient (P_{app}) was calculated using the following equation:

$$P_{app} = \frac{-ln\left(1 - \frac{C_A}{C_{equilibrium}}\right)}{S \times \left(\frac{1}{V_D} + \frac{1}{V_A}\right) \times t} \tag{8}$$

where V_D is the donor volume; V_A is the acceptor volume; and $C_{equilibrium}$ is the equilibrium concentration, where $C_{equilibrium} = \frac{C_D \times V_D + C_A \times V_A}{V_D + V_A}$, S is the membrane area and t is the incubation time (in seconds). Compounds that have a $P_{app} < 0.1 \times 10^{-6}$ cm/s are referred as ones with low permeability, compounds found to have medium permeability have a 0.1×10^{-6} cm/s $\leq P_{app} < 1 \times 10^{-6}$ cm/s, and compounds with a $P_{app} \geq 1 \times 10^{-6}$ cm/s are classified as ones with high permeability [38].

3. Results and Discussion

3.1. Physicochemical Characterization of Mesoporous Carbon Carriers

Small-angle XRD patterns of OMCs synthesized by hard and soft template methods before and after oxidation with APS are displayed in Figure 1. The diffractogram of the pristine $C_{KIT\text{-}6}$ sample shows a strong peak at $2\Theta \approx 1°$ and less intensive reflections in the range $2\Theta \approx 1.5$–$2.3°$, indicating the presence of an ordered cubic structure with Ia3d symmetry (Figure 1a). On the other hand, in the case of the XRD profile of the carbon $C_{SBA\text{-}15}$, an intensive peak at $2\Theta \approx 1°$ characteristic for hexagonal pore arrangement is noted. Moreover, the reflections at $2\Theta \approx 1.7$–$2.5°$, corresponding to the planes (100), (110), and (200) of p6mm structure, are also observed (Figure 1b). It was established that the use of a gentle oxidant, ammonium persulfate, for functionalization of materials, does not significantly affect the ordering of the cubic and hexagonal mesoporous structure of $C_{KIT\text{-}6}$ and $C_{SBA\text{-}15}$ samples, respectively. Pristine and oxidized carbons obtained by soft templating are characterized by a less ordered mesoporous structure, as evidenced by a low-intensity peak at the angle $2\Theta \approx$ between 0.5 and 1° (Figure 1c). The expected ordering of the 2D mesoporous structure of C_{ST} and C_{ST}-APS is hexagonal; however, it is not possible to determine the symmetry group from the XRD data.

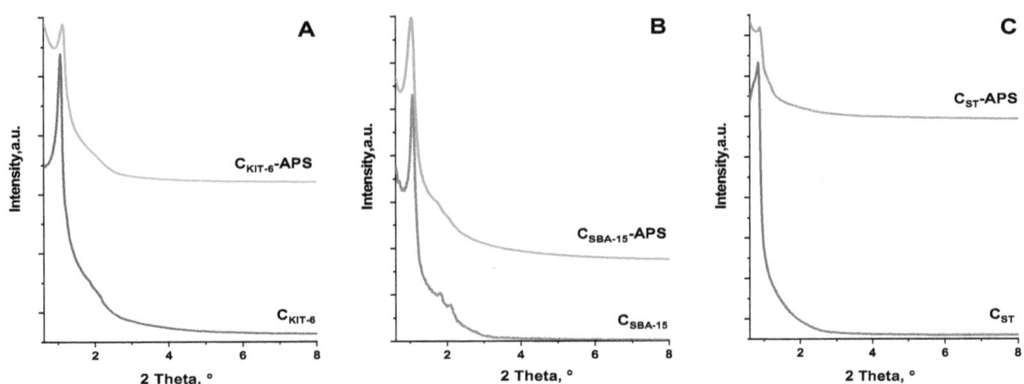

Figure 1. Small-angle X-ray diffraction (XRD) patterns of pristine and oxidized ordered mesoporous carbons (OMCs), (**a**) $C_{KIT\text{-}6}$ and $C_{KIT\text{-}6}$-APS, (**b**) $C_{SBA\text{-}15}$ and $C_{SBA\text{-}15}$-APS, (**c**) C_{ST} and C_{ST}-APS.

The textural features of nanomaterials have a major impact on the mass transport, accessibility of adsorption sites for different active pharmaceutical ingredients, and their adsorption capacity. The data on the specific surface area, pore volume, and size of all mesoporous carbon carriers are collected in Table 2. According to these results, the synthesis of ordered mesoporous carbons $C_{KIT\text{-}6}$ and $C_{SBA\text{-}15}$ on the basis of silica matrices KIT-6 and SBA-15, respectively, provides materials with a well-developed BET surface area ($S_{CKIT\text{-}6}$—1003 m^2/g, $S_{CSBA\text{-}15}$—986 m^2/g) and total pore volume ($V_{CKIT\text{-}6}$—1.15 cm^3/g, $V_{CSBA\text{-}15}$—1.47 cm^3/g). The carbon C_{ST} obtained by the soft templating is characterized by a much smaller specific surface area (526 m^2/g) and pore volume (0.49 cm^3/g). It should be noted that, regardless of the synthesis method used, all materials contain micropores in the structure whose surface area is 306 m^2/g for $C_{KIT\text{-}6}$, 545 m^2/g for $C_{SBA\text{-}15}$, and 231 m^2/g for C_{ST}. They are probably located within the walls of the mesopores. As follows from Table 2, although the mesostructural regularity of the carbonaceous carriers is preserved, after oxidation with APS, their textural parameters deteriorate considerably in comparison with the non-functionalized materials. It is assumed that the modification process with a gentle oxidation agent takes place primarily inside micropore/small mesopore, which may be due to their high potential to easily attach oxygen-containing functional groups. Consequently, the oxygen-containing groups can partially block the pores in the structure of carbon materials, leading to decreasing their volume and surface area.

Table 2. Textural parameters of pristine and oxidized ordered mesoporous carbons (OMCs). BET, Brunauer–Emmett–Teller; APS, ammonium persulfate solution.

Material	BET Surface Area (m^2/g)	Total Pore Volume (cm^3/g)	Average Pore Diameter (nm)	Micropores Surface Area (m^2/g)	Micropore Volume (cm^3/g)
C_{KIT-6}	1003	1.15	5.78	306	0.34
C_{KIT-6}-APS	656	0.89	5.49	252	0.26
C_{SBA-15}	986	1.47	6.54	545	0.61
C_{SBA-15}-APS	689	0.95	5.49	380	0.44
C_{ST}	526	0.49	4.12	231	0.14
C_{ST}-APS	248	0.29	4.67	178	0.12

The surface chemistry of materials has a direct impact on their sorption capacities towards active pharmaceutical ingredients. Figure 2 depicts the content of oxygen functional groups of an acidic and basic nature on the surface of mesoporous carbon carriers determined using the Boehm method [30]. The oxidation of C_{KIT-6}, C_{SBA-15}, and C_{ST} samples with APS causes a significant increase in the amount of acidic groups, which are favorable especially for the adsorption of guest molecules from polar solvents. Interestingly, the total number of acidic groups on the surface of C_{KIT-6}-APS (4.03 mmol/g) and C_{SBA-15}-APS (4.00 mmol/g) materials is similar. The oxidized carbon C_{ST}-APS synthesized by the soft template method contains a lower number of acidic groups (2.11 mmol/g) compared with other oxidized samples. Moreover, it was established that C_{SBA-15}, C_{KIT-6}-APS, and C_{ST}-APS samples do not possess oxygen groups of a basic nature on the surface. In the case of the C_{SBA-15}-APS carbon sample, during the oxidation process with APS solution, a small amount of chromene and pyrone-like groups was generated on its surface. Therefore, an increase in the content of basic functional groups was observed.

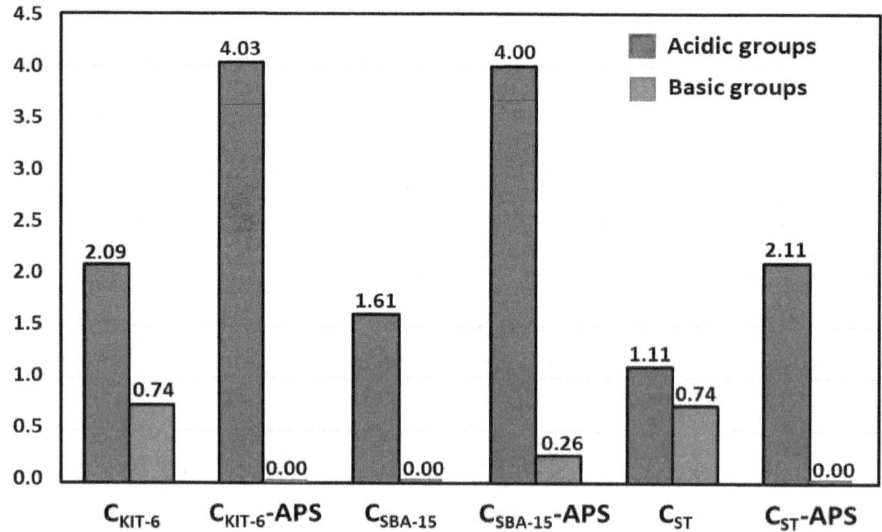

Figure 2. Acid–base properties of pristine and oxidized OMCs.

3.2. Paracetamol Adsorption and Release Studies

For the purpose of setting the time required for reaching equilibrium between the paracetamol molecules and OMCs, the kinetics of adsorption was thoroughly analyzed. As presented in Figure 3, the uptake of the drug molecules was very fast in the first 10 min of the process. This demonstrates that, on the surface of carbonaceous carriers, a large number of vacant adsorption sites occurred, and paracetamol could be adsorbed with ease. With the extending contact time, drug molecules penetrated further and deeper within the pores. They also came across a greater resistance if the process was continued. The adsorption process slowed down considerably. After 60 min, no increase in the amount of adsorbed paracetamol was noted, which means that a state of equilibrium was reached and the limited number of active sites on the OMC samples' surface were engaged. In this study, the experimental data were fitted to the pseudo-first-order kinetic model of Lagergren and pseudo-second-order kinetic model of Ho and McKay [33,34]. The values of k_1 and k_2 constants, correlation coefficients (R^2), and the theoretical amounts of the paracetamol adsorbed ($q_{e(cal)}$) on the surface of carbon materials are collected in Table 3. The k_1 constants were estimated from the plots of $\ln(q_e - q_t)$ versus t, while those of k_2 were estimated from the plots of t/q_t versus t. The low correlation coefficients for the pseudo-first-order model (R^2 = 0.927–0.987; Table 3) exclude the possibility of its application to describe the mechanism of paracetamol adsorption onto mesoporous carbon samples. Moreover, the $q_{e(cal)}$ values calculated on the basis of the linear plots are significantly lower than those corresponding experimental $q_{e(exp)}$ values. The experimental data revealed better consent with the pseudo-second-order kinetic model, suggested by higher correlation coefficient values (R^2 = 0.999; Table 3). It signifies that this kinetic model can be used to predict the amount of drug adsorbed at different contact time intervals by OMCs obtained via hard and soft template methods. It should be mentioned that, according to this model, chemisorption takes place in addition to physisorption. These processes depend on the properties of both the adsorbents and the adsorbates.

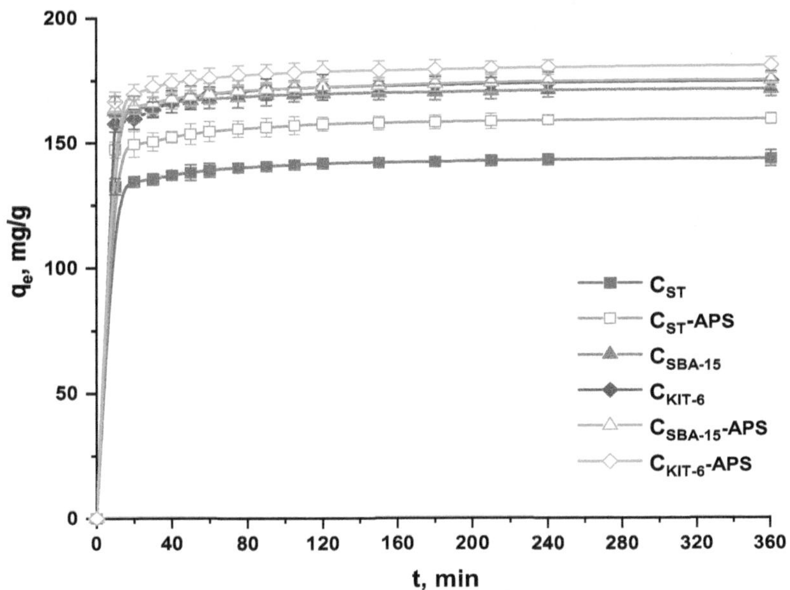

Figure 3. Amount of paracetamol adsorbed on the surface of OMCs as a function of contact time (initial solution concentration of drug—75 mg/L).

Table 3. Pseudo-first-order and pseudo-second-order kinetic model parameters.

Material	$q_{e(exp)}$ (mg/g)	Pseudo-First-Order Model			Pseudo-Second-Order Model		
		$q_{e(cal)}$ (mg/g)	k_1 (min^{-1})	R^2	$q_{e(cal)}$ (mg/g)	k_2 (g/mg·min)	R^2
C_{ST}	143	6.18	0.016	0.942	144	0.003	0.999
C_{ST}-APS	159	9.94	0.019	0.939	161	0.003	0.999
C_{SBA15}	171	7.35	0.018	0.927	172	0.004	0.999
C_{SBA-15}-APS	174	11.93	0.022	0.925	175	0.003	0.999
C_{KIT-6}	174	11.44	0.026	0.987	175	0.003	0.999
C_{KIT-6}-APS	181	10.72	0.023	0.969	182	0.003	0.999

Figure 4 depicts the equilibrium adsorption isotherms of paracetamol onto pristine and ox-OMCs in aqueous solution. It was observed that the amount of paracetamol adsorbed significantly increases with an increasing initial concentration of its solutions until the adsorption reaches a saturation point. This may be due to the occurrence of the dynamic interplay between the adsorbate and the carbon adsorbents taking place on active sites characterized by a progressive affinity for the drug species.

Among the pristine mesoporous carbons, C_{KIT-6} and C_{SBA-15} exhibited higher sorption capacity towards paracetamol than the C_{ST} sample, which is related to their better developed specific surface area and larger pore volume. The type of mesoporous structure does not considerably affect the drug adsorption process. According to the results, the oxidation of carbon materials with the use of APS leads to an increase in their sorption capacity towards paracetamol. Similar results were observed by Liang et al. [39], who detected that, when activated carbon had an acidic character and contained a high concentration of oxygen groups on the surface, more acetaminophen could be loaded into these materials. Therefore, probably the most important factor determining the amount of the adsorbed drug is the content of the oxygen functionalities on the OMC surfaces. During the adsorption of paracetamol, acceptor–donor complexes can be formed between the groups containing free electron pairs (e.g., oxygen in phenolic/carboxylic groups) that are present on the surface of OMCs and the electropositive nitrogen in paracetamol molecules. The paracetamol exhibits proton acceptor and donor groups. However, the resonance-generated changes result in nitrogen passing from the proton acceptor to the donor [40]. Therefore, hydrogen bond interactions can also occur during the drug adsorption process. They will be more intense in mesoporous carbons possessing a higher concentration of proton acceptor functional groups.

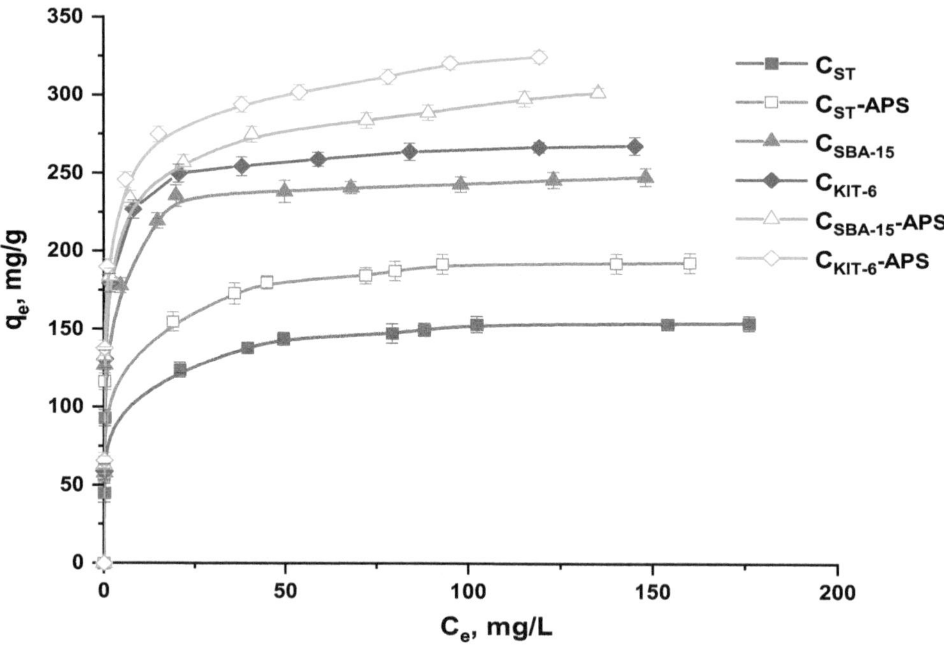

Figure 4. Adsorption isotherms of paracetamol onto pristine and oxidized OMCs.

At the equilibrium of the adsorption process, the adsorption isotherm can be used to estimate the distribution of adsorbate molecules between the liquid and solid phases. In this work, analysis of the experimental results was performed with the use of the Langmuir and Freundlich adsorption models [31,32]. All parameters—q_m, K_L, $1/n$, and K_F—and correlation coefficients R^2 are listed in Table 4. They were computed from the intercept and linear gradient of the graphs of C_e/q_e and C_e for the Langmuir isotherm (Figure 5a) and from the plots of $ln(q_e)$ against $ln(C_e)$ for the Freundlich model (Figure 5b). On the basis of the values of the R^2 correlation coefficient (0.999), it was established that the Langmuir isotherm appropriately describes the results obtained for the adsorption of paracetamol on the surface of pristine and oxidized mesoporous carbon materials. The experimental data revealed that the maximum sorption capacity (q_e) of all synthesized samples towards drug is slightly lower from those estimated theoretically (q_m). On the basis of these results, it can be stated that paracetamol molecules were adsorbed on the surface of carbon materials by forming a homogenous monolayer. The factor $1/n$

Oxidative stress leads the formation of reactive oxygen species (ROS) against the endogenous and exogenous stimuli. Under physiological conditions, ROS are repeatedly generated and eliminated through ROS scavenging systems in order to maintain redox homeostasis. Change in redox balance

Table 4. The parameters calculated from fitting the results of the adsorption isotherms of paracetamol onto pristine and oxidized carbon carriers to the Langmuir and Freundlich models.

Material	Langmuir			Freundlich		
	q_m (mg/g)	K_L (L/mg)	R^2	K_F (mg/g (L/mg)$^{1/n}$)	1/n	R^2
C_{ST}	154	0.602	0.999	81	0.137	0.856
C_{ST}-APS	196	0.369	0.999	102	0.137	0.856
C_{SBA15}	250	0.727	0.999	120	0.170	0.799
C_{SBA-15}-APS	303	0.493	0.999	142	0.172	0.861
C_{KIT-6}	270	0.787	0.999	128	0.178	0.801
C_{KIT-6}-APS	323	0.574	0.999	153	0.178	0.860

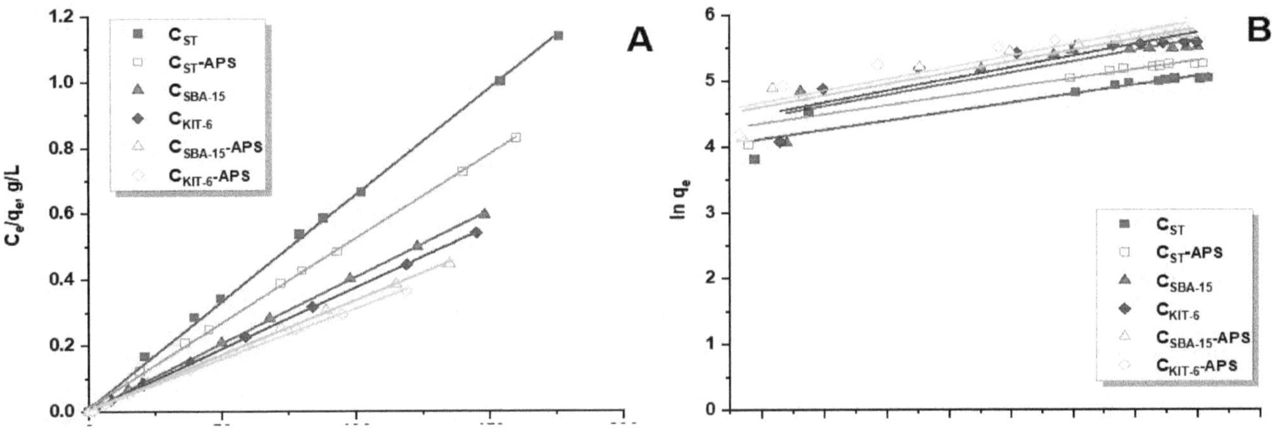

Figure 5. The fit of experimental data concerning adsorption of paracetamol onto pristine and oxidized OMCs to the (**a**) Langmuir and (**b**) Freundlich models.

The effectiveness of the paracetamol adsorption process on the surface of ordered mesoporous carbon materials was also studied by infrared spectroscopy (Figure 6). The FT-IR spectra of pristine and functionalized OMCs were discussed in our previous paper [41]. They clearly demonstrate that the process of oxidation with an acidic solution of ammonium persulfate leads to the generation of a high density of carboxylic, ketone, phenolic, and etheric groups (Figure 6a). After drug loading, the significant differences in the FT-IR spectra of nanomaterials were detected. The absorption bands at wavenumbers around 3100–3700 cm^{-1} can be assigned to overlapped N-H and O-H stretching vibrations present in the adsorbed molecules of paracetamol. The C=O stretching vibrations were observed at 1660 cm^{-1}, while C-H bending vibration was detected at 1400 cm^{-1}. Moreover, C_{Ar}-N stretching vibrations were identified at 1232 cm^{-1}. Additionally, the vibrations of the aromatic ring (C_{Ar}-C_{Ar}) were found at 1600–1500 cm^{-1} [42–44]. The absorption bands at 2300 cm^{-1} corresponded to N-H/C-O stretching vibrations that appeared as a result of the interactions between paracetamol and mesoporous carbon materials (Figure 6b).

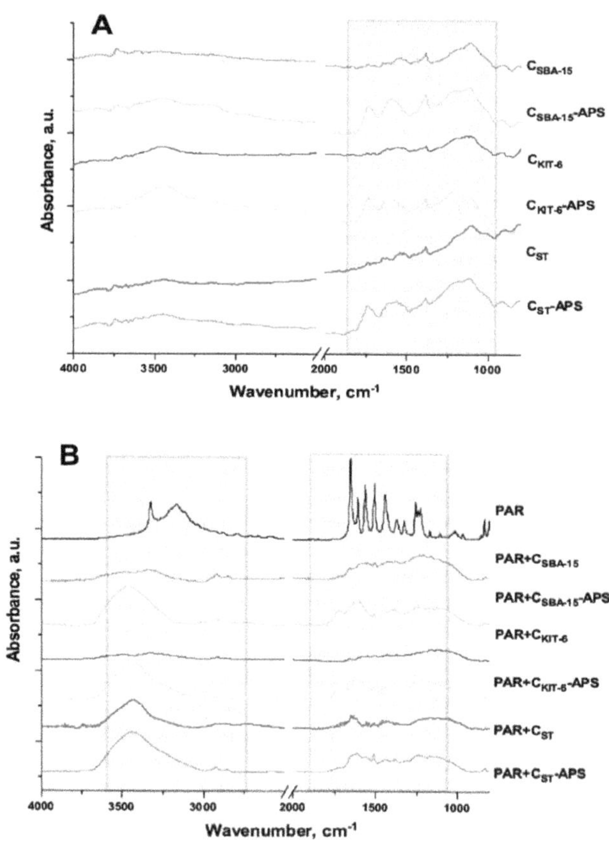

Figure 6. FT-IR spectra of C_{SBA-15}, C_{SBA-15}-APS, C_{KIT-6}, C_{KIT-6}-APS, C_{ST}, and C_{ST}-APS (**a**) before and (**b**) after adsorption of paracetamol (PAR).

The paracetamol release studies were performed in simulated gastric fluid (pH 1.2). Primarily, the drug release profiles from gelatin capsule and ordered mesoporous carbon systems were compared. Figure 7 presents the dissolution profile of pure paracetamol from a gelatin capsule. After 10 min of the analysis, ca. 100% of acetaminophen was detected in the medium, so immediate drug release was observed. On the other hand, the sustained release pattern was identified when paracetamol was diffused from non-functionalized ordered mesoporous carbon materials (Figure 8). The quantity of drug released within 2 h diminished in the following sequence $C_{ST} > C_{KIT-6} > C_{SBA-15}$. Paracetamol molecules were mostly loaded inside the pores of materials during the adsorption process and could not be freely liberated to acceptor medium. This phenomenon was most noticeable for C_{SBA-15}, in which case ca. 28% of drug was released within 120 min. This sample showed the largest pore diameter (6.54 nm) compared with other materials C_{KIT-6} (5.78 nm) and C_{ST} (4.12 nm) (Table 2). On the basis of these parameters, it could be stated that the amount of paracetamol released decreased as the pore diameter increased. It should be highlighted that C_{SBA-15} also exhibited the largest micropore surface area and the highest micropore volume, which allowed the drug molecules to be loaded inside, and as a consequence, they were not easily desorbed. These results proved that the textural parameters and the structure of carbon materials influenced the percentage of acetaminophen that was diffused to acceptor medium. Similar conclusions were reached when the paracetamol was released from activated and pristine carbon powders. The properties of these materials such as mesopore and micropore volume sizes determined the drug release pattern [45]. These observations were consistent with other studies in which porous materials such as zirconia/silica hybrids were applied as paracetamol carriers. The data obtained in this study proved that the amount of drug diffused to receptor medium was determined by chemical compositions of these materials (ZrO_2-SiO_2) and their textural parameters [46]. Moreover, it was established that the porosity of nanocarrier and the quantity of functional groups on its surface had an influence on the drug release ability.

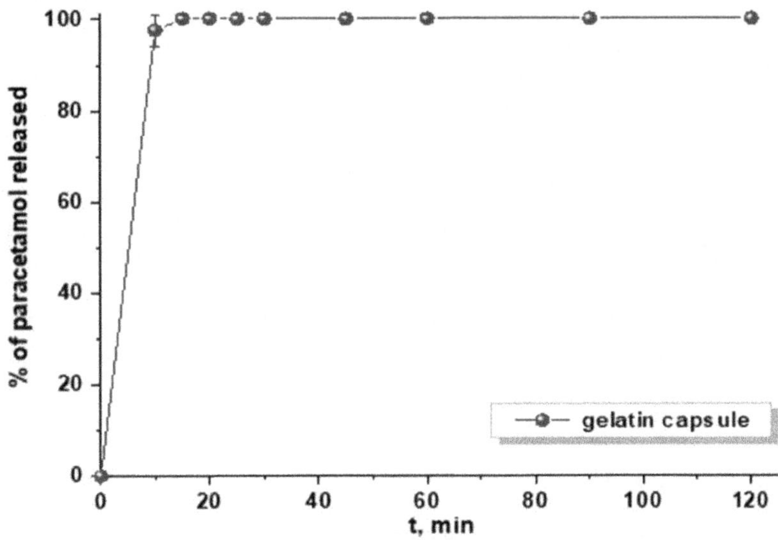

Figure 7. Dissolution profile of pure paracetamol from a gelatine capsule.

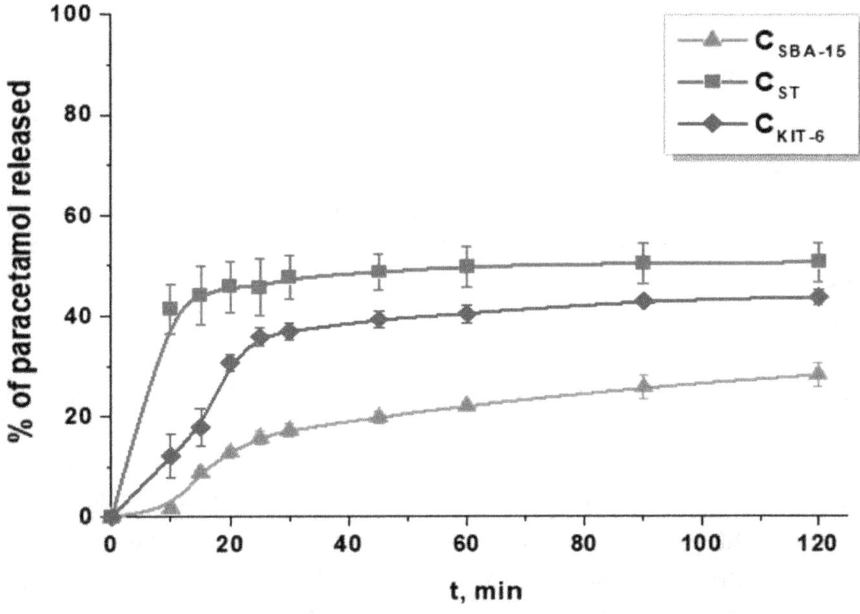

Figure 8. Release profiles of paracetamol from pristine OMCs.

Therefore, the paracetamol was also released from functionalized mesoporous carbon vehicles. In order to compare the data obtained, the dissolution profiles of paracetamol from pristine and oxidized OMCs are presented in Figure 9A–C. The results proved that all functionalized materials showed a higher percentage of drug release than the pristine samples. Owing to the oxidation of ordered mesoporous carbons, the paracetamol molecules were gathered mostly on the external surface of these materials, thus they could be easily desorbed from the modified materials.

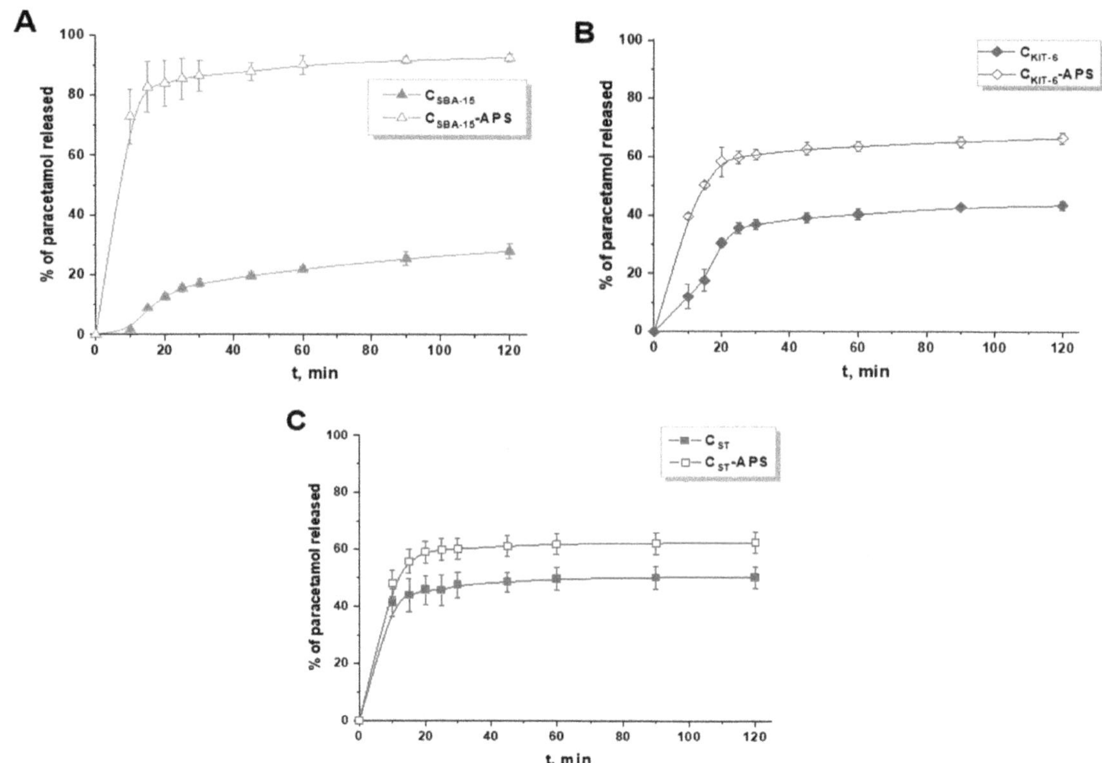

Figure 9. Release profiles of paracetamol from pristine and oxidized OMCs: (**A**) C_{SBA-15} and C_{SBA-15}-APS, (**B**) C_{KIT-6} and C_{KIT-6}-APS, and (**C**) C_{ST} and C_{ST}-APS.

The most significant difference in the amount of acetaminophen released was observed between C_{SBA-15} and C_{SBA-15}-APS. For C_{SBA-15}-APS, the initial burst release of around 73% was detected in the first 10 min of the analysis, and afterwards, the amount of drug increased steadily to reach ca. 92%. Meanwhile, for C_{KIT-6}-APS in the beginning of the analysis, ca. 40% of paracetamol was detected in the acceptor fluid to achieve 67% after 120 min. The difference between the drug release from modified and non-modified C_{KIT-6} is mainly because of various acid–base properties of both materials. Therefore, in this case, the textural parameters are not as important as the number and types of groups attached to the surface of the material. The total number of acidic groups on the surface of C_{KIT-6}-APS was almost two times higher compared with C_{KIT-6}. It could be suggested that, for carbon material decorated with functional groups, host–guest interactions were different compared with that of pristine material, which had influence on the drug release pattern. A much lower difference in the percentage of drug released between the pristine and functionalized sample was observed for C_{ST} and C_{ST}-APS samples. This could be justified by a similar total content of oxygen functional groups on the surface of the pristine material (1.85 mmol/g) and functionalized one (2.11 mmol/g). Two distinctive release steps were also observed when metal–organic frameworks (MIL-53(Fe) congruous and MIL-101) were applied as carriers for paracetamol. The drug was released slowly in a diffusion-controlled manner from MIL-53 (Fe) in 6 days. Because of the larger pore diameter and poorer host–guest interactions, the release of paracetamol from MIL-101 was faster than from MIL-53(Fe). However, the quickest diffusion of acetaminophen (in less than one hour) was observed from SBA-15 [47]. This phenomenon was associated with the large pore diameter of mesopores and competition between the paracetamol molecules and water during the adsorption process [48]. It was proved that drug release is dependent not only on its diffusion from the pores of materials, but also on host–guest interactions that occurred between the carrier and active compound. Mesoporous silica nanomaterials were also suggested as vehicles that could deliver the drug in a controlled, sustained pattern. Paracetamol was added at the beginning of the synthesis of these materials to bind drug to the silica network by van der Waals interactions. The drug release kinetics proceeded in two release stages, a fast release observed in the first hours and then sustained release. The amount of paracetamol diffused from SiO_2 was 60% after 3 h and 80% after 200 h [49]. On the other hand, only 27% of paracetamol in 12 h was released from activated carbon powder, the drug loading capacity of which was 281 mg/g [39]. In another study, activated carbon was also applied as a vehicle for paracetamol [50]. The complete drug release was observed after 10 min of the analysis (1% of SDS, sodium dodecyl sulfate was added to the buffer solution). However, the experiment was carried out only in buffer medium at pH 5.8 and pH 7.2. There was no analysis performed in simulated gastric fluid.

In order to understand the paracetamol diffusion mechanism from carbon nanocarriers, the results were fitted to five different kinetic models that are the most commonly applied in drug release studies (Table 5). The results proved that, for all pristine carbon samples, the highest values of R^2 were detected for the Higuchi model. Therefore, it can be assumed that paracetamol release was controlled by diffusion for C_{SBA-15}, C_{KIT-6}, and C_{ST}. Meanwhile, for oxidized materials, the drug release was the most consistent with the Korsmeyer–Peppas model. On the basis of the release exponent (n value), it is possible to characterize which type of diffusion follows the drug ($n < 0.45$ corresponds to Fickian diffusion, $0.45 < n < 0.89$ is related to non-Fickian diffusion, $n = 0.89$ corresponds to case II transport—zero order release, and $n > 0.89$ is associated with super case II transport) [51]. For C_{SBA-15}-APS and C_{ST}-APS, the paracetamol release was driven by Fickian diffusion as a result of chemical potential gradient. Meanwhile, for C_{KIT-6}-APS, the n value was higher than 0.45, which indicated the non-Fickian diffusion mechanism.

Table 5. Kinetics models applied to describe the release mechanism from pristine and oxidized OMCs.

Material	Zero Order	First Order	Higuchi	Hixson–Crowell	Korsmeyer–Peppas	n
C_{SBA-15}	0.935	0.951	0.989	0.946	0.939	0.972
C_{SBA-15}-APS	0.800	0.899	0.895	0.871	0.955	0.075
C_{KIT-6}	0.667	0.647	0.969	0.629	0.737	0.197
C_{KIT-6}-APS	0.864	0.913	0.936	0.880	0.953	0.510
C_{ST}	0.953	0.960	0.976	0.958	0.955	0.069
C_{ST}-APS	0.734	0.766	0.860	0.756	0.948	0.096

The behavior of paracetamol release from ordered mesoporous carbons was compared with the dissolution profiles of pure paracetamol by the determination of f_1 and f_2 factors (Table 6). The release profiles are considered to be similar when f_1 (difference factor) is close to 0 (range 0–15) and f_2 (similarity factor) is close to 100 (range 50–100). The f_1 and f_2 factors determined for paracetamol in combination with the selected ordered mesoporous carbon carriers indicate that the release profiles obtained differ from the dissolution profiles of pure paracetamol. It proved that the drug was released in a modified pattern.

Table 6. The two-factor values for paracetamol (PAR) systems based on mesoporous carbon materials.

Systems	f_1	f_2
PAR + C_{KIT-6}	72.8	7.2
PAR + C_{KIT-6}-APS	70.3	12.7
PAR + C_{SBA-15}	86.6	3.5
PAR + C_{SBA-15}-APS	25.4	28.3
PAR + C_{ST}	55.9	12.9
PAR + C_{ST}-APS	47.9	16.5

Additionally, the parallel artificial membrane permeability assay was applied as an in vitro model of passive transcellular transport of the active compound (Figure 10). According to the literature, the results obtained correlate well with in vivo drug absorption [52]. For all system based on oxidized mesoporous carbon materials, the values of P_{app} were higher than 1.0×10^{-6} cm/s, which classified them as highly permeable.

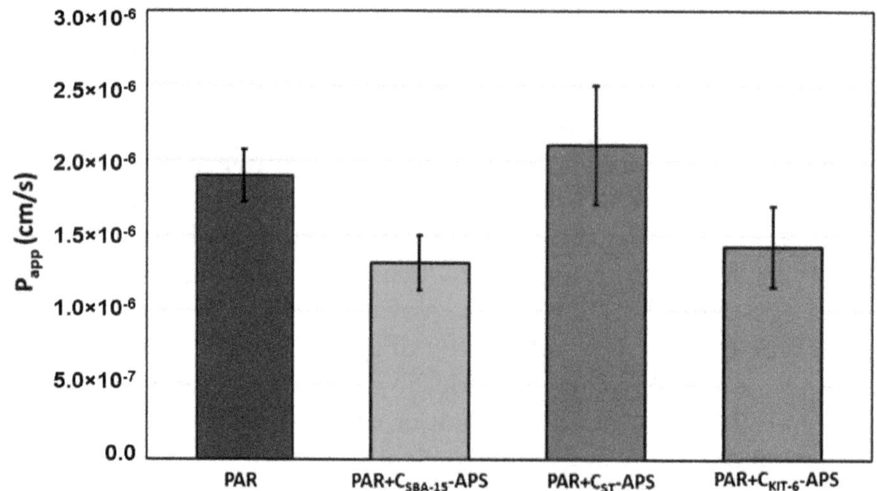

Figure 10. Gastrointestinal mean permeability of paracetamol from oxidized mesoporous carbons using the parallel artificial membrane permeability assay (PAMPA).

4. Conclusions

In this study, new delivery systems for paracetamol were designed. They were based on non-toxic ordered mesoporous carbons of cubic and hexagonal structure obtained via hard and soft template methods. The carbon materials were oxidized with an acidic solution of APS at 60 °C for 6 h. The functionalization brought about a considerable depletion of the specific surface area and pore volume of materials, but it concomitantly led to the generation of acidic oxygen-containing functionalities. It was suggested that functional groups are attached primarily inside micropores/small mesopores, which are partially blocked. The OMCs modified in the previously mentioned manner turned out to be a very efficient adsorbents of paracetamol from aqueous solutions. The adsorption of drug on their surfaces occurred by donor–acceptor complexes and hydrogen bond formation. They were more intense in materials containing a higher concentration of functional groups. Our investigation data referring to the adsorption of paracetamol were consistent with the model of Langmuir isotherm, indicating that the drug molecules form homogeneous monolayer coverage on the surface of the carbon carriers. The pseudo-second-order model exhibited the best correlation to the kinetic results. It was shown that the amount and rate of drug release were influenced by the porosity of the materials and the total number of surface functionalities. The difference between the drug release from modified and non-modified nanocarriers was mainly because of the various acid–base properties of materials. Among all the samples tested in this study, the best material for paracetamol loading and release is C_{SBA-15}-APS. This ordered mesoporous carbon exhibited optimal drug loading capacity. Moreover, a high amount of paracetamol was released within 1 h of the analysis, which was desirable. All paracetamol delivery systems based on oxidized mesoporous carbon materials exhibited high permeability through the artificial membrane.

Our future plan is to design new carbon materials decorated with other functional groups. It is assumed that, because of the introduction of different modifications onto the surface of nanomaterials, the release process may be modulated in order to obtain either sustained or immediate diffusion of paracetamol. Owing to the introduction of functional groups, the drug could be liberated in the specific site in the human body.

Author Contributions: J.G.—Conceptualization, Investigation, Writing—Original Draft Preparation, Visualization; A.E.—Investigation, Visualization; A.O.—Writing—Original Draft Preparation; D.L.—Investigation; A.S.—

Investigation; J.C.-P.—Conceptualization, Writing—Review & Editing. All authors have read and agreed to the published version of the manuscript.

References

1. Wang, S. Ordered mesoporous materials for drug delivery. *Microporous Mesoporous Mater.* **2009**, *117*, 1–9. [CrossRef]
2. Vallet-Regi, M.; Ramila, A.; Del Real, R.P.; Pérez-Pariente, J. A new property of MCM-41: Drug delivery system. *Chem. Mater.* **2001**, *13*, 308–311. [CrossRef]
3. Luo, Z.; Fan, S.; Gu, C.; Liu, W.; Chen, J.; Li, B.; Liu, J. Metal–organic framework (MOF)-based nanomaterials for biomedical applications. *Curr. Med. Chem.* **2019**, *26*, 3341–3369. [CrossRef]
4. Nkansah, P.; Antipas, A.; Lu, Y.; Varma, M.; Rotter, C.; Rago, B.; El-Kattan, A.; Taylor, G.; Rubio, M.; Litchfield, J. Development and evaluation of novel solid nanodispersion system for oral delivery of poorly water-soluble drugs. *J. Control. Release* **2013**, *169*, 150–161. [CrossRef]
5. Goscianska, J.; Olejnik, A.; Pietrzak, R. In vitro release of L-phenylalanine from ordered mesoporous materials. *Microporous Mesoporous Mater.* **2013**, *177*, 32–36. [CrossRef]
6. Goscianska, J.; Olejnik, A.; Nowak, I.; Marciniak, M.; Pietrzak, R. Ordered mesoporous silica modified with lanthanum for ibuprofen loading and release behaviour. *Eur. J. Pharm. Biopharm.* **2015**, *94*, 550–558. [CrossRef]
7. Saha, D.; Warren, K.E.; Naskar, A.K. Controlled release of antipyrine from mesoporous carbons. *Microporous Mesoporous Mater.* **2014**, *196*, 327–334. [CrossRef]
8. Saha, D.; Moken, T.; Chen, J.; Hensley, D.K.; Delaney, K.; Hunt, M.A.; Nelson, K.; Spurri, A.; Benham, L.; Brice, R. Micro-/mesoporous carbons for controlled release of antipyrine and indomethacin. *RSC Adv.* **2015**, *5*, 23699–23707. [CrossRef]
9. Wang, L.; Zheng, M.; Xie, Z. Nanoscale metal-organic frameworks for drug delivery: A conventional platform with new promise. *J. Mater. Chem. B* **2018**, *6*, 707–717. [CrossRef] [PubMed]
10. Abánades Lázaro, I.; Forgan, R.S. Application of zirconium MOFs in drug delivery and biomedicine. *Coord. Chem. Rev.* **2019**, *380*, 230–259. [CrossRef]
11. Liang, C.; Li, Z.; Dai, S. Mesoporous carbon materials: Synthesis and modification. *Angew. Chemie Int. Ed.* **2008**, *47*, 3696–3717. [CrossRef]
12. Ryoo, R.; Joo, S.H.; Kruk, M.; Jaroniec, M. Ordered mesoporous carbons. *Adv. Mater.* **2001**, *13*, 677–681. [CrossRef]
13. Jun, S.; Joo, S.H.; Ryoo, R.; Kruk, M.; Jaroniec, M.; Liu, Z.; Ohsuna, T.; Terasaki, O. Synthesis of new, nanoporous carbon with hexagonally ordered mesostructure. *J. Am. Chem. Soc.* **2000**, *122*, 10712–10713. [CrossRef]
14. Ma, X.; Yuan, H.; Hu, M. A simple method for synthesis of ordered mesoporous carbon. *Diam. Relat. Mater.* **2019**, *98*, 107480. [CrossRef]
15. Carboni, M.; Abney, C.W.; Taylor-Pashow, K.M.L.; Vivero-Escoto, J.L.; Lin, W. Uranium sorption with functionalized mesoporous carbon materials. *Ind. Eng. Chem. Res.* **2013**, *52*, 15187–15197. [CrossRef]
16. Jun, S.; Choi, M.; Ryu, S.; Lee, H.-Y.; Ryoo, R. Ordered mesoporous carbon molecular sieves with functionalized surfaces. In *Studies in Surface Science and Catalysis*; Elsevier: Amsterdam, The Netherlands, 2003; Volume 146, pp. 37–40. ISBN 0167-2991.
17. Goscianska, J.; Malaika, A. A facile post-synthetic modification of ordered mesoporous carbon to get efficient catalysts for the formation of acetins. *Catal. Today* **2019**, in press. [CrossRef]
18. Li, X.; Zhu, H.; Liu, C.; Yuan, P.; Lin, Z.; Yang, J.; Yue, Y.; Bai, Z.; Wang, T.; Bao, X. Synthesis, modification, and application of hollow mesoporous carbon submicrospheres for adsorptive desulfurization. *Ind. Eng. Chem. Res.* **2018**, *57*, 15020–15030. [CrossRef]
19. Jeong, Y.; Cui, M.; Choi, J.; Lee, Y.; Kim, J.; Son, Y.; Khim, J. Development of modified mesoporous carbon (CMK-3) for improved adsorption of bisphenol-A. *Chemosphere* **2020**, *238*, 124559. [CrossRef]
20. Nazir, A.; Yu, H.; Wang, L.; Haroon, M.; Ullah, R.S.; Fahad, S.; Elshaarani, T.; Khan, A.; Usman, M. Recent progress in the modification of carbon materials and their application in composites for electromagnetic interference shielding. *J. Mater. Sci.* **2018**, *53*, 8699–8719. [CrossRef]

21. Marciniak, M.; Goscianska, J.; Pietrzak, R. Physicochemical characterization of ordered mesoporous carbons functionalized by wet oxidation. *J. Mater. Sci.* **2018**, *53*, 5997–6007. [CrossRef]
22. Viswanathan, P.; Muralidaran, Y.; Ragavan, G. Challenges in oral drug delivery: A nano-based strategy to overcome. In *Nanostructures for Oral Medicine*; Elsevier: Amsterdam, The Netherlands, 2017; pp. 173–201.
23. Niu, X.; Wan, L.; Hou, Z.; Wang, T.; Sun, C.; Sun, J.; Zhao, P.; Jiang, T.; Wang, S. Mesoporous carbon as a novel drug carrier of fenofibrate for enhancement of the dissolution and oral bioavailability. *Int. J. Pharm.* **2013**, *452*, 382–389. [CrossRef]
24. Zhang, Y.; Zhi, Z.; Li, X.; Gao, J.; Song, Y. Carboxylated mesoporous carbon microparticles as new approach to improve the oral bioavailability of poorly water-soluble carvedilol. *Int. J. Pharm.* **2013**, *454*, 403–411. [CrossRef] [PubMed]
25. Zhu, W.; Zhao, Q.; Sun, C.; Zhang, Z.; Jiang, T.; Sun, J.; Li, Y.; Wang, S. Mesoporous carbon with spherical pores as a carrier for celecoxib with needle-like crystallinity: Improve dissolution rate and bioavailability. *Mater. Sci. Eng. C* **2014**, *39*, 13–20. [CrossRef] [PubMed]
26. Zhao, P.; Jiang, H.; Jiang, T.; Zhi, Z.; Wu, C.; Sun, C.; Zhang, J.; Wang, S. Inclusion of celecoxib into fibrous ordered mesoporous carbon for enhanced oral bioavailability and reduced gastric irritancy. *Eur. J. Pharm. Sci.* **2012**, *45*, 639–647. [CrossRef] [PubMed]
27. Upfal, J. *The Australian Drug Guide: Every Person's Guide to Prescription and Over-the-Counter Medicines, Street Drugs, Vaccines, Vitamins and Minerals*; Black Inc.: Melbourne, Australia, 2006; ISBN 1863951741.
28. Fusi-Schmidhauser, T.; Preston, N.J.; Keller, N.; Gamondi, C. Conservative management of Covid-19 patients—Emergency palliative care in action. *J. Pain Symptom Manag.* **2020**, *60*, e27–e30. [CrossRef]
29. Sohrabi, C.; Alsafi, Z.; O'Neill, N.; Khan, M.; Kerwan, A.; Al-Jabir, A.; Iosifidis, C.; Agha, R. World Health Organization declares global emergency: A review of the 2019 novel coronavirus (COVID-19). *Int. J. Surg.* **2020**, *76*, 71–76. [CrossRef]
30. Boehm, H.P. Some aspects of the surface chemistry of carbon blacks and other carbons. *Carbon N. Y.* **1994**, *32*, 759–769. [CrossRef]
31. Langmuir, I. The adsorption of gases on plane surfaces of glass, mica and platinum. *J. Am. Chem. Soc.* **1918**, *40*, 1361–1403. [CrossRef]
32. Freundlich, H.M.F. Over the adsorption in solution. *J. Phys. Chem* **1906**, *57*, 1100–1107.
33. Lagergren, S.K. About the theory of so-called adsorption of soluble substances. *Sven. Vetenskapsakad. Handingarl* **1898**, *24*, 1–39.
34. Ho, Y.-S.; McKay, G. Sorption of dye from aqueous solution by peat. *Chem. Eng. J.* **1998**, *70*, 115–124. [CrossRef]
35. Goscianska, J.; Nowak, I.; Olejnik, A. Sorptive properties of aluminium ions containing mesoporous silica towards l-histidine. *Adsorption* **2016**, *22*, 571–579. [CrossRef]
36. Olejnik, A.; Nowak, I.; Schroeder, G. Functionalized polystyrene beads as carriers in release studies of two herbicides: 2, 4-dichlorophenoxyacetic acid and 2-methyl-4-chlorophenoxyacetic acid. *Int. J. Environ. Sci. Technol.* **2019**, *16*, 5623–5634. [CrossRef]
37. Prior, A.; Frutos, P.; Correa, C.P. Comparison of dissolution profiles: Current guidelines. In Proceedings of the VI Congreso SEFIG, Granada, Spain, 9–11 February 2003; Volume 3, pp. 507–509.
38. Fischer, H.; Kansy, M.; Avdeef, A.; Senner, F. Permeation of permanently positive charged molecules through artificial membranes—Influence of physico-chemical properties. *Eur. J. Pharm. Sci.* **2007**, *31*, 32–42. [CrossRef]
39. Liang, D.; Lu, C.; Li, Y.L.; Li, Y.H. Adsorption of paracetamol by activated carbon and its release in vitro. *Xinxing Tan Cailiao* **2006**, *21*, 144–150.
40. Bernal, V.; Erto, A.; Giraldo, L.; Moreno-Piraján, J.C. Effect of solution pH on the adsorption of paracetamol on chemically modified activated carbons. *Molecules* **2017**, *22*, 1032. [CrossRef]
41. Goscianska, J.; Olejnik, A.; Nowak, I.; Marciniak, M.; Pietrzak, R. Stability analysis of functionalized mesoporous carbon materials in aqueous solution. *Chem. Eng. J.* **2016**, *290*, 209–219. [CrossRef]
42. Milczewska, K.; Voelkel, A.; Zwolińska, J.; Jędro, D. Preparation of hybrid materials for controlled drug release. *Drug Dev. Ind. Pharm.* **2016**, *42*, 1058–1065. [CrossRef]

43. Mallah, M.A.; Sherazi, S.T.H.; Bhanger, M.I.; Mahesar, S.A.; Bajeer, M.A. A rapid Fourier-transform infrared (FTIR) spectroscopic method for direct quantification of paracetamol content in solid pharmaceutical formulations. *Spectrochim. Acta A Mol. Biomol. Spectrosc.* **2015**, *141*, 64–70. [CrossRef]
44. Refat, M.S.; Mohamed, G.G.; El-Sayed, M.Y.; Killa, H.M.A.; Fetooh, H. Spectroscopic and thermal degradation behavior of Mg (II), Ca (II), Ba (II) and Sr (II) complexes with paracetamol drug. *Arab. J. Chem.* **2017**, *10*, S2376–S2387. [CrossRef]
45. McCary, S.E.; Rybolt, T.R. Storage and timed release of acetaminophen from *Porous carbonaceous* materials. *Open J. Phys. Chem.* **2013**, *3*, 76–88. [CrossRef]
46. Ciesielczyk, F.; Goscianska, J.; Zdarta, J.; Jesionowski, T. The development of zirconia/silica hybrids for the adsorption and controlled release of active pharmaceutical ingredients. *Colloids Surfaces A Physicochem. Eng. Asp.* **2018**, *545*, 39–50. [CrossRef]
47. Gordon, J.; Kazemian, H.; Rohani, S. MIL-53 (Fe), MIL-101, and SBA-15 porous materials: Potential platforms for drug delivery. *Mater. Sci. Eng. C* **2015**, *47*, 172–179. [CrossRef] [PubMed]
48. Mellaerts, R.; Jammaer, J.A.G.; Van Speybroeck, M.; Chen, H.; Van Humbeeck, J.; Augustijns, P.; Van den Mooter, G.; Martens, J.A. Physical state of poorly water soluble therapeutic molecules loaded into SBA-15 ordered mesoporous silica carriers: A case study with itraconazole and ibuprofen. *Langmuir* **2008**, *24*, 8651–8659. [CrossRef]
49. López, T.; Álvarez, M.; Ramírez, P.; Jardón, G.; López, M.; Rodriguez, G.; Ortiz, I.; Novaro, O. Sol-gel silica matrix as reservoir for controlled release of paracetamol: Characterization and kinetic analysis. *J. Encapsul. Adsorpt. Sci.* **2016**, *6*, 47. [CrossRef]
50. Miriyala, N.; Ouyang, D.; Perrie, Y.; Lowry, D.; Kirby, D.J. Activated carbon as a carrier for amorphous drug delivery: Effect of drug characteristics and carrier wettability. *Eur. J. Pharm. Biopharm.* **2017**, *115*, 197–205. [CrossRef]
51. Siepmann, J.; Peppas, N.A. Modeling of drug release from delivery systems based on hydroxypropyl methylcellulose (HPMC). *Adv. Drug Deliv. Rev.* **2012**, *64*, 163–174. [CrossRef]
52. Bermejo, M.; Avdeef, A.; Ruiz, A.; Nalda, R.; Ruell, J.A.; Tsinman, O.; González, I.; Fernández, C.; Sánchez, G.; Garrigues, T.M. PAMPA—A drug absorption in vitro model: 7. Comparing rat in situ, Caco-2, and PAMPA permeability of fluoroquinolones. *Eur. J. Pharm. Sci.* **2004**, *21*, 429–441. [CrossRef]

2

Effectiveness of Diverse Mesoporous Silica Nanoparticles as Potent Vehicles for the Drug L-DOPA

Sumita Swar, Veronika Máková * and Ivan Stibor

Department of Nanomaterials in Natural Science, Institute for Nanomaterials, Advanced Technologies and Innovation, Technical University of Liberec, Studentská 1402/2, 46117 Liberec, Czech Republic; dearsumita@gmail.com (S.S.); ivan.stibor@tul.cz (I.S.)

* Correspondence: veronika.makova@tul.cz

Abstract: Our study was focused on the synthesis of selective mesoporous silica nanoparticles (MSNs: MCM-41, MCM-48, SBA-15, PHTS, MCF) that are widely studied for drug delivery. The resulting mesoporous surfaces were conveniently prepared making use of verified synthetic procedures. The MSNs thus obtained were characterized by Brunauer-Emmett-Teller (BET) analysis and scanning electron microscopy (SEM). The selected MSNs with various pore diameters and morphologies were examined to evaluate the capability of L-DOPA drug loading and release. L-DOPA is a well-known drug for Parkinson's disease. The L-DOPA drug loading and release profiles were measured by UV-VIS spectroscopy and SBA-15 was proved to be the most effective amongst all the different types of tested mesoporous silica materials as L-DOPA drug vehicle.

Keywords: mesoporous silica; nanoparticles; characterisation; electron microscopy; nitrogen adsorption; drug loading and release

---

1. Introduction

The worldwide market for CNS therapeutics is steadily increasing, with the prognosis that in 2025 it could reach a value of 128.9 billion USD [1]. Among others, one cause of this rapid increase could be that the incidence of many CNS disorders increases exponentially after the age of 65 and the number of people in the world over 65 is increasing sharply. It takes longer to get a CNS drug to the market (12–16 years) compared with a non-CNS drug (10–12 years). The reason for this may lie in the complexity of the brain, the liability of CNS drugs to cause CNS side effects, and the requirement of CNS drugs to cross the blood-brain barrier (BBB) [2]. A major reason for the lack of progress in treating chronic neurodiseases is due to the presence of the BBB, a physical barrier between the CNS parenchyma and vasculature that plays a critical role in maintaining homeostasis within the CNS. Tight junctions exist between endothelial cells that inhibit paracellular diffusion of polar molecules, macromolecules and cells. These forces solute transport into the CNS to occur primarily across individual endothelial cells. Currently, 98% of small-molecule therapeutics and essentially 100% of large-molecule therapeutics, including monoclonal antibodies, proteins and gene therapies, cannot cross the BBB [3]. Numerous multidisciplinary-based strategies for transporting therapeutics from the blood into the brain through the blood-brain barrier have been proposed [3,4], including the use of receptor-mediated transcytosis in combination with different types of inorganic or organic nanoparticles (NPs) [3]. In 2013, Wiley et al. reported the use of gold NPs with transferrin in the delivery of a wide variety of therapeutics, some of which have already reached the clinical testing stage in humans [3–5]. Lamanna et al. designed, synthesised and characterised superparamagnetic iron oxide (SPIO) nanoparticles bearing different functional groups [6]. Progress in using iron oxide NPs for biological and biomedical applications [7,8] has advanced rapidly thanks to the tremendous work achieved in the synthesis and functionalization of these nanomaterials [9,10]. However, these NPs have some limitations in use such as stability in biological solutions at pH 7.4 close to the physiological blood.

The design of nanoparticles for biomedical applications is still challenging [6]. Moreover, several problems related to targeted nanoparticles are always observed. These include agglomeration, distribution, transport efficiency, too-early or too-late degradation, cytotoxicity, biocompatibility etc. Particles with average hydrodynamic sizes of 10–100 nm are optimal for in vivo delivery. Due to the reasons mentioned above, very promising materials in these areas seem to be the mesoporous silica nanoparticles (MSNs). In general, the mesoporous materials are defined by IUPAC as materials with pore sizes between 2 to 50 nm [11]. These materials belong to the nanoporous material family having a pore size of the materials less than 100 nm. The microporous (pore size less than 2 nm) and macroporous (pore size more than 50 nm) materials also come under the classification of nanoporous materials. Mesoporous silica nanoparticles (MSNs) are among the best known and most widely used porous materials [11–16]. Thanks to their morphologies including high surface area, tunable pore sizes and large pore volumes that find these material's diverse applications in catalysis, sorption, separations, sensing, optics and drug delivery [17]. The surfactant micelle-templated mesoporous silica materials are mainly classified as: mobile crystalline materials (MCM-41, MCM-48, MCM-50), Santa Barbara amorphous type materials (SBA-15, SBA-16), Michigan State University materials (MSU), Korean Advanced Institute of Science and Technology material (KIT-1, KIT-16), plugged hexagonal templated silica (PHTS), mesostructured cellular foam (MCF) and (FSM-16) [11,15].

The use of mesoporous material MCM-41 for a drug delivery system was firstly proposed in 2007 by Vallet-Regi et al. Biocompatible MSN-based controlled release systems have been demonstrated to be able to deliver different guest molecules (drugs) [14,15]. With the rapid development of silica-based drug delivery systems over the past decades, the use of pure mesoporous silica suffers from limitations such as targeted drug delivery mechanisms' study, drug kinetics marker in pharmacological research, and track/evaluate the efficiency of the drug release in disease diagnosis and therapy [14]. Therefore, functionalized mesoporous silica materials with luminescence or magnetism have emerged with time [12]. The smart combination of different functional groups with MSNs has been investigated for the development of multifunctional medical platforms aiming simultaneous targeted delivery, fast diagnosis, and efficient therapy [12,18,19]. Very recently, the redox-responsive mesoporous organosilica nanoparticles containing disulfide bridges have been developed with higher efficacy for drug delivery system [20]. Therefore, more researches are being attracted to exploring new possibilities for MSN application in drug delivery.

The synthetic methods that were applied to produce the specific MSNs in this work are well verified by various other researches [11,12,15]. Our research was focused on the potential of using mesoporous nanoparticles for specifically L-DOPA drug loading and release. Mentioned nanoparticles have been studied and evaluated with the aim to find the most convenient combination of these nanoparticles and L-DOPA for needs Parkinson's disease treatments.

2. Materials and Methods

2.1. Materials

Cetyltrimethylammonium bromide (99%, CTAB), tetraethyl orthosilicate (98%, TEOS), fumed silica powder (0.2–0.3 μm average particle size, SiO_2), poly(ethylene glycol)-block-poly(propylene glycol)-block-poly(ethylene glycol)—P123 (Mw = 5800 g/mol), 1,12-dibromododecane (≥96%), *N,N*-dimethylhexadecylamine (≥95%, GC) and mesitylene (98%) were supplied by Merck (Darmstadt, Germany). Tetraethylammonium hydroxide (25% in water, TEAOH) and pyridine (99.5%) were purchased from ACROS Organics (Geel, Belgium). Ammonium fluoride (NH_4F, 99.2%) was supplied by Lach:Ner (Neratovice, Czech Republic). Ethanol (99.9%, EtOH), methanol (99%, MeOH), ammonium hydroxide (NH_4OH, 25%), hydrochloric acid (HCl, 35%) and sodium hydroxide (NaOH) were supplied by Penta (Prague, Czech Republic). Milli-Q water was used for nanoparticle synthesis and purification. 3-(3,4-Dihydroxyphenyl)-L-alanine (>98%, L-DOPA) was purchased from TCI EUROPE N.V. (Zwijndrecht, Belgium). Liquid nitrogen 5.0 (N_2, 99.99% purity) was obtained from Linde (Liberec, Czech Republic).

2.2. *Synthesis of Mesoporous Silica (SiO_2) Nanoparticles (MSNs)*

2.2.1. MCM-41 (Spherical—S)

CTAB (3.75 g) was added to Milli-Q water (70.71 g) in a round bottom flask (250 mL) and stirred at 500 rpm/1 h/45 °C. Then NH_4OH 25% solution (25.74 g) and EtOH (90 g) were added at 500 rpm/30 min. TEOS (7.05 g) was introduced dropwise into the stirring solution at 500 rpm for 3 h. The mixture was stirred at 300 rpm/12 h/25 °C. Finally, the mixture was filtrated under vacuum and thus obtained product was washed with distilled water and methanol (150 mL). The particles were dried at 90 °C/20 h and the post-treatment was achieved by calcination at 550 °C/5 h with a heating rate of 1°C/min in an ambient atmosphere.

2.2.2. MCM-41 (Highly Ordered—HO)

NH_4OH 22.7% solution (106.5 g) was mixed with Milli-Q water (116.5 g) of to form a homogeneous solution in a round bottom flask (250 mL). Subsequently, CTAB (1 g) was added at 500 rpm/45 °C until a homogeneous solution was obtained. When the solution reached to room temperature (r.t.), TEOS (4.67 g) was added and the mixture was stirred at 500 rpm/2 h/room temperature. The resulting precipitate was collected using vacuum filtration, washed with distilled water until neutralization and dried at 90 °C overnight. Finally, the product was calcined at 550 °C/6 h.

2.2.3. MCM-48

Milli-Q water (120 g) and NaOH (0.69 g) were added to Gemini 16-12-16 surfactant (5.8 g) in a round bottom flask (250 mL). The Gemini surfactant was prepared according to the procedure mentioned in the literature [10]. The solution was stirred at 700 rpm/room temperature until the surfactant was dissolved. Fumed silica (4 g) was added and the mixture was stirred at 700 rpm/2 h. The sealed flask was aged in an oven at 130 °C/3 days. Thereafter, the product was filtered, washed 4 times with deionized water (100 mL) and centrifuged at 10,000 rpm/5 min. Particles were heated in an oven at 130 °C/24 h. Finally, the product was recovered by vacuum filtration and further washed thrice with 150 mL distilled water. The obtained product was calcined at 550 °C/6 h.

2.2.4. SBA-15

P123 (4 g) was added into the solution of Milli-Q water (130 g) and HCl 35% (21 mL) in a round bottom flask (250 mL). The solution was stirred at 800 rpm/3 h/room temperature. TEOS (8.53 g) was introduced and the mixture was stirred overnight at 45 °C. Ageing of the white precipitate was carried out at 80 °C/24 h, in the sealed flask without stirring. The product was collected by vacuum filtration, washed thrice with 50 ml of distilled water, then dried overnight at 80 °C and finally calcined at 550 °C/6 h.

2.2.5. PHTS (Plugged Hexagonal Templated Silica)

P123 (4 g) was added into the solution of Milli-Q water (130 g) and HCl 35% (21 mL) in a round bottom flask (250 mL). The solution was stirred at 800 rpm/3 h/room temperature. Then TEOS (14.93 g) was added into the mixture and the mixture was continuously stirred at 60 °C/overnight. The product aging was carried out for at 80 °C/24 h, then collected by vacuum filtration, washed thrice with 50 mL of distilled water, dried overnight at 80 °C and finally calcined at 550 °C/6 h.

2.2.6. MCF (Mesostructured Cellular Foam)

P123 (4 g) was added into the solution of Milli-Q water (130 g) and HCl 35% (21 mL) in a round bottom flask (250 mL) stirred at 700 rpm/room temperature until the surfactant was dissolved. NH_4F (47 mg) and mesitylene (4.6 mL) were introduced into the flask. The temperature was raised to 40 °C and stirring was continued at 800 rpm/1 h. Then, TEOS (8.53 g) was added and stirred at 40 °C/20 h. The mixture was transferred to an autoclave and kept at 100 °C/24 h. The product was collected by vacuum filtration, washed thrice with 50 mL of water and finally calcined at 550 °C/6 h. Yields of all the prepared samples are summarised in the Table 1.

Table 1. Yields of all the synthetized particles.

Sample	Yield (g)	Yield (%)
MCM-41(S)	2 ± 0.4	~28
MCM-41(HO)	0.9 ± 0.1	~20
MCM-48	3 ± 0.3	~75
SBA-15	2.8 ± 0.2	~32
PHTS	4.2 ± 0.7	~28
MCF	2.3 ± 0.5	~27

2.3. Analyses

2.3.1. Scanning Electron Microscopy (SEM)

Size distribution and shape homogeneity of MSNs were examined by SEM (ZEISS, Jena, Germany) images. Samples were prepared by taking small quantities of MSNs dispersed in distilled water. Then the solution was dropped on the carbon-coated copper grid and dried under vacuum to ensure the complete removal of the solvent. MSNs were sputtered with 2 nm platinum layer, subsequently were viewed as secondary electron images (2 kV).

2.3.2. Nitrogen Adsorption

The gas sorption analyser (Autosorb®iQ, Quantachrome Instruments, Ashland, OR, USA) was employed to examine the surface areas and pore size distributions of prepared MSNs. The surface areas and pore size distributions were calculated using ASiQwin software (version for Windows XP) based on adsorption-desorption isotherms. The pristine samples were degassed at 300 °C/3 h. Then N_2 adsorption and desorption isotherms were measured at the temperature of −196 °C. Multipoint BET (Brunauer-Emmett-Teller) analysis was applied for the total surface area calculation. Models of DFT (Density Functional Theory) were used to determine pore size distribution and also compared to relatively old BJH (Barret-Joyner-Halenda) model.

2.4. Drug Loading on and Releasing from MSNs

2.4.1. Preparation of L-DOPA Solution

Milli-Q water (50 mL) was added to L-DOPA (50 mg) in an Erlenmeyer flask (100 mL) covered with aluminium foil and sonicated for 1 h/18 °C for complete dissolution. The solution was used for drug loading and calibration.

2.4.2. L-DOPA Loading

The drug L-DOPA was loaded by soaking silica (10 mg) in 1 mg/mL of L-DOPA solution (in Milli-Q water) for 2 h, 4 h, 6 h, 15 h and 24 h. The drug-loaded MSNs were stored into the refrigerator (4 °C) covered with aluminium foil as L-DOPA solution is sensitive towards heat and light. The drug-loaded samples were centrifuged at 10,000 rpm/10 min and the clear solution above the precipitate was collected for examining the loading profiles each of the samples. The L-DOPA loaded solid samples were collected after filtration and dried in the desiccator.

2.4.3. L-DOPA Release

L-DOPA loaded samples (100 mg) were dispersed in a phosphate buffer solution (10 mL) with pH 7.2 (PBS, K_2HPO_4 and KH_2PO_4) and kept at 37 °C using an incubator in order to simulate the body temperature during 15 min, 30 min, 1 h, 2 h and 3 h. A higher amount of drug was expected to be released into the intestine at pH range 7–8 [20]. Monitoring of drug loading and releasing was accomplished by UV spectrophotometry.

Both the drug loading and releasing profiles for each of the samples were determined by monitoring the absorbance change using the UV-VIS spectrophotometer (DR 6000, HACH®, Prague, Czech Republic, wavelength range: 190–1100 nm, scanning speed: 900 nm/min). The calibration curve (for drug loading profile) was prepared by measuring the absorbance at various suitable concentrations of L-DOPA solution in water and absorption peaks were recorded at 290 nm for L-DOPA. Similarly, for drug releasing profile, the calibration curve was also obtained for L-DOPA solution in PBS.

2.5. Statistical Analyses

The experiments were performed three times and standard deviation (SD) was calculated using Excel (Office Professional Plus 2016, Microsoft). Student's t test ($\alpha = 0.05$) was used to evaluate whether the difference was statistically significant.

3. Results and Discussion

3.1. Synthesis of Mesoporous Silica Nanoparticles

The schematic overview of the synthetic approach to mesoporous silica materials is shown in Figure 1. The synthesis of templated mesoporous silica follows a few steps: dissolution of template molecules (CTAB or P123) in the solvent (usually water); addition of the silica source (TEOS or fumed silica); stirring at required conditions to allow the hydrolysis and pre-condensation; recovery of the product and the final stage of template removal by calcination [11]. Hydrolysis may occur both in acidic or basic medium [13].

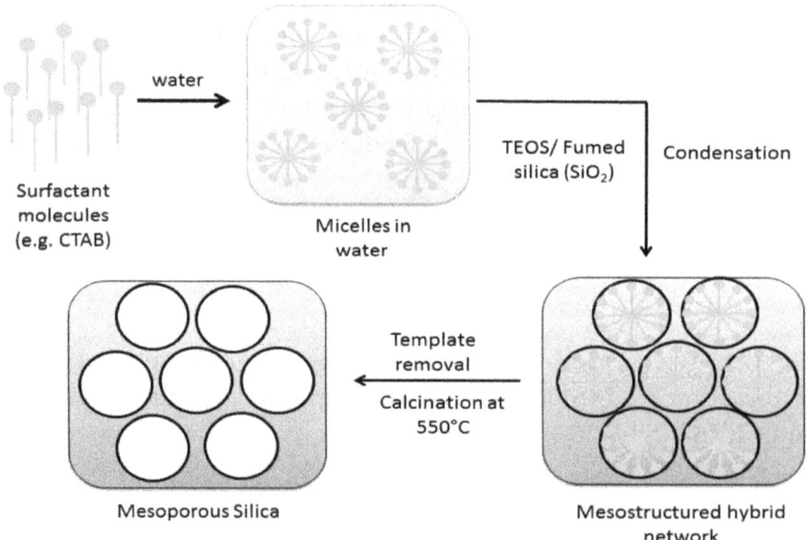

Figure 1. Overview of a synthetic approach to the mesoporous silica formation.

Soft templating, including micelle templating, offers an alternative facile and environmentally friendly approach for MSN preparation. The structural transformation of amphiphilic surfactant organizations can be understood by the surfactant packing factor/parameter, $g = V/l.a_0$, where V is the volume of the hydrophobic chains in surfactant, l is the surfactant chain length, and a_0 is the effective area of the hydrophilic head group of the surfactant at the interface [17]. Generally, surfactants with lower critical micelle concentration (CMC) are more favoured to obtain ordered structure. According to the classical micelle chemistry, above a critical value, g-packing factor increases and therefore, mesophase transitions occur. When $g < 1/3$, particles tend to form Pm3n cubic structures and mixed 3D hexagonal and cubic structures; when $1/3 < g < 1/2$, particles tend to form p6mm hexagonal structures; when $1/2 < 2/3$, particle tend to form Ia3d cubic structures; when $g \sim 1$, lamellar structures are favoured [11,17].

3.2. Characterisation Methods

3.2.1. Morphology of the Samples

The SEM micrographs in Figure 2a–f reveal that the obtained samples have different morphologies, with various shapes and sizes (see Table 2). MCM-41(HO) and MCM-41(S) showed highly ordered conical disc-shaped and spherical nanosized particles, respectively, with a polydispersity of particle size (Figure 2a,b) [11,16,21].

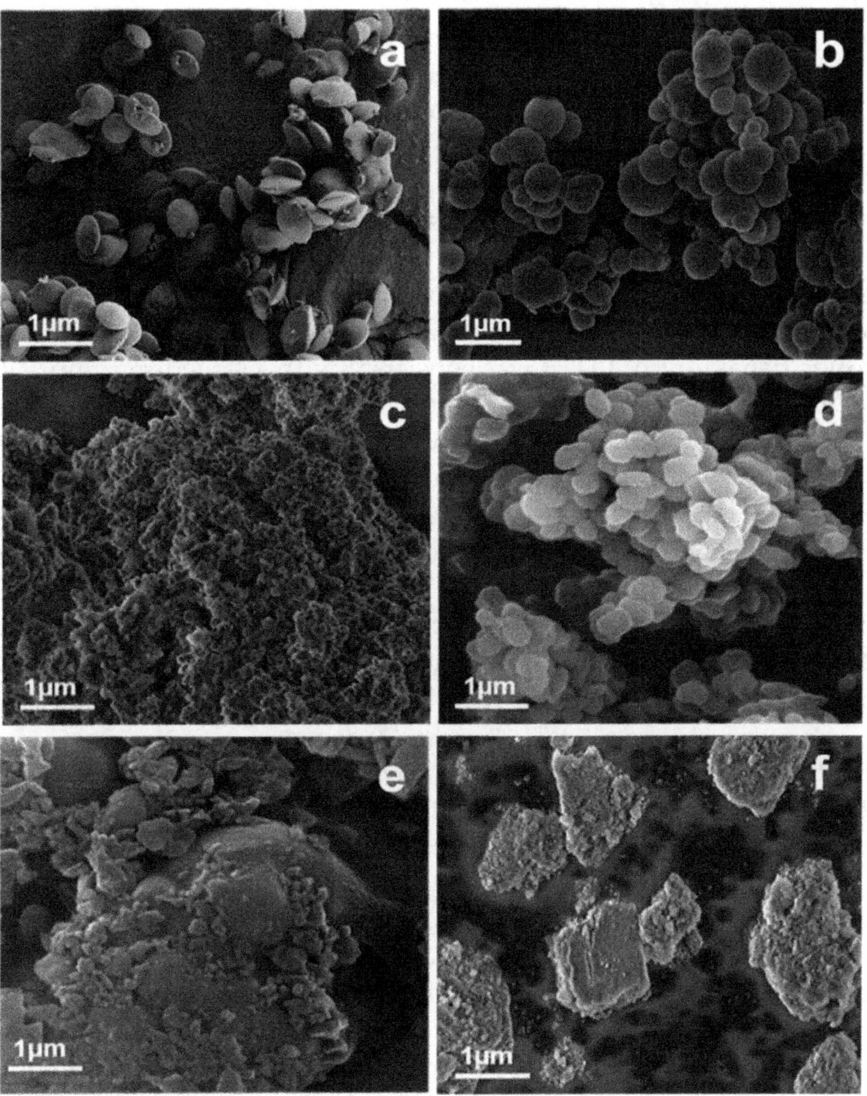

Figure 2. SEM images of MSNs: MCM-41(HO) (**a**); MCM-41(S) (**b**); MCM-48 (**c**); SBA-15 (**d**); PHTS (**e**) and MCF (**f**).

Table 2. The range of particle size and geometry of the particles obtained via SEM.

Sample	Geometry	Particle Size (nm)
MCM-41(S)	spheres	200–900
MCM-41(HO)	cone discs	400–600
MCM-48	agglomerated	>1000
SBA-15	bagel-shaped (short rods)	300–500
PHTS	agglomerated	>1000
MCF	agglomerated	>1000

MCM-41(HO) exhibited more uniform nanoparticles with sizes between 400–600 nm. On the contrary to this, the particle sizes of MCM-41(S) were observed in the range of 200–900 nm. Figure 2c,e,f (MCM-48, PHTS and MCF, respectively) show the agglomeration of the MSNs into clusters (>1 μm) where the smaller particles are also clearly visible. SBA-15 (Figure 2d) revealed comparatively uniform bagel-shaped particles about the size 300–500 nm [21]. The morphology of mesopores in the silica particles could not be evaluated by SEM. The nature of the porous structures was examined by BET analysis.

3.2.2. Surface area and Porosity of the Prepared Samples

Figure 3 shows nitrogen adsorption and desorption isotherms of the six different types MSNs: MCM-41(S); MCM-41(HO); MCM-48; SBA-15; PHTS and MCF. All the samples can be classified as type IV isotherms according to the IUPAC classification and that is typical to the mesoporous silica materials [22]. MCM-41(S) and MCM-41(HO) exhibited similar N_2 sorption isotherms where an increase in adsorption took place above $P/P_0 = 0.2$, suggesting the capillary condensation of N_2 within the pores and confirmed the presence of mesopores [21]. MCM-48 demonstrated adsorption isotherm at a higher relative pressure ($P/P_0 > 0.9$) that corresponds to N_2 condensation in the interparticle voids and also reflects the small size of mesoporous material [23]. SBA-15 exhibited H1 hysteresis loop starting from $P/P_0 = 0.6$, that is characteristic of SBA-15 with highly ordered pores [23]. The adsorption-desorption behaviour of PHTS was consistent with a structure comprising both open and blocked cylindrical mesopores [22]. PHTS showed two-step desorption where the first desorption step was similar to that of SBA-15, indicating the open mesopores. The second desorption step of PHTS was attributed to the plugs (NPs) within the mesoporous. For the plugged pores, desorption was delayed resulting in second desorption [11]. The hysteresis loop was appeared at $P/P_0 = 0.4$–0.75. The MCF N_2 sorption isotherm with characteristic long H2 hysteresis loop was in a good agreement with other article [24].

Figure 4 depicts the difference between usual mesoporous material such as SBA-15 and PHTS with plugged pores. PHTS mesopores are narrowed by nanoparticles (plugs) to create inkbottle-like sections. On the contrary, SBA-15 has open mesopores [11]. Usually, small micropores are also exhibited on the walls of MSNs.

The characteristics of calcined mesoporous silica materials were analysed by BET for examining their specific surface areas. The pore size distributions were determined by the BJH model that was further verified by DFT model. All the results are summarised in Table 3. The previously widely used BJH model is no longer recommended for such applications in micro-mesoporous materials examination as it can significantly underestimate the pore size for narrow mesopores (for pore diameter smaller than 10 nm the pore size may be underestimated even by 30%). However, BJH modelling was used to compare the synthesised materials with the specifications found in the literature [11]. All the MCM-41 samples exhibited high specific surface area lying between 700–1120 m^2/g. The pore diameters were in the range of ~2–4 nm, although their morphologies were different. MCM-48 showed relatively low surface area (470 m^2/g) compared to other MSNs, although the pore diameter is similar to the MCM-41(S) sample. The specific surface area of SBA-15 was 1020 m^2/g with larger pore diameter (~8 nm) compared to MCM series. PHTS also displayed high surface area with 940 m^2/g and the pore diameter of open pores was between 5–7.5 nm, whereas the plugged pores were less than 2 nm. In this case, the DFT was considered a more reliable method than BJH as there was a significant difference in adsorption-desorption pore diameter for plugged pores. MCF displayed the highest pore size of 15–10 nm with 760 m^2/g surface area. SBA-15 and MCF exhibited comparatively higher pore volumes (2.34, 1.17 and surface area 1.88 cm^3/g respectively). On the other hand, MCM-41(S), MCM-41(HO), MCM-48 and PHTS possessed the pore volumes ~0.7–0.8 and surface area only 88 cm^3/g.

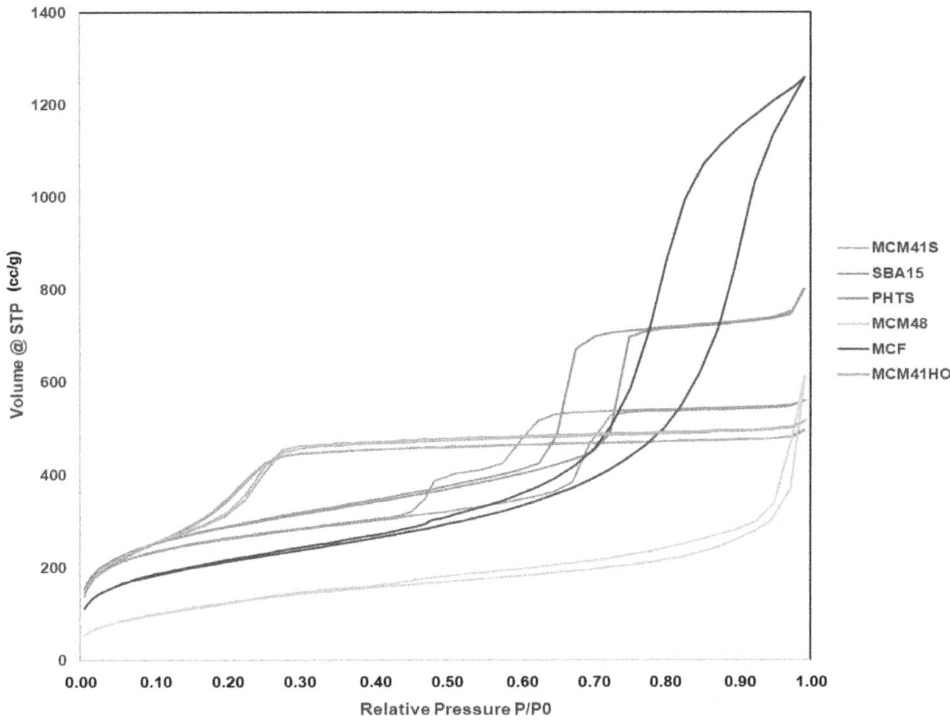

Figure 3. Nitrogen adsorption-desorption isotherms at −196 °C for MCM-41(S); MCM-41(HO); MCM-48; SBA-15; PHTS and MCF.

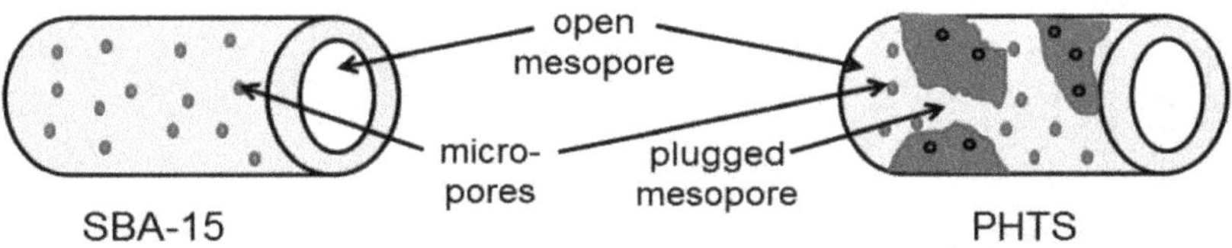

Figure 4. Schematic representation of the pore structure: SBA-15 and PHTS.

Table 3. Calcined MSN samples evaluated via N_2 adsorption.

Sample	BET Specific Surface Area (m^2/g)	Pore Volume (cm^3/g) [DFT model]	Pore Diameter (nm)		
			DFT Model	BJH Model	
				Adsorption Branch	Desorption Branch
MCM-41(S)	880	0.72	3.18	2.12	2.14
MCM-41(HO)	1120	0.75	3.30	2.25	2.26
MCM-48	470	0.77	3.18	2.12	2.22
SBA-15	1020	1.17	7.59	8.97	6.33
PHTS	940	0.83	5.06; 1.64	7.12; 0.89	5.23; 3.87
MCF	760	1.88	11.68	15.43	10.19

For all the synthesized MSNs, N_2 sorption isotherms, BET and BJH (verified by DFT) data regarding pore sizes, surface areas and pore volumes were compatible with the verified once given in the literature [11]. Therefore, the pore structures (morphologies) are suggested to be the same as demonstrated in various literature mentioned earlier [15,17].

The morphological properties such as high surface area, large pore volume and the narrow particle size distribution are well suited for the application of nano-encapsulation in drug delivery systems. Moreover, different types of prepared mesoporous silica allowed us for precise comparison of their properties (high polydispersity in particle size, different porosity, particle morphology and pore structure) for L-DOPA drug release [25]. For the evaluation of L-DOPA delivery profile, MSNs with same pore sizes but different morphologies (MCM-41(S); MCM-41(HO)) and MSNs with various pore sizes (MCM-48, SBA-15, PHTS and MCF), illustrated in Figure 5, were chosen to understand the effect of pore size along with particle morphology on drug loading and release profile.

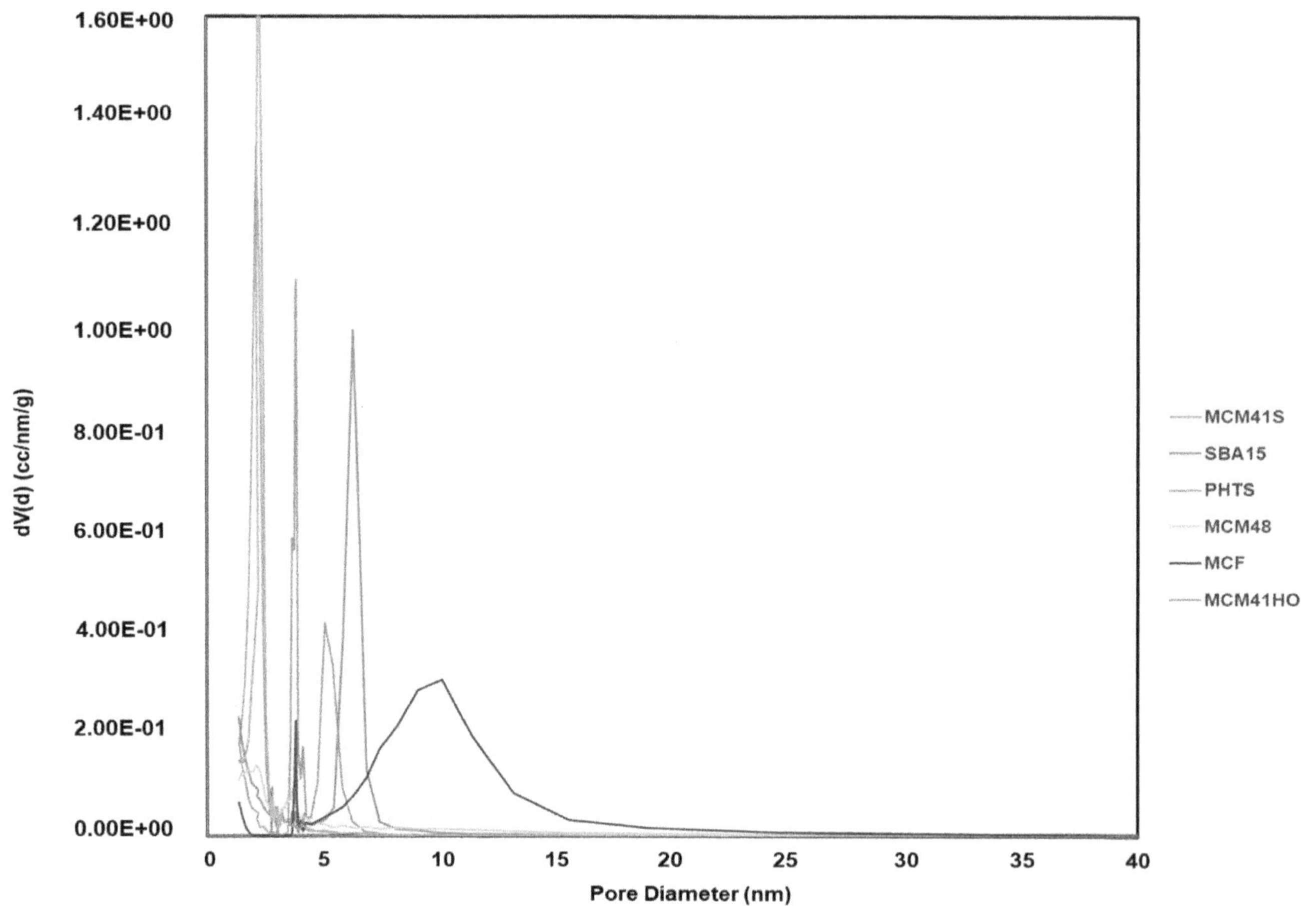

Figure 5. Pore size distribution of the prepared nanoparticles.

3.3. L-DOPA Loading and Release

L-DOPA is an amino acid that is made and used as part of the normal human body as well as some animals and plants. It can cross the protective blood-brain barrier, unlike dopamine. Therefore, L-DOPA increases dopamine concentration for the common Parkinson disease treatment. This treatment was proven clinically by Nicholson and his group [26]. MSNs were widely explored for drug delivery using various types of drugs, whereas L-DOPA was not given any importance to having MSNs as the potential carriers [25,27]. In our research, the potential of using MSNs for specifically L-DOPA drug loading and release has been studied and evaluated. The illustration of the whole process for drug loading and release is given in Figure 6.

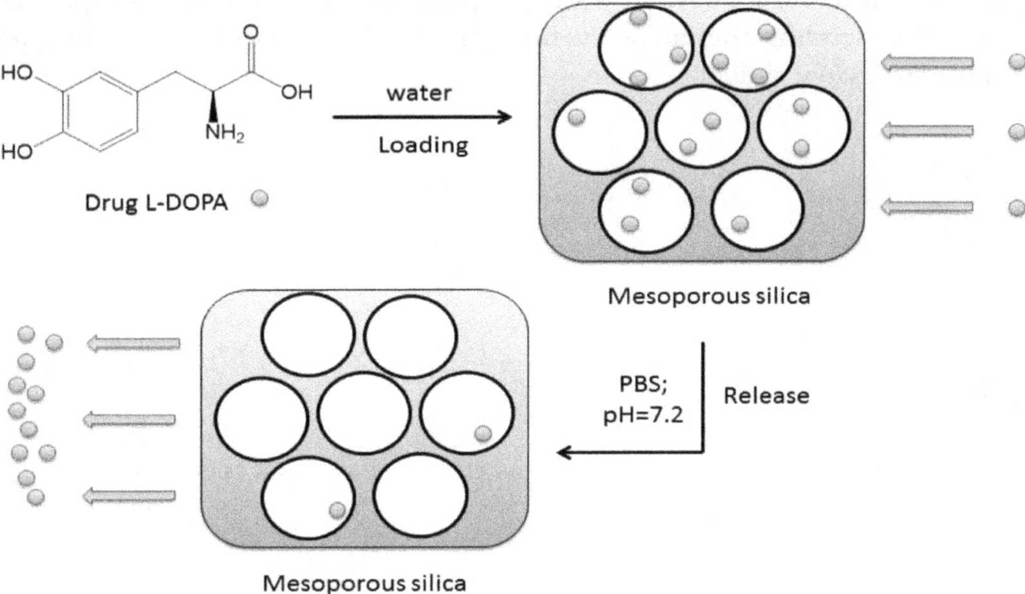

Figure 6. The illustration for L-DOPA drug loading to and release from mesoporous silica.

The calculations for loading and release of drugs using mesoporous particles have been widely discussed in many research works [28,29].

3.3.1. L-DOPA Drug Loading

L-DOPA drug loading was monitored by UV-VIS spectrophotometer and the calibration curve see Figure 7 was plotted to calculate the concentration change with respect to time using the absorbance spectra for evaluating the L-DOPA loading.

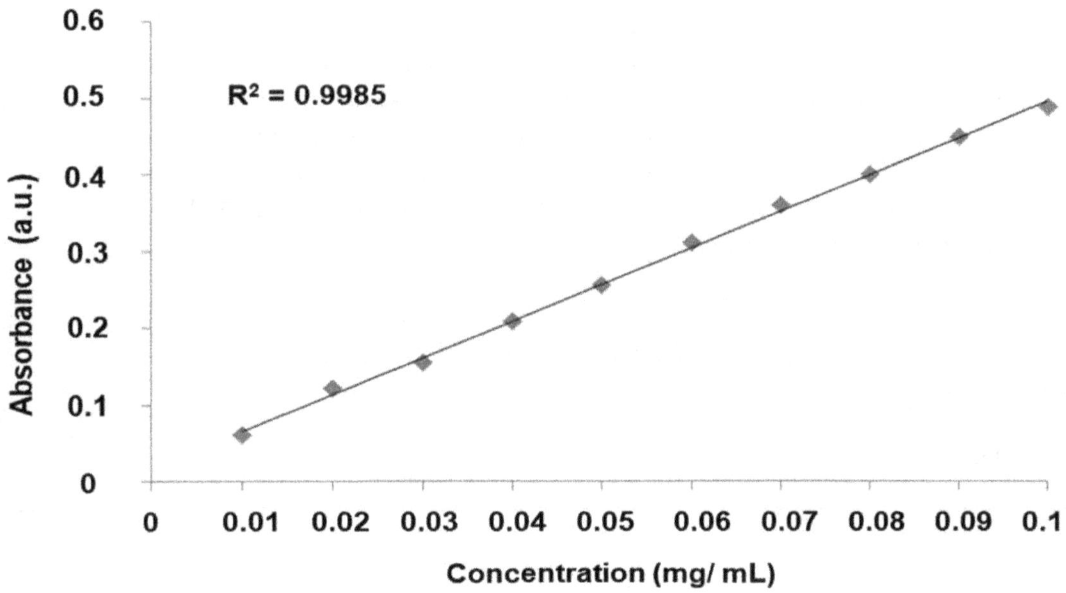

Figure 7. The standard calibration curve of L-DOPA in water.

The loading profiles of L-DOPA for MSNs are presented in Figure 8. We expected to observe the differences in drug loading amount as the mentioned MSNs had different surface morphologies although the pore sizes were similar.

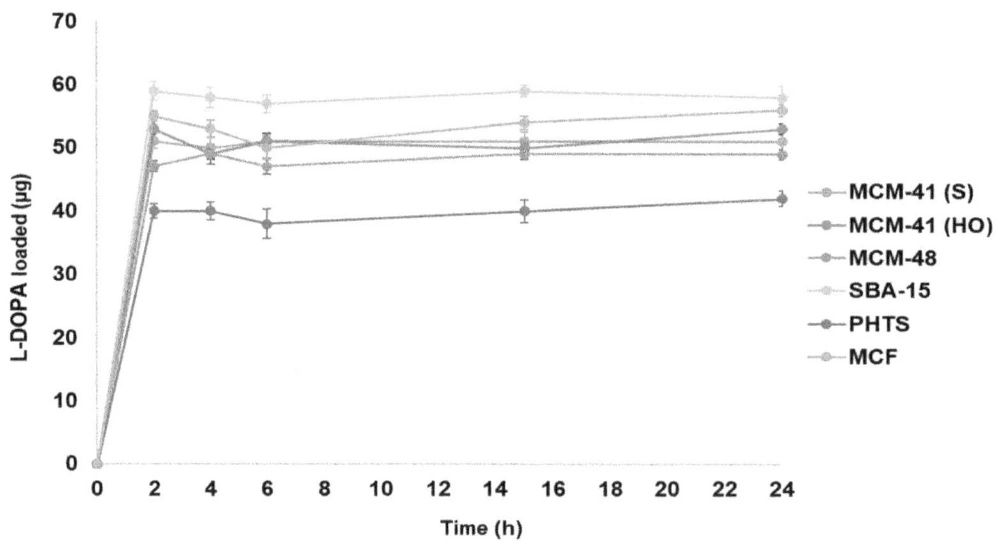

Figure 8. The L-DOPA loading profiles for all six types of mesoporous silica particles.

The curves show the drug loading (in µg) per 10 mg of the prepared mesoporous silica materials. Maximum loading was allowed by SBA-15 (59 µg) amongst all the mesoporous silica materials. SBA-15 is widely used for drug delivery and the obtained comparative results also support SBA-15 as the best mesoporous silica material. MCM-41(S), MCM-41(HO) and MCM-48 showed the narrow difference in loaded drug (51 µg, 53 µg and 49 µg respectively) as the pore diameters of all MCM materials were found to be similar. Highly ordered MCM-41(HO) exhibited more loading compared to other MCM series materials due to uniformity of porosity as well as surface morphology. The MCM-41(S) had spherical morphology, but particle sizes were less uniform than MCM-41(HO), therefore loading was less than MCM-41(HO). Due to large pore sizes of MCF, the loading performance of it (56 µg) was very close to SBA-15 and PHTS demonstrated minimum loading (42 µg), probably due to the presence of plugged pores. The L-DOPA loading was observed to be fast (2 h). The loadings were not continued more than 24 h as L-DOPA aqueous solution is very sensitive to light and heat. Moreover, the solution turns black as a result of degradation in solution [30]. The amounts of L-DOPA (wt.%) drug loaded in different samples are summarised in Table 4.

Table 4. L-DOPA loaded within the samples.

Sample	MCM-41 (S)	MCM-41 (HO)	MCM-48	SBA-15	PHTS	MCF
L-DOPA loaded (wt.%)	5.1 ± 0.3	5.3 ± 0.5	4.9 ± 0.3	5.9 ± 0.3	4.2 ± 0.6	5.6 ± 0.2

3.3.2. L-DOPA Drug Release

Like L-DOPA drug loading, L-DOPA drug release in PBS was also monitored by UV-VIS spectrophotometer. The calibration curve (Figure 9) was plotted using the absorbance spectra to measure the released drug concentration directly with respect to time for L-DOPA in PBS at pH 7.2.

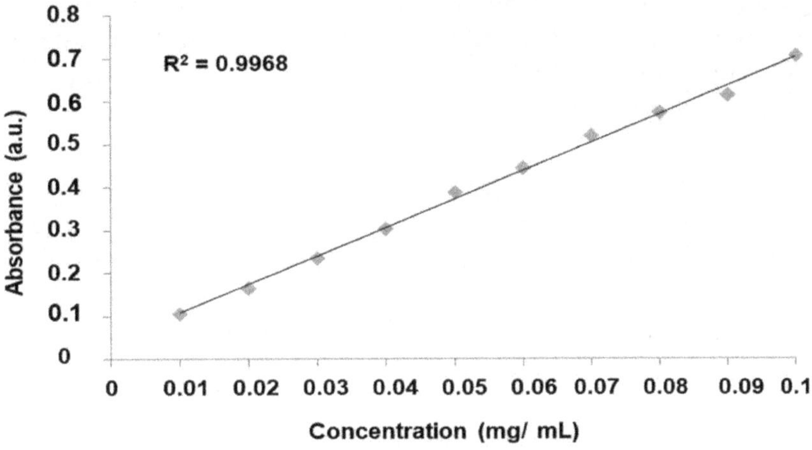

Figure 9. The standard calibration curve of L-DOPA in PBS.

The absorbance spectra recorded during the release of L-DOPA drug in different time intervals were used in order to prepare a plot indicating the release profile. The release profiles are depicted in Figure 10.

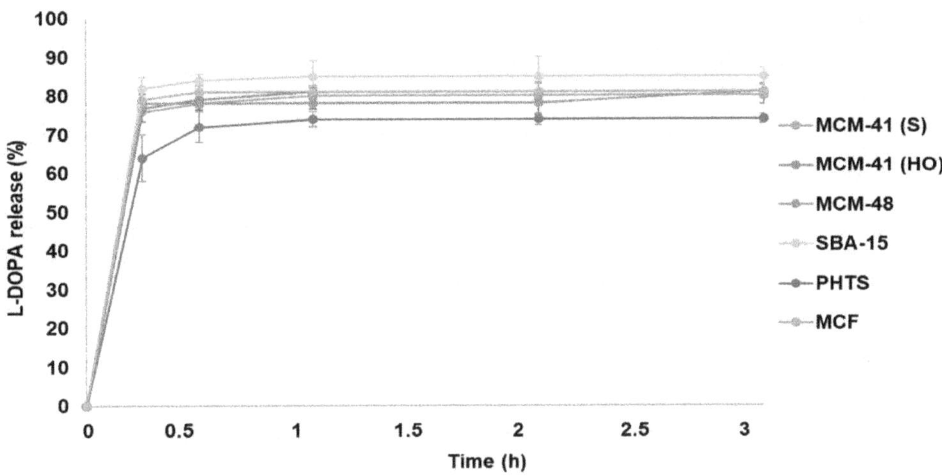

Figure 10. The L-DOPA drug release profiles for all six types of mesoporous silica particles.

The results established that the release is sustained rather than prolonged [27]. The release profiles of all tested materials were quite similar. SBA-15 with high surface area and pore volume (pore diameter ~7.6 nm) achieved highest release amount with ~85% in 1h whereas, PHTS revealed the lowest release (~74%). In MCM series, MCM-41 (HO) showed more drug release capacity (~81%) than others and all the results were compatible with the drug loading profiles. MCM-48 released ~78% of loaded L-DOPA, but MCM-41 (S) released ~80%. MCF having comparatively large pores (~12 nm) achieved ~83% drug release.

The comparative studies of drug loading and release revealed that surface morphologies, specific surface area, pore volumes and pore diameters played an important role in drug loading and release profiles of different MSNs. Amongst all the tested mesoporous silica materials, SBA-15 was found to be the best for L-DOPA drug loading and release. The analyses of drug loading and release profiles revealed that MSNs can be used for effective L-DOPA drug delivery choosing suitable mesoporous silica.

3.4. Up and Coming Outcomes Related to Biocompatibility Assessments

Numerous research papers are focused on the biocompatibility of various types MSNs [31,32]. Moreover, the chemo-physical properties of particles including their size, shape, surface area, structure and the route of drug administration have proved to play significant roles in their biocompatibility. For example, small MSNs (50 nm) exhibited effective drug delivery from the aspect of cellular uptake. On the contrary, large submicron particles (1220 nm) showed less cytotoxicity than nanoparticles (190 nm and 420 nm) [32]. Unfortunately, the attempts are limited by less understanding of particle interactions with cells in circulation. Current knowledge related to the biocompatibility for MSNs does not match with the rapid pace of research and sometimes is misleading [31]. With the rapid development of biomaterials, the original concept of "biocompatibility" has widely deviated. The biocompatibility may include all damaging as well as beneficial biological effects caused by MSNs [31,33,34]. Therefore, an appropriate protocol for an effective biocompatibility evaluation should be always chosen concerning all the important parameters, which are necessary for safety evaluation, mainly in case, of drug delivery systems.

4. Conclusions

Six different mesoporous silica materials were successfully prepared. The SEM and BET techniques were applied to evaluate the morphology and particle characteristics (surface areas, pore volumes and pore size distributions) of the prepared materials. A comparative study focused on the efficiency of L-DOPA drug loading and release among all the prepared mesoporous silica samples, analysed via UV-VIS absorption spectroscopy, confirmed SBA-15 as the most promising material for further experiments related to the kinetics of L-DOPA drug delivery system. We assume that the pore size of MSNs plays much more important role than their surface morphologies as all the MCM-41 (S/HO) samples, with nearly similar pore size, demonstrated almost same delivery profiles, although their surface morphologies were very different. The successful L-DOPA loading is highly encouraging for the continuation of further studies on in vitro and in vivo biocompatibility for evaluating the potential of clinical application.

Author Contributions: Conceptualization, I.S.; methodology, I.S.; software, V.M.; validation, V.M. and S.S.; formal analysis, S.S.; investigation, S.S.; resources, S.S.; data curation, S.S.; writing—original draft preparation, V.M.; writing—review and editing, V.M.; visualization, V.M.; supervision, I.S.

References

1. Central Nervous System (CNS). Therapeutic Market Report, 2018–2025. Available online: https://www.grandviewresearch.com/industry-analysis/central-nervous-system-cns-therapeutic-market (accessed on 7 September 2019).
2. Wilhelm, I.; Krizbai, I.A. In Vitro Models of the Blood–Brain Barrier for the Study of Drug Delivery to the Brain. *Mol. Pharm.* **2014**, *11*, 1949–1963. [CrossRef] [PubMed]
3. Wiley, D.T.; Webster, P.; Gale, A.; Davis, M.E. Transcytosis and Brain Uptake of Transferrin-Containing Nanoparticles by Tuning Avidity to Transferrin Receptor. *Proc. Natl. Acad. Sci. USA* **2013**, *110*, 8662–8667. [CrossRef]
4. Kamaly, N.; Xiao, Z.; Valencia, P.M.; Radovic-Moreno, A.F.; Farokhzad, O.C. Targeted Polymeric Therapeutic Nanoparticles: Design, Development and Clinical Translation. *Chem. Soc. Rev.* **2012**, *41*, 2971–3010. [CrossRef]
5. Davis, M.E.; Zuckerman, J.E.; Choi, C.H.J.; Seligson, D.; Tolcher, A.; Alabi, C.A.; Yen, Y.; Heidel, J.D.; Ribas, A. Evidence of RNAi in Humans from Systemically Administered SiRNA via Targeted Nanoparticles. *Nature* **2010**, *464*, 1067–1070. [CrossRef]
6. Lamanna, G.; Kueny-Stotz, M.; Mamlouk-Chaouachi, H.; Ghobril, C.; Basly, B.; Bertin, A.; Miladi, I.; Billotey, C.; Pourroy, G.; Begin-Colin, S.; et al. Dendronized Iron Oxide Nanoparticles for Multimodal Imaging. *Biomaterials* **2011**, *32*, 8562–8573. [CrossRef]
7. Fang, C.; Zhang, M. Multifunctional Magnetic Nanoparticles for Medical Imaging Applications. *J. Mater. Chem.* **2009**, *19*, 6258–6266. [CrossRef] [PubMed]
8. Qiao, R.; Yang, C.; Gao, M. Superparamagnetic Iron Oxide Nanoparticles: From Preparations to in Vivo MRI Applications. *J. Mater. Chem.* **2009**, *19*, 6274–6293. [CrossRef]

9. Berry, C.C. Progress in Functionalization of Magnetic Nanoparticles for Applications in Biomedicine. *J. Phys. D Appl. Phys.* **2009**, *42*, 224003. [CrossRef]
10. Thanh, N.T.K.; Green, L.A.W. Functionalisation of Nanoparticles for Biomedical Applications. *Nano Today* **2010**, *5*, 213–230. [CrossRef]
11. Meynen, V.; Cool, P.; Vansant, E.F. Verified Syntheses of Mesoporous Materials. *Microporous Mesoporous Mater.* **2009**, *3*, 170–223. [CrossRef]
12. Yang, P.; Gai, S.; Lin, J. Functionalized Mesoporous Silica Materials for Controlled Drug Delivery. *Chem. Soc. Rev.* **2012**, *41*, 3679–3698. [CrossRef]
13. Brinker, C.J. Hydrolysis and Condensation of Silicates: Effects on Structure. *J. Non-Cryst. Solids* **1988**, *100*, 31–50. [CrossRef]
14. Wang, Y.; Zhao, Q.; Han, N.; Bai, L.; Li, J.; Liu, J.; Che, E.; Hu, L.; Zhang, Q.; Jiang, T.; et al. Mesoporous Silica Nanoparticles in Drug Delivery and Biomedical Applications. *Nanomed. Nanotechnol. Biol. Med.* **2015**, *11*, 313–327. [CrossRef]
15. Douroumis, D.; Onyesom, I.; Maniruzzaman, M.; Mitchell, J. Mesoporous Silica Nanoparticles in Nanotechnology. *Crit. Rev. Biotechnol.* **2013**, *33*, 229–245. [CrossRef]
16. Deng, X.; Chen, K.; Tüysüz, H. Protocol for the Nanocasting Method: Preparation of Ordered Mesoporous Metal Oxides. *Chem. Mater.* **2017**, *29*, 40–52. [CrossRef]
17. Wu, S.H.; Mou, C.Y.; Lin, H.P. Synthesis of Mesoporous Silica Nanoparticles. *Chem. Soc. Rev.* **2013**, *42*, 3862–3875. [CrossRef] [PubMed]
18. He, Y.; Luo, L.; Liang, S.; Long, M.; Xu, H. Amino-Functionalized Mesoporous Silica Nanoparticles as Efficient Carriers for Anticancer Drug Delivery. *J. Biomater. Appl.* **2017**, *32*, 524–532. [CrossRef] [PubMed]
19. Xu, X.; Wu, C.; Bai, A.; Liu, X.; Lv, H.; Liu, Y. Folate-Functionalized Mesoporous Silica Nanoparticles as a Liver Tumor-Targeted Drug Delivery System to Improve the Antitumor Effect of Paclitaxel. *J. Nanomater.* **2017**, *2017*, 2069685. [CrossRef]
20. Maggini, L.; Cabrera, I.; Ruiz-Carretero, A.; Prasetyanto, E.A.; Robinet, E.; Cola, L.D. Breakable Mesoporous Silica Nanoparticles for Targeted Drug Delivery. *Nanoscale* **2016**, *8*, 7240–7247. [CrossRef]
21. Zukal, A.; Šiklová, H.; Čejka, J.; Thommes, M. Preparation of MCM-41 Silica Using the Cationic Surfactant Blend. *Adsorption* **2007**, *13*, 247–256. [CrossRef]
22. Vazquez, N.I.; Gonzalez, Z.; Ferrari, B.; Castro, Y. Synthesis of Mesoporous Silica Nanoparticles by Sol–Gel as Nanocontainer for Future Drug Delivery Applications. *Bol. Soc. Esp. Ceram. Vidr.* **2017**, *56*, 139–145. [CrossRef]
23. Yu, J.; Shen, L.; Cao, Y.; Lu, G. Preparation of Pd-Diimine@SBA-15 and Its Catalytic Performance for the Suzuki Coupling Reaction. *Catalysts* **2016**, *6*, 181. [CrossRef]
24. Hermida, L.; Abdullah, A.Z.; Mohamed, A.R. Synthesis and Characterization of Mesostructured Cellular Foam (MCF) Silica Loaded with Nickel Nanoparticles as a Novel Catalyst. *Mater. Sci. Appl.* **2013**, *4*, 52–62. [CrossRef]
25. Rahmani, S.; Durand, J.O.; Charnay, C.; Lichon, L.; Férid, M.; Garcia, M.; Gary-Bobo, M. Synthesis of Mesoporous Silica Nanoparticles and Nanorods: Application to Doxorubicin Delivery. *Solid State Sci.* **2017**, *68*, 25–31. [CrossRef]
26. Nicholson, G.; Pereira, A.C.; Hall, G.M. Parkinson's Disease and Anaesthesia. *Br. J. Anaesth.* **2002**, *89*, 904–916. [CrossRef] [PubMed]
27. Sevimli, F.; Yılmaz, A. Surface Functionalization of SBA-15 Particles for Amoxicillin Delivery. *Microporous Mesoporous Mater.* **2012**, *158*, 281–291. [CrossRef]
28. Jangra, S.; Girotra, P.; Chhokar, V.; Tomer, V.K.; Sharma, A.K.; Duhan, S. In-Vitro Drug Release Kinetics Studies of Mesoporous SBA-15-Azathioprine Composite. *J. Porous Mater.* **2016**, *23*, 679–688. [CrossRef]
29. Jangra, S.; Duhan, S.; Goyat, M.S.; Chhokar, V.; Singh, S.; Manuja, A. Influence of Functionalized Mesoporous Silica in Controlling Azathioprine Drug Release and Cytotoxicity Properties. *Mater. Res. Innov.* **2017**, *21*, 413–425. [CrossRef]
30. Pulikkalpura, H.; Kurup, R.; Mathew, P.J.; Baby, S. Levodopa in *Mucuna pruriens* and Its Degradation. *Sci. Rep.* **2015**, *5*, 11078. [CrossRef]

31. Behzadi, S.; Serpooshan, V.; Tao, W.; Hamaly, M.A.; Alkawareek, M.Y.; Dreaden, E.C.; Brown, D.; Alkilany, A.M.; Farokhzad, O.C.; Mahmoudi, M. Cellular Uptake of Nanoparticles: Journey inside the Cell. *Chem. Soc. Rev.* **2017**, *46*, 4218–4244. [CrossRef]
32. Tang, F.; Li, L.; Chen, D. Mesoporous Silica Nanoparticles: Synthesis, Biocompatibility and Drug Delivery. *Adv. Mater. Weinh.* **2012**, *24*, 1504–1534. [CrossRef] [PubMed]
33. Zhao, Y.; Sun, X.; Zhang, G.; Trewyn, B.G.; Slowing, I.I.; Lin, V.S.Y. Interaction of Mesoporous Silica Nanoparticles with Human Red Blood Cell Membranes: Size and Surface Effects. *ACS Nano* **2011**, *5*, 1366–1375. [CrossRef] [PubMed]
34. Narayan, R.; Nayak, U.Y.; Raichur, A.M.; Garg, S. Mesoporous Silica Nanoparticles: A Comprehensive Review on Synthesis and Recent Advances. *Pharmaceutics* **2018**, *10*, 118. [CrossRef] [PubMed]

3

Utilization of Ethylcellulose Microparticles with Rupatadine Fumarate in Designing Orodispersible Minitablets with Taste Masking Effect

Katarzyna Wasilewska [1], Patrycja Ciosek-Skibińska [2], Joanna Lenik [3], Stanko Srčič [4], Anna Basa [5] and Katarzyna Winnicka [1,*]

1 Department of Pharmaceutical Technology, Medical University of Białystok, Mickiewicza 2c, 15-222 Białystok, Poland; katarzyna.wasilewska@umb.edu.pl

2 Chair of Medical Biotechnology, Warsaw University of Technology, Noakowskiego 3, 00-664 Warsaw, Poland; pciosek@ch.pw.edu.pl

3 Department of Analytical Chemistry and Instrumental Analysis, Faculty of Chemistry, Maria Curie-Skłodowska University, M. Curie-Skłodowska Sq. 3, 20-031 Lublin, Poland; j.lenik@poczta.umcs.lublin.pl

4 Department of Pharmaceutical Technology, University of Ljubljana, Aškerčeva c. 7, 1000 Ljubljana, Slovenia; stanko.srcic@ffa.uni-lj.si

5 Department of Physical Chemistry, Faculty of Chemistry, University of Białystok, Ciołkowskiego 1K, 15-245 Białystok, Poland; abasa@uwb.edu.pl

* Correspondence: kwin@umb.edu.pl

Abstract: Minitablets in orodispersible form constitute a flexible drug delivery tool for paediatric and geriatric population as they eliminate the risk of chocking and do not require drinking water in the application. Due to their direct contact with taste buds, taste sensation is an important factor. Preparing microparticles with taste masking polymers utilizing spray drying is an efficient technique for reducing the bitterness of drugs. Ethylcellulose is a hydrophobic polymer widely used as a taste masking material. Rupatadine fumarate, one of the newest antihistamines, features an intensive bitter taste, hence in designing orodispersible formulations, achieving an acceptable taste is a crucial issue. The main objective of this work was to formulate orodispersible minitablets containing taste masked ethylcellulose-based microparticles with rupatadine fumarate and evaluation of their quality, especially in terms of taste masking efficacy. The accessed data indicated that all obtained minitablets were characterized by beneficial pharmaceutical properties. Three independent methods: in vivo with healthy volunteers, in vitro drug dissolution, and "electronic tongue" confirmed that all designed formulations provided satisfactory taste masking rate and that formulation F15 (prepared with Pearlitol® Flash and Surelease® microparticles with rupatadine fumarate) was characterized by the lowest bitterness score.

Keywords: ethylcellulose; spray drying; microparticles; rupatadine fumarate; orodispersible minitablets; taste masking

1. Introduction

The challenge of modern pharmaceutical technology is designing easy-to-administer drug dosage forms where the dose is sufficiently flexible to enable proper application and dose titration both to paediatric and adult patients. The currently available formulations that might be used in any age population are primarily liquids. However, the barrier of their utilization are difficulties in effective taste masking of bitter active pharmaceutical ingredients (API), the necessity of applying a large volume of medical preparation to adults, as well as low physicochemical and microbiological stability. Therefore, new technological solutions and strategies are being sought, as the appropriate drug formulation should be acceptable for a wide age group, in terms of organoleptic properties (taste, smell, appearance) to ensure regular intake of medicine, even while prolonged therapy. In case of solids, a crucial element that decides if they are swallowed, is their size—the smaller the unit, the easier application [1–4].

The solid drug dosage form, which connects the advantages of liquids (flexibility of dosing, ease of swallowing) with the qualities of solids (taste masking, stability), as well as enables individual dose adjustments for patients of all ages are minitablets (MT). MT are created for those encountering difficulties with application of larger tablets or as a form providing the possibility of dose titration by "multiplication", which allows the use of one product for the entire age population. The appropriate dose is determined by the number of MT administered (e.g., children of different ages will take different number of MT as one dose). MT are characterized by small sizes of one to three millimeters and mass of 5–25 mg. They are produced like traditional tablets, using existing technologies and production lines, as well as standard tableting blends. A promising type of MT are orodispersible minitablets (ODMT), which are characterized by very short disintegration and dissolution rates. ODMT are particularly recommended for patients with swallowing problems, by eliminating the risk of choking to a minimal [5–11].

The major limitation in designing orodispersible formulations is unpleasant taste of API. Insufficient taste masking effect of medicine is the most common reason for refusing of taking the preparation [12]. Taste masking techniques can be divided in two main groups: chemical modifications of API to reduce its solubility or creating a physical barrier between drug molecules and taste receptors. The first group includes primarily conversion into a prodrug (ester, salt), complexation with cyclodextrins, or ion exchange resins. The second mechanism involves designing microparticles or coatings using polymers having limited solubility in the oral cavity environment. A useful method of decreasing unsavory taste of a medicine is obtaining microparticles utilizing taste masking polymers. There are several technologies for preparing microparticles, among which spray drying is one of the most effective and efficient [12–16].

The aim of the following paper was to create ODMT containing microparticles with rupatadine fumarate (RUP) as a model bitter drug. Microparticles were obtained employing the spray-drying, utilizing ethylcellulose as a barrier forming polymer. In our previous work, microparticles prepared using different forms of EC were compared. The microparticles prepared with an aqueous dispersion of EC were found to have better properties in terms of taste masking effectiveness and morphology [17], therefore they were used to formulate ODMT. ODMT were evaluated regarding their morphological structure utilizing scanning electron microscopy (SEM), uniformity of weight and thickness, mechanical properties, drug content, and potential interactions occurring using differential scanning calorymetry. Disintegration time was evaluated in vivo by healthy volunteers on petri dishes and with texture analyzer usage. The crucial test—assessment of taste masking effect was carried out according to three alternative approaches: in vivo, by the drug dissolution and with electronic tongue utilization.

2. Materials and Methods

2.1. Materials

Aquacoat® ECD was donated from FMC BioPolymer, Newark, NJ, USA. Surelease® E-7-19040 was given from Colorcon Inc., Harleysville, PA, USA. Parteck® ODT was received from Merck KGaA, Darmstadt, Germany. SmartEx® QD-50 was handed over from Shin-Etsu Chemical Co., Ltd., Tokyo, Japan. F-Melt C was purchased from Fuji Chemical Industry Co., Ltd., Toyama, Japan. Pearlitol® Flash was a gift from Roquette, Lestrem, France. Magnesium stearate and methylene blue were acquired from POCh, Piekary Śląskie, Poland. RUP was procured from Xi'An Kerui Biotechnology Co., Ltd., Xi'An, China.

2.2. Preparation of ODMT

A traditional tablet presser (Type XP1, Korsch, Berlin, Germany) with 3-mm punches was employed to manufacture ODMT by direct compression. In tableting bulk preparation, optimized spray dried microparticles with RUP prepared with EC aqueous dispersions selected during preliminary studies—urelease® and Aquacoat® ECD as a barrier coatings were utilized [17]. The conditions of the spray drying process were established experimentally: 85 °C, aspirator flow 98%, rate of flow 3.5 mL/min. Efficient barrier for masking the bitterness of drug enclosed in microparticles was obtained utilizing RUP:polymer ratio (0.5:1) with 6% EC concentration and this formulation was used for designing ODMT. ODMT with a mass of 14 mg and amount of microparticles corresponding to 0.5 mg of RUP per single tablet were assumed. The compositions of designed tableting masses utilized in the study are shown in Table 1. Prepared tableting blends were mixed manually for 30 s. To determine relevant conditions of the tableting process, various pressure force grades ranging from 0.6 to 1.2 kN were tested. Tablets with optimal properties that did not have a damaged surface of microparticles were obtained using a 0.9 kN (± 0.1) force. To simplify the formulation of ODMT, multifunctional co-processed mixtures were utilized. Co-processed mixtures are designed by processing several excipients to possess advantages that cannot be achieved by the simple physical mixtures of their components [18–24].

Table 1. Composition of orodispersible minitablets (ODMT) formulations.

Ingredient [%]	Formulation															
	F1	F2	F3	F4	F5	F6	F7	F8	F9	F10	F11	F12	F13	F14	F15	F16
RUP	-	3.5			-	3.5			-	3.5			-	3.5		
SUR MP RUP *[corresponding to 0.5 mg RUP per one tablet]*	-		7.15		-	-	7.15		-	-	7.15		-	-	7.15	
AQ MP RUP *[corresponding to 0.5 mg RUP]*	-			8.65	-	-		8.65	-	-		8.65	-	-		8.65
Parteck® ODT	99	95.5	91.85	90.35	-	-			-	-			-	-		
SmartEx® QD-50	-				99	95.5	91.85	90.35	-	-			-	-		
F-Melt C	-				-	-			99	95.5	91.85	90.35	-	-		
Pearlitol® Flash	-				-	-			-				99	95.5	91.85	90.35
Magnesium stearate	1	1	1	1	1	1	1	1	1	1	1	1	1	1	1	1

2.3. Flow Properties of Powders

The tableting blends (Table 1) were subjected to preformulative quality assessment in accordance with pharmacopoeial requirements [25]. Each study was carried out in triplicate. A tapping apparatus (Electrolab ETD-1020, Mumbai, India) was utilized for the compressibility studies. The bulk and tapped densities were calculated as quotients of the weight of the powder to its volumes occupied before and after tapping and then the powder density index (Index Carr) and the powder flow index (Hausner's ratio) were calculated. To investigate powder flow time, 50 g of the sample was placed in the funnel with the outlet closed and after opening the valve, the flow of the whole sample through the funnel was measured [25].

2.4. Evaluation of Morphology of ODMT

Morphological structure was assessed utilizing scanning electron microscopy (Inspect™S50, FEI Company, Hillsboro, OR, USA). Swatches were placed on adhesive tapes fixed to the surface of a special stand and gold sprayed. Tests were performed at room temperature, using various magnifications.

2.5. *Quality Assessment of ODMT*

2.5.1. Uniformity of Weight and Thickness

Twenty randomly chosen ODMT were weighted individually, employing analytical balance (Radwag, Radom, Poland) [25]. The thickness was tested with calibrated digital caliper utilization (Beta 1651DGT, Milan, Italy).

2.5.2. Mechanical Properties

Tests were conducted with friability tester (EF-1 W, Electrolab, Mumbai, India) according to pharmacopoeial monograph for a quantity of ODMT corresponding to 6.5 g [25]. The crushing strength of ODMT was tested utilizing a hardness tester (5Y, Pharmaton AG, Thun, Switzerland) and a Texture Analyzer TA.XT. Plus (Stable Microsystems, Godalming, UK) with a steel cylinder of 6 mm diameter and 0.1 mm/s pre-speed [25]. The minimum force (N) needed to crush the ODMT was measured by vertically applying pressure along its diameter. Ten randomly selected tablets from the batch were used for hardness assessment in both methods.

2.5.3. Drug Content

HPLC apparatus (Agilent Technologies 1200) equipped with Waters Spherisorb® 5 μm ODS1 4.6 × 250 mm column (Waters Corporation, Milford, CT, USA) was applied to evaluate RUP content uniformity for individual ODMT. As a mobile phase methanol:phosphate buffer pH = 3.0 (35:65, v/v) was utilized (isocratic elution). Flux was established as 1.0 mL/min and wavelength as 245 nm. Buffer was composed of NaH_2PO_4 and water, adjusted to pH = 3.0 by H_3PO_4. Standard calibration curve was linear in the range of 1–100 μg/mL and the correlation coefficient R^2 was 0.999. The studies were carried out in triplicate [26–28].

2.6. *Disintegration Time Assessment*

2.6.1. In Vivo

The study was carried out by six probands (Research Ethics Committee at Medical University of Białystok approval number R-I-002/438/2016) in the following stages: oral cavity rinsing with water, placing ODMT in the mouth without chewing until disintegration, splitting out. The time needed for the total disintegration in the mouth was recorded.

2.6.2. Petri Dish

Petri dish having a diameter of 7 cm was filled with 4 mL of phosphate buffer pH = 6.8 imitating natural spit (composing of Na_2HPO_4; KH_2PO_4 and water; adjusted to pH 6.8 by 1-M NaOH) [17] and single ODMT was put in the center. The test was repeated for 6 tablets from each batch. Time for the tablet to completely disintegrate into fine particles was measured.

2.6.3. Texture Analyzer

The study was conducted with a texture analyzer (Stable Microsystems, Godalming, UK) with an ODT disintegration time rig (Figure 1). Single ODMT was attached to the bottom of the probe with double-side adhesive tape. The ODMT was immersed in the medium (4 mL of phosphate buffer pH = 6.8 imitating natural spit) until it comes in contact with the perforated bottom of the container. The test was repeated for 6 tablets from each batch.

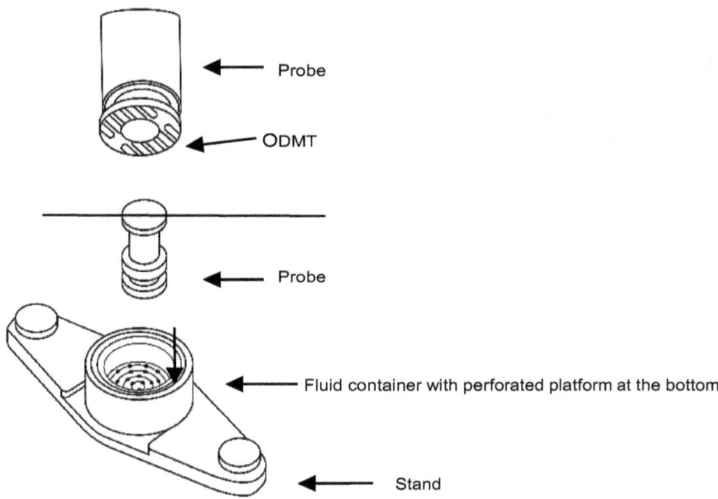

Figure 1. Schematic illustration of disintegration time rig of the texture analyzer.

2.6.4. Wettability

The wettability test was carried out according to Stoltenberg and Breitkreutz [29]. A 96-well plate (Biologix Group Limited, Lenexa, KS, USA) was used and a cellulose filter disc was placed in each well, which was then moistened by adding 20 μL of 0.3% aqueous solution of methylene blue. The time from placing the ODMT on moistened paper to complete coloring of the MT matrix was noted.

2.6.5. Differential Scanning Calorimetry

RUP raw material (API), microparticles placebo (MP AQ placebo, MP SUR placebo), microparticles (MP AQ RUP, MP SUR RUP), ODMT placebo (F1, F5, F9, F13), ODMT with pure RUP (F2, F6, F10, F14) and ODMT with RUP enclosed in SUR MP (F3, F7, F11, F15) and AQ MP (F4, F8, F12, F16) were tested using thermal analyzer system (DSC Mettler Toledo, Greifensee, Switzerland). Swatches were accurately weighed (5 mg), inserted in pans made of aluminum, then warmed up to 300 °C with 10 °C/min rate with 20 mL/min flow of nitrogen.

2.7. Evaluation of Taste Masking Effectiveness

2.7.1. In Vivo

The study was conducted in accordance with the Declaration of Helsinki and the protocol was approved by the Ethics Committee of Medical University of Białystok approval number R-I-002/438/2016. The efficiency of taste masking level was tested by six probands undergoing a test conducted as follows: five ODMTs were placed in the oral cavity for 30 s (the maximum time to dissolve/disintegrate in accordance to FDA guidelines [30]), spitted and mouth were rinsed with water. Sensory evaluation was marked as follows: 0—no bitterness, 1—slightly bitterness, 2—moderately bitterness, 3—significant bitterness. Before the experiment was carried out, the participants were chosen on the basis of sensory sensitivity test, utilizing four main flavors [31].

2.7.2. RUP Dissolution

RUP dissolution was carried out in apparatus II (paddle) (Erweka Dissolution Tester DT 600HH, Heusenstamm, Germany) with phosphate buffer (pH 6.8, 50 mL) imitating natural spit in following conditions: 75 rpm and 37 °C (+/−0.5). The quantity of dissolved RUP was assessed as pointed in 2.5.3.

2.7.3. Electronic Tongue

Reagents and Membrane Materials

Analytical reagent grade chemicals and purified water with 0.07 μS/cm conductivity (Elix Advantage System Mili-Q plus Milipore, Spittal an der Drau, Austria) were used. The membrane consisted of poly(vinylchloride) (PVC) (Tarwinyl, Tarnów, Poland); bis(2-ethylhexyl) sebacate (DOS), and o-nitrophenyl octyl ether (o-NPOE) (Fluka, St. Gallen, Switzerland); potassium tetrakis [3,5-bis(trifluoromethyl)phenyl]-borate (KTFPB), tridodecylmethylammonium chloride (TDMAC), 1-dodecylpyridinium chloride (DDPC), (Sigma—Aldrich, St. Luis, MO, USA), and potassium tetrakis(p-chlorophenyl)borate (KTpCPB) (Fluka, St. Gallen, Switzerland); calix[6]arene-hexaacetic acid hexaethylester (amine ionophore I) (Fluka, St. Gallen, Switzerland), and 3-mercapto-5-/2′-hydroxynaphthyl-azo-triazole (METRIAN) (Department of Drug Chemistry, Medical University of Lublin, Poland).

Membrane Preparation

Each solid contact electrode consists of a conventional body and an exchange Teflon holder in which the two phases are placed. The interior lamina (1) contains PVC with plasticizer in which the Ag/AgCl electrode is inserted and the exterior lamina (2) contains the ion-sensitive component and inner layer components. The exterior lamina is in contact with the tested solutions. The steps of the membrane phase preparation:

(1) weighing inner layer components: 30% (*w/w*) PVC, 70% (*w/w*) of plasticizers, DOS or o-NPOE,
(2) mixing and deaerating of obtained mixture,
(3) filling the Teflon holder with mixture to cover the silver-silver chloride electrode,
(4) gelating inner layer (1) at 373 K for 30 min, cooling of the gelled layer,
(5) weighing outer layer components, 27–33% (*w/w*) of PVC, 64–68% (*w/w*) of plasticizers, 1–5% of electroactive components (2) (Table 2),
(6) dissolving of obtained mixture in THF,
(7) placing drops on the inner layer (1),
(8) gelating outer layer (2) in result of evaporation THF at 293 K; repeating the steps several times.

Table 2. Electrodes forming sensor array of the electronic tongue.

Electrode Number no.	Electrode Type	Ionophore (%, *w/w*)	Lipophilic Salt (%, *w/w*)	Plasticizer (%, *w/w*)	Polymer (%, *w/w*)
1–2	CSF-D	–	KTFPB (1%)	DOS (66%)	PVC (33%)
3–4	CSF-N	–	KTFPB (1%)	o-NPOE (66%)	PVC (33%)
5–6	CSC-D	–	KTpCPB (3%)	DOS (64%)	PVC (33%)
7–8	CSC-N	–	KTpCPB (3%)	o-NPOE (64%)	PVC (33%)
9–10	AM-D	Amine ionophore I (5%)	–	DOS (68%)	PVC (27%)
11–12	MET-N	METRIAN (4%)	–	o-NPOE (66%)	PVC (30%)
13–14	PC-N	–	DDPC (3%)	o-NPOE (64%)	PVC (33%)
15–16	AN-N	–	TDMAC (4%)	o-NPOE (66%)	PVC (30%)

Potentiometric Measurements

EMF electrochemistry interface system (Lawson Labs. Inc., Malvern, PA, USA) and IBM PC were used for potentiometric measurements. The potentiometric sensor array of the system contains 16 solid contact ion-selective electrodes (two sensors of each type) differing active substances and plasticizers each other. The constructed solid contact electrodes were stored for 24 h in RUP solutions before the first measurement. As a standard, Ag/AgCl electrode (Orion 90-02, Thermo Electron Corporation, Beverly, MA, USA) was used. The electrodes calibration curves were performed in 10^{-5}–10^{-3} mol L^{-1} RUP solutions because of the poor solubility of RUP in water. Previously developed measurement protocol for electronic tongue analysis of pharmaceutical samples [32] was applied to test taste masking and API dissolution from designed ODMTs. First, the sensors were immersed in deionized water (50 mL) to obtain 5 min signal stabilization. Then adequate samples were added and released API and excipients influenced electrodes' signals, that were recorded as the changes of potentials (ΔEMF) of particular electrodes in sensor array in a function of time. The release measurements were carried out for solutions of pure API (RUP), all studied ODMTs and respective placebos. The signals of the sensors were registered during 15 min (5 min stabilization, 10 min release), in 5 repetition for each sample type. The sensors were water rinsed and dried between assays.

Data Analysis

Data matrix was composed of data vectors assigned to every investigated formulation (16 variables for every time-point, responding to 16 ΔEMF signals of 16 potentiometric sensors). The data matrixes were processed by chemometric procedures: Principal Component Analysis (PCA) or Partial Least Squares (PLS). These calculations as well as data analysis and presentation were performed in SOLO® software (Eigenvector Research Inc., Manson, WA, USA).

3. Results and Discussion

3.1. *Pharmaceutical Evaluation of ODMT*

An attempt was made to design and develop ODMT as an innovative drug dosage form, utilizing RUP enclosed in ethylcellulose microparticles to reduce bitterness. In preparation of ODMT, mainly spherical, homogenous, smooth surfaced microparticles based on EC aqueous dispersions were used (Figure 2). The mean size of microparticles made from Surelease® was 3.2 +/− 1.1 μm and from Aquacoat® ECD was 3.6 +/− 1.5 μm

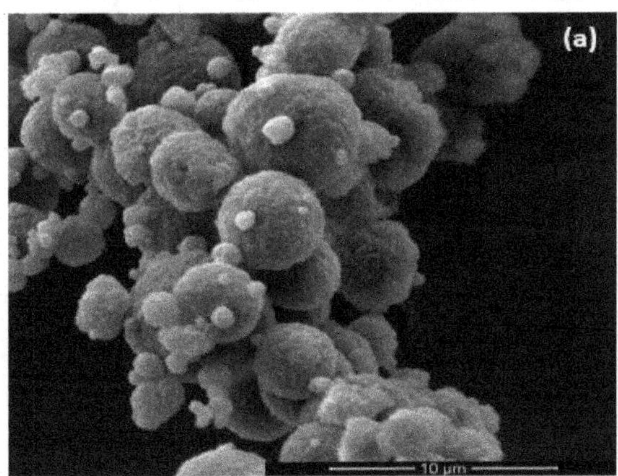

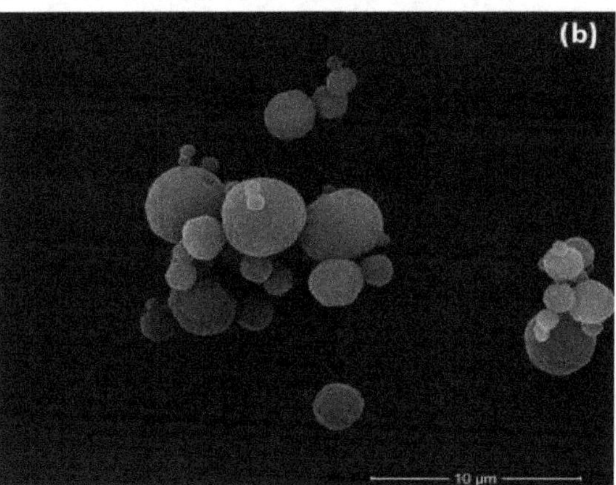

Figure 2. SEM picture of microparticles prepared using: (**a**) Surelease®, (**b**) Aquacoat® ECD under magnification 10,000×.

As a model drug with bitter taste, RUP (a long-acting second generation antihistamine showing anti-allergic and demulcent effect applied both in children and adults) was utilized. RUP is the histamine receptor selective antagonist and receptor for platelet activating factor (PAF), which highlights it from drugs belonging to this group and clarifies its unique mechanism of action. RUP binds to the H_1 receptor permanently and firmly, acting as an inverse agonist, which prolongs duration of its action. It was indicated that RUP is characterized by far greater affinity to H_1 receptor than fexofenadine or levocetirizine. Furthermore, by binding to PAF receptors, RUP causes their blockade, what is clinically relevant to PAF allergic inflammatory processes and bronchial hyperreactivity symptoms. RUP has not only been shown to reduce the amount of erythema (which is characteristic of all antihistamines), but also reduces PAF-induced platelet aggregation. The third component of RUP activity is its additional anti-inflammatory effect consisting in: inhibition of mast cell degranulation and release of histamine and cytokines (e.g., IL-4,5,6,8, TNF α), inhibition of eosinophil and neutrophil chemotaxis, inhibition of expression of adhesive molecules (CD18, CD11b) and transcription factors [33–39]. Commercially it is available in traditional tablets form [40] and due to its unpleasant taste, there is no orodispersible drug dosage forms on the pharmaceutical market.

To reduce bitterness of RUP, ethylcellulose (EC), a hydrophobic polymeric material widespread applied in masking the unpleasant aroma and taste was applied. It belongs to the GRAS (generally regarded as safe) and FDA Inactive Ingredients [41]. Moreover, EC is considered not to carry any health risks, therefore its daily intake has not been explicated by the World Health Organization (WHO) [42]. It is an ethyl ether of cellulose, in the form of a free-flowing, odorless, tasteless, biocompatible, non-allergenic, and nonirritant white to light-tan powder dissolving only in organic media, thus creating a polymeric barrier that allows for temporary isolation of a bitter drug from the oral cavity environment [43–45]. EC is accepted to be utilized in paediatric medicinal products, as well as in non-parenteral formulations authorized in Europe [41,46,47]. EC is available in organic form (e.g., Ethocel®) and as aqueous dispersions (e.g., Surelease®, Aquacoat ECD®). Surelease® contains a 25% of solid EC and dibutyl sebacate and oleic acid as plasticizers. In Aquacoat® ECD there is 27% EC, sodium lauryl sulfate, and cetyl alcohol. The dispersions are accepted for pharmaceutical use in the Europe, United States, and Japan [48,49].

ODMT were prepared by direct compression method, using commercially available mixtures: Parteck® ODT, SmartEx® QD-50, FMelt® C, Pearlitol® Flash. The amount of API was set as 0.5 mg per one ODMT. The dose selection was related to the fact that by multiplication, the dose of 2.5 mg required for children weighting from 10 to 25 kg can be easily achieved. No significant technological problems were observed during tableting process. It was connected with low API content in the tablet masses, so it did not affect the flowing properties of powders. The similar composition of all mixtures based mainly on mannitol caused all the obtained formulations to be characterized by similar physical parameters (Table 3). The best flowability was noted for blends with FMelt® C and Pearlitol® Flash.

Table 3. Characteristics of tableting blends.

Powder Mixture	Density [g/mL]		Flow Properties	
	Bulk	Tapped	Hausner's Ratio	Carr's Index [%]
F1	0.58	0.72	20.45	1.26
F2	0.58	0.71	20.45	1.26
F3	0.56	0.70	20.40	1.27
F4	0.57	0.68	20.20	1.24
F5	0.51	0.65	15.38	1.28
F6	0.52	0.65	15.38	1.28
F7	0.50	0.63	15.39	1.29
F8	0.49	0.62	15.25	1.30
F9	0.56	0.67	13.25	1.16
F10	0.56	0.66	13.24	1.16
F11	0.54	0.62	13.23	1.17
F12	0.52	0.61	13.22	1.15
F13	0.48	0.57	13.10	1.15
F14	0.48	0.58	13.10	1.15
F15	0.45	0.54	13.05	1.19
F16	0.44	0.53	13.13	1.16

Physical parameters of prepared tablets might be described as relatively good as the balance between the mechanical properties (sufficient hardness, friability <1%) and the quick disintegration time was captured. The obtained ODMT were hard enough that they did not crush while handling, and simultaneously, the formulations were characterized by the desired rapid disintegration time (below 30 s) (Table 4). The weight and thickness uniformity of ODMT is essential as it impacts dosing accuracy. The average masses of obtained formulations had values from 12.5 mg to 14.1 mg. Thickness of obtained ODMT was in the range from 1.80 mm to 2.01 mm. The optimal mechanical characteristics and rapid dissolution time are key aspects in orodispersible formulations depending on the conditions applied during the process. Appropriate tensile force is particularly important while tableting microparticles. Too high a value of tensile force could result in cracking microparticles, which has an undesirable effect in the case of taste masking. No microparticles crushing occurred at the applied pressure (Figure 3). The tensile force value 0.9 kN was determined experimentally as optimal. While lower pressure was applied, the tablets were too brittle to handle with, while higher disintegration time was insufficient (>30 s). Friability (in every formulation < 1%) and hardness tests have proven that obtained ODMTs were characterized by mechanical properties adequate enough so as not to be damaged during the manufacturing process or packing. However, the hardness of tablets prepared with microparticles utilization was smaller in comparison to placebo or formulations with pure RUP. RUP loading was in the range from 0.4 to 0.5 mg—the lowest values were marked for F8, F12, F16 and they did not meet pharmacopoeial requirements (<85%) [25].

Table 4. Physicochemical characteristics of prepared ODMT.

Parameter / Formulation	F1	F2	F3	F4	F5	F6	F7	F8	F9	F10	F11	F12	F13	F14	F15	F16
Weight [mg] *	13.4 ± 0.2	13.7 ± 0.3	14.0 ± 0.7	13.6 ± 0.5	14.1 ± 0.3	12.6 ± 0.9	12.9 ± 0.6	12.5 ± 0.7	13.8 ± 0.3	13.4 ± 0.2	13.5 ± 0.4	13.4 ± 0.5	14.1 ± 0.2	13.4 ± 0.5	13.9 ± 0.3	13.70 ± 0.4
Thickness * [mm]	2.01 ± 0.1	2.01 ± 0.1	1.96 ± 0.2	1.94 ± 0.3	1.94 ± 0.1	1.96 ± 0.2	1.82 ± 0.2	1.80 ± 0.3	2.0 ± 0.1	1.98 ± 0.1	1.97 ± 0.3	1.95 ± 0.3	1.97 ± 0.1	1.95 ± 0.1	1.95 ± 0.3	1.93 ± 0.4
Hardness [N] ** *(by hardness tester)*	15.4 ± 3.4	14.4 ± 2.4	8.40 ± 4.5	8.20 ± 4.7	16.8 ± 2.2	16.2 ± 2.5	8.1 ± 2.1	7.8 ± 2.3	15.9 ± 2.5	15.1 ± 2.1	8.1 ± 2.7	7.8 ± 2.9	16.1 ± 1.2	15.8 ± 2.1	8.1 ± 3.7	7.5 ± 4.2
Hardness [N] ** *(by texture analyzer)*	15.1 ± 3.9	14.6 ± 2.3	8.1 ± 4.0	8.0 ± 4.4	16.7 ± 2.2	16.5 ± 2.4	8.1 ± 1.5	7.8 ± 2.5	16.0 ± 2.2	15.0 ± 2.0	8.2 ± 2.5	8.0 ± 2.8	16.1 ± 1.1	15.9 ± 2.3	8.0 ± 3.5	7.6 ± 4.1
Friability [%]	0.1	0.1	0.1	0.2	0.1	0.45	0.1	0.1	0.1	0.1	0.1	0.3	0.1	0.1	0.1	0.2
Drug content * [mg]**	-	0.47 ± 0.1	0.48 ± 0.3	0.43 ± 0.4	-	0.45 ± 0.1	0.43 ± 0.2	0.42 ± 0.3	-	0.47 ± 0.1	0.45 ± 0.3	0.41 ± 0.4	-	0.49 ± 0.1	0.5 ± 0.1	0.40 ± 0.2
% of declared dose	-	94	96	86	-	90	86	84	-	94	90	82	-	98	100	0.80

*—the test was performed for 20 tablets [25]; **—the test was performed for 10 tablets in triplicate; ***—the test was performed for 10 tablets [25].

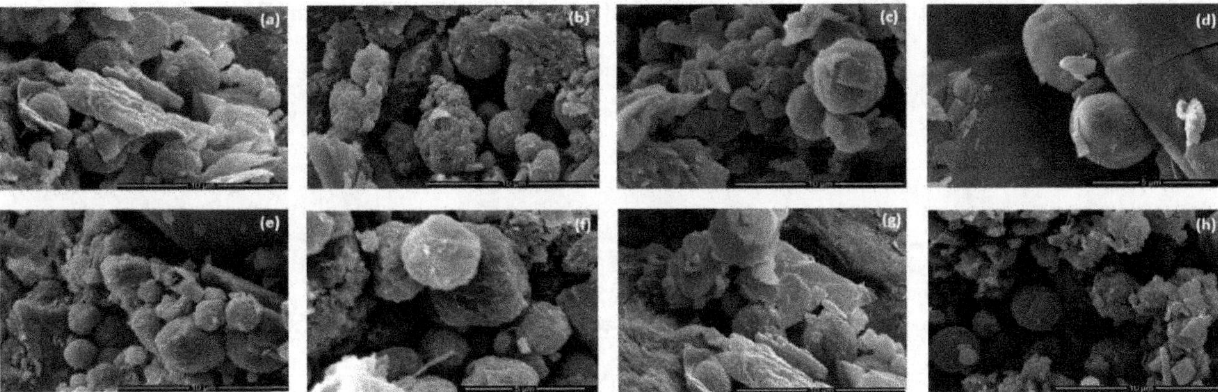

Figure 3. SEM pictures of ODMT cross-sections: (**a**) formulation F3, (**b**) formulation F4, (**c**) formulation F7 under magnification 10,000×, (**d**) formulation F8 under magnification 50,000×, (**e**) formulation F11 under magnification 10,000×, (**f**) formulation F12 under magnification 50,000×, (**g**) formulation F15, (**h**) formulation F16 under magnification 10,000×.

Disintegration time tests, conducted under conditions imitating those prevailing in the oral cavity (2–7 mL) are recommended [50–53], therefore tests in vivo with healthy volunteers, on petri dishes and using a texture analyzer were utilized. Regardless of the method, disintegration time of all ODMT formulations was below 30 s, and most formulations disintegrated even below 15 s. The longest disintegration time was recorded for F13, F14, F15, F16—19–24 s. In all tablets, wetting time below 30 s was noted.

An appropriate selection of pharmaceutical excipients is a key issue in creating drug dosage forms, as the excipients might affect physicochemical properties of API. Differential scanning calorimetry (DSC) is one of the analytical techniques frequently applied to determine drug physical properties, as well as to investigate potential incompatibilities with other components. The procedure provides detailed information about the presence of impurities and energetic properties of substances pointing to the differences in the heat flow generated or absorbed by the sample. To evaluate possible interactions, RUP raw material (API), microparticles placebo (MP AQ placebo, MP SUR placebo), microparticles (MP AQ RUP, MP SUR RUP), ODMT placebo (F1, F5, F9, F13), ODMT with pure RUP (F2, F6, F10, F14) and ODMT with RUP enclosed in SUR MP (F3, F7, F11, F15) and AQ MP (F4, F8, F12, F16) (Figure 4) were assessed. RUP chemical nomenclature is 8-chloro-6,11-dihydro-11-[1-[(5-methyl-3-pyridyl)methyl]-4-piperidylidene]-5H-benzo[5,6]cyclohepta[1,2-b]pyridine fumarate [54]. Its melting point should range from 194 to 201 °C. In the literature, there are no polymorphic forms reported for RUP [54,55]. The thermogram of pure RUP presents endothermic event at 196.44 °C characterized by a sharp pick, corresponding to its melting point. Sample decomposition after melting can be observed. Exothermic event transition is shown at 210.35 °C. Both melting and decomposition was noted in a constricted range of temperatures. No additional thermal events connected with decomposition or loss of surface water were observed. Thermograms of microparticles show that there are no thermal events for AQ MP and SUR MP placebo, which indicates that used aqueous dispersion of EC are in an amorphous state. Converting RUP into microparticle form by the spray drying did not significantly change solid state nature of the drug; however, some changes in its melting point occurred—in case of AQ MP RUP the peak has been shifted to 190.67 °C and for SUR MP RUP to 210.1 °C, which indicates that its melting point decreased about 6 °C or increased about 14 °C in microparticle samples, respectively. This is probably due to the fact that excipients used can slightly change physicochemical properties of API during spray drying. In all ready-made co-processed mixtures, the main ingredient is D-mannitol, whose melting point ranges from 155 °C to 165 °C, what was confirmed in the obtained thermogram. There is also a peak in 87 °C of magnesium stearate. No changes in the position of melting peaks and their specific heats were observed in the thermograms of ODMT. There are no further peaks of RUP as

API dissolves at the mannitol melting point. No distinct interactions between RUP and used excipients were observed.

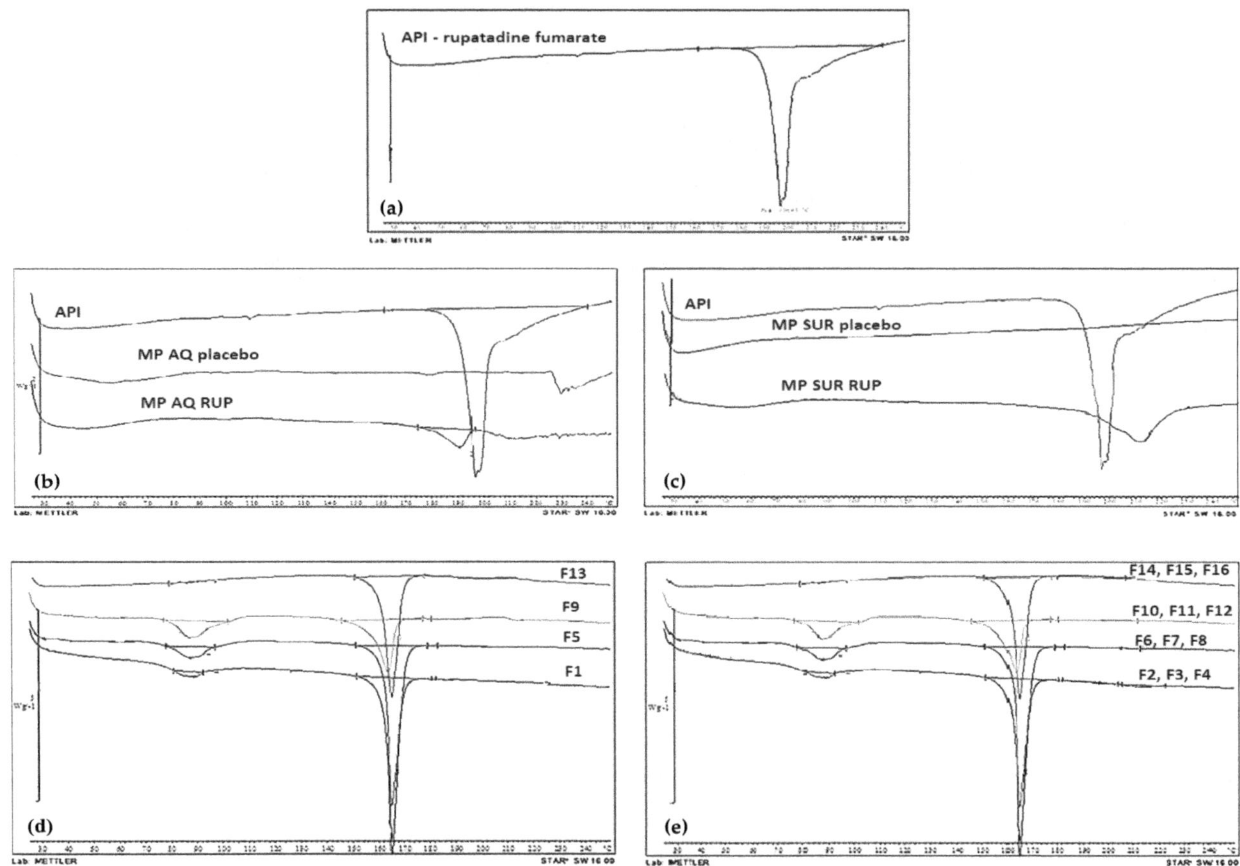

Figure 4. DSC thermograms of RUP - rupatadine fumarate (**a**) microparticles placebo obtained with Aquacoat® or Surelease® (MP AQ placebo MP SUR placebo) and with RUP (MP AQ RUP MP SUR RUP) (**b**,**c**) ODMT placebo (F1, F5, F9, F13) (**d**) ODMT with pure RUP (F2, F6, F10, F14) and with RUP enclosed in microparticles (F3, F4, F7, F8, F11, F12, F15, F16) (**e**).

3.2. *Taste-Masking Efficiency Evaluation*

Evaluation of taste masking effectiveness is a significant issue, as there are no pharmacopoeial and universal methods to assess the taste. To determine taste masking degree, in vivo (human taste panel) and various in vitro methods (e-tongue, drug release) can be utilized. Human taste panel is the most frequently used strategy of taste evaluation as it is widely available; however, it presents a certain challenge. There are high variances in human taste receptors expression and differences in taste perception (e.g., smoking or taking medicines have an impact). As well, children's participation in such a study is considered to be unethical, in turn the results obtained in adults are difficult to extrapolate to the entire population due to the different perception of taste sensations. Nevertheless, the predominant approach of assessing the taste of raw medicines and drug dosage forms is by human volunteers. An alternative approach is electronic tongues utilization. It is an analytical gustatory tool for automatic analysis of drug taste. Its essential element is the sensor array composed of chemical sensors with various selectivity. Potentiometric signals recorded in the tested sample do not provide direct information about the composition of the sample, but create its specific digital chemical image, whose interpretation allows to identify a sample or the content of its individual components, including those responsible for generating the taste. Evaluation of bitter taste can also be correlated to the drug release rate. It seems to be the simplest way to determine taste-masking efficacy based mainly on the quantification of drug concentration [56–59].

3.2.1. In Vivo Taste Evaluation

Initially, six selected healthy volunteers assessed ODMT formulations containing microparticles (F3, F4, F7, F8, F11, F12, F15, F16) as non-bitter or slightly bitter in comparison to those with pure RUP (F2, F6, F10, F14), which were determined as moderately or very bitter (Table 5). It should be also mentioned that mannitol—the main component of obtained ODMT—besides being a sweetening agent, while dissolving in the mouth maintains an impression of cooling, which has a favorable effect on taste sensation during the application [31].

Table 5. Sensory evaluation of designed ODMT formulations, estimated as follows: 0—no bitterness, 1—slightly bitterness, 2—moderately bitterness, 3—significantly bitterness.

Volunteer	Score											
	F2	**F3**	**F4**	**F6**	**F7**	**F8**	**F10**	**F11**	**F12**	**F14**	**F15**	**F16**
A	3	0	0	2	0	0	2	0	1	2	0	1
B	3	1	1	3	1	1	3	1	1	3	1	1
C	2	1	0	2	0	0	2	0	1	2	0	1
D	2	0	1	2	0	0	2	0	0	2	0	0
E	3	0	1	3	1	1	3	1	1	3	0	1
F	2	1	0	2	0	0	2	0	0	2	0	0

3.2.2. In Vitro RUP Release

Taste masking was also evaluated by RUP release from obtained formulations. Slowing the release of a drug is associated with better efficacy of masking the taste. ODMT made with microparticles (F3, F4, F7, F8, F11, F12, F15, F16) released RUP significantly slower compared to ODMT with pure RUP (F2, F6, F10, F14), where immediate release of RUP occurred (Figure 5). After one minute of dissolution test, maximum 15% of RUP was released, which indicates satisfactory taste masking effect considering very quick disintegration time (about 20 s) and short residence time in the oral cavity.

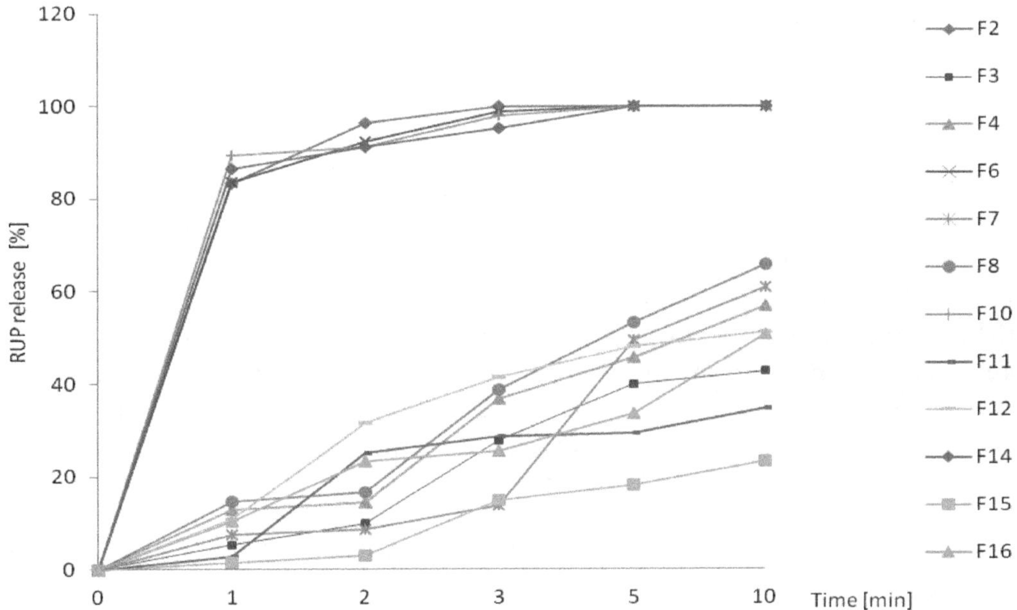

Figure 5. RUP release from designed ODMT performed in paddle apparatus.

3.2.3. Electronic Tongue

To investigate in detail taste masking efficiency for the studied formulations, human panel responses were processed by means of a multivariate technique—PCA. This data analysis method helps to find the most significant information hidden in the multidimensional data structure. As a result, a score plot in principal components (PC) coordinates is obtained, which shows clusters of samples based on their similarity. The more similar multidimensional characteristics are, the closer are the objects in the PC1-PC2 space. PCA scores plot (Figure 6) presents PCA processed data of human panel responses shown in Table 5.

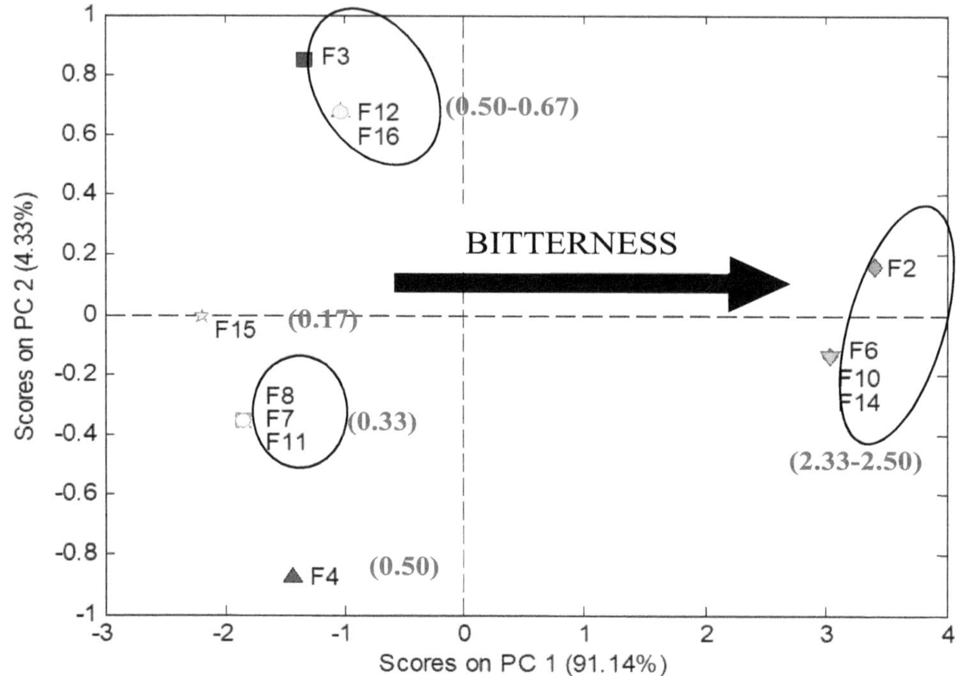

Figure 6. PC1, PCA of human panel responses showing similarity of sensed bitterness for the studied minitablets. Values in brackets show mean values of bitterness score calculated from Table 5.

The formulations form various clusters according to the sensed bitterness. The most bitter formulations: F2, F6, F10, F14, that reached mean score higher than 2, are placed close to each other and are characterized by high value of PC1. F6, F10, and F14 were evaluated identically by all volunteers, therefore they are overlapping, having the same coordinates PC1-PC2. Only one volunteer (a) estimated F2 as very bitter in contrast to F6, F10, F14 scored by him/her as moderately bitter, therefore F2 is similar to F6, F10, F14 PC1-PC2 scores, but not the same. ODMT F15 are placed in the highest distance from F2, F6, F10, and F14 cluster, having the lowest value of PC1, because they were estimated as not bitter by 5 out of 6 volunteers (the lowest mean value of bitterness). All remaining formulations were scored as very slightly bitter (mean values of bitterness from 0.33 to 0.67), and accordingly, they exhibit moderate PC1 values. All these observations perfectly match the dissolution tests (Figure 5), where formulations F2, F6, F10, F14 show high dynamics of RUP release, whereas the slowest release in the first two minutes is observed in the case of F15 minitablets.

Before the measurements of pharmaceutical formulations, an important stage of research was optimization of the sensor array. For this purpose, calibration curves of electrodes towards RUP were determined. As it results from Figure 7, for all electrodes containing various active substances and plasticizers in the membrane, different sensitivity towards RUP was achieved. Sensitivity ranged from about 10 mV decade^{-1} to about 51 mV decade^{-1} of 10^{-5}–10^{-3} mol L^{-1}.

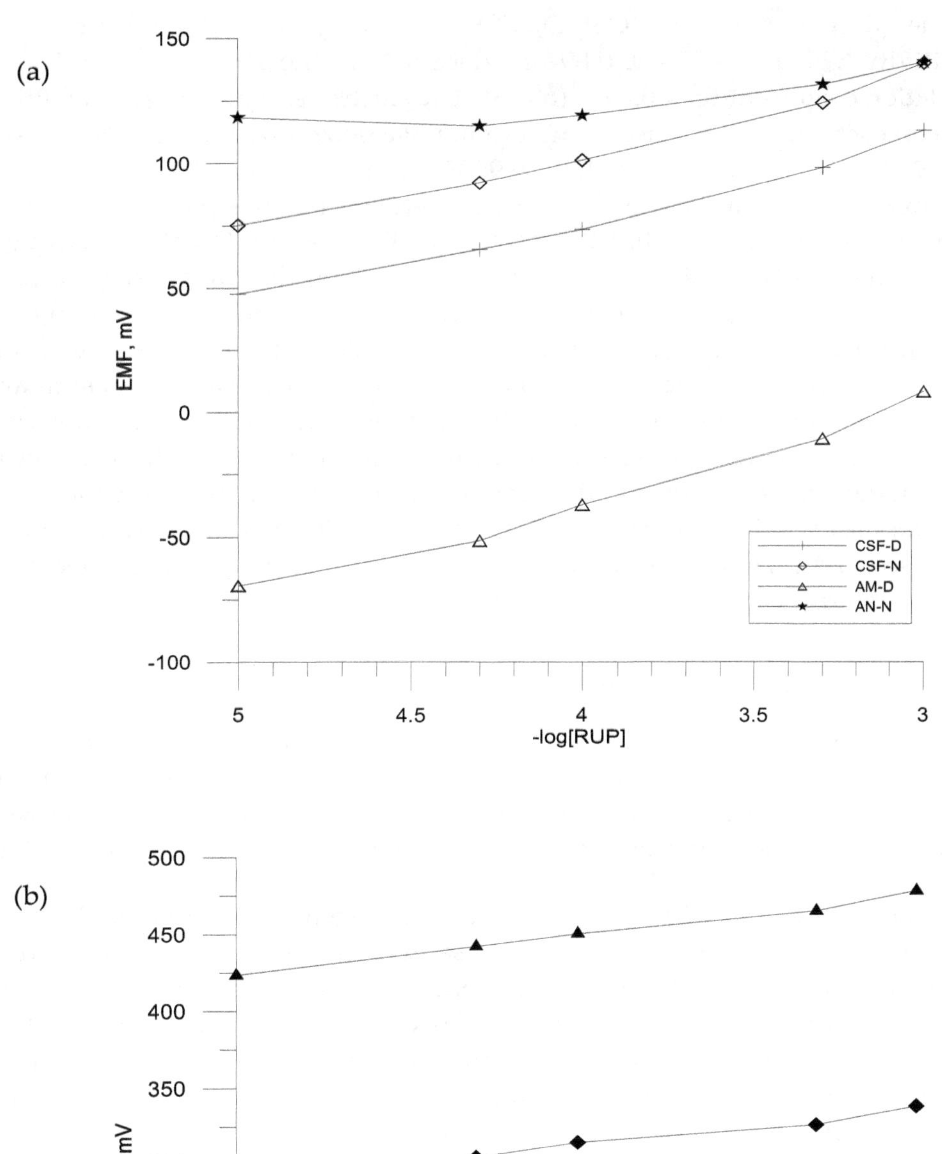

Figure 7. PC2, calibration curves of ion-selective electrodes with CSF, AM, AN (**a**) and CSC, MET, PC (**b**) in 10^{-5}–10^{-3} mol L^{-1} RUP solutions.

The electrodes based on KTFPB (CSF-D, CSF-N) displayed very similar calibration curves, with mean sensitivity 29.2 ± 4.3–32.4 ± 0.89 mV $decade^{-1}$ in the 10^{-5}–10^{-3} mol L^{-1} linear range, good mean correlation coefficient R^2 = 0.9944 (n = 3). The electrodes containing KTpCPB reveal visible differences between each other; the sensor's membrane plasticized with DOS (CSC-D) showed lower mean sensitivity 23.1 ± 4.4 mV $decade^{-1}$ (R^2 = 0.9983) than electrode with o-NPOE. This electrode exhibited linear range with slope close to the near Nernstian 51.5 ± 4.0 mV $decade^{-1}$ and good correlation coefficient R^2 = 0.9993. Slightly lower sensitivity exhibited the electrode with amine ionophore, mean response 41.5 ± 4.6 mV $decade^{-1}$. Moreover, the lowest slope of characteristics was obtained for electrodes prepared with ammonium and pyridinium ion exchangers. The slope coefficient of linear range of characteristic amounts 10 mV $decade^{-1}$ for PC-N electrode and 6 mV $decade^{-1}$ for AN-N electrode. The sensor based on metrian (MET-N) showed a similar response to electrodes CSF. All electrodes possessed lower or higher sensitivity to ionic RUP molecules (carboxyl groups, protonated nitrogen atom) as a result of the interaction of RUP with the active components of the polymeric membrane. Concluding, the prepared electrodes of electronic tongue sensor array exhibited satisfactory sensitivity towards studied API. According to our previous studies [17,60,61], such sensors are also cross-sensitive, responding to various excipients, which is a necessary condition for electronic tongue study.

3.2.4. Electronic Tongue—Taste Evaluation

The prepared sensor array was applied to check taste masking efficiency of all prepared ODMT. The procedure of measurements are presented in the experimental section. According to it, the responses of every sensor was given as ΔEMF in a function of time. Taste evaluation was performed for signals recorded after two minutes of release and resulting PCA score plot is presented in Figure 8.

All placebos formed a distinct cluster; they are grouped together even though their composition is different. On the opposite side of the plot, pure RUP samples are observed. All studied formulations take place between placebos and API, showing moderate taste between the two, which is correct and was expected. The clusters of formulations are partially overlapping, however similarity between electronic tongue study and human panel evaluation can be noticed. There is a cluster formed by F2, F6, and F14 ODMT in the closest distance to pure RUP, therefore their bitterness is most similar to pure API. Moreover, in proximity of this cluster, F10 can be seen. These four formulations showed the highest bitterness according to human panel (Figure 6) and highest dynamic of RUP release (Figure 8). The closest to RUP samples are F2 minitablets, which were evaluated as the most bitter, having a mean value of bitterness score equal to 2.5. The formulation that was the closest to placebo (not bitter) was F15, having the lowest bitterness score (0.17) and this fact also correlates well with human panel results and dissolution study. However, cluster of F15 is not distinct, it is spread out between other formulations, overlapping, e.g., F3 and F11 minitablets. Generally, samples having similar taste sensed by the human panel are considered similar also in terms of electronic tongue response, e.g., F8 is close to F7, and F12 is close to F16. The correlation is not perfect—the most surprising is the position of F11, in high distance from F7 and F8 minitablets. Nevertheless, the results of electronic tongue study reveal highest efficiency of taste masking for formulation F15 and lowest for formulations F2, F6, F10, and F14, which was confirmed by dissolution tests (Figures 5 and 9) and human panel results.

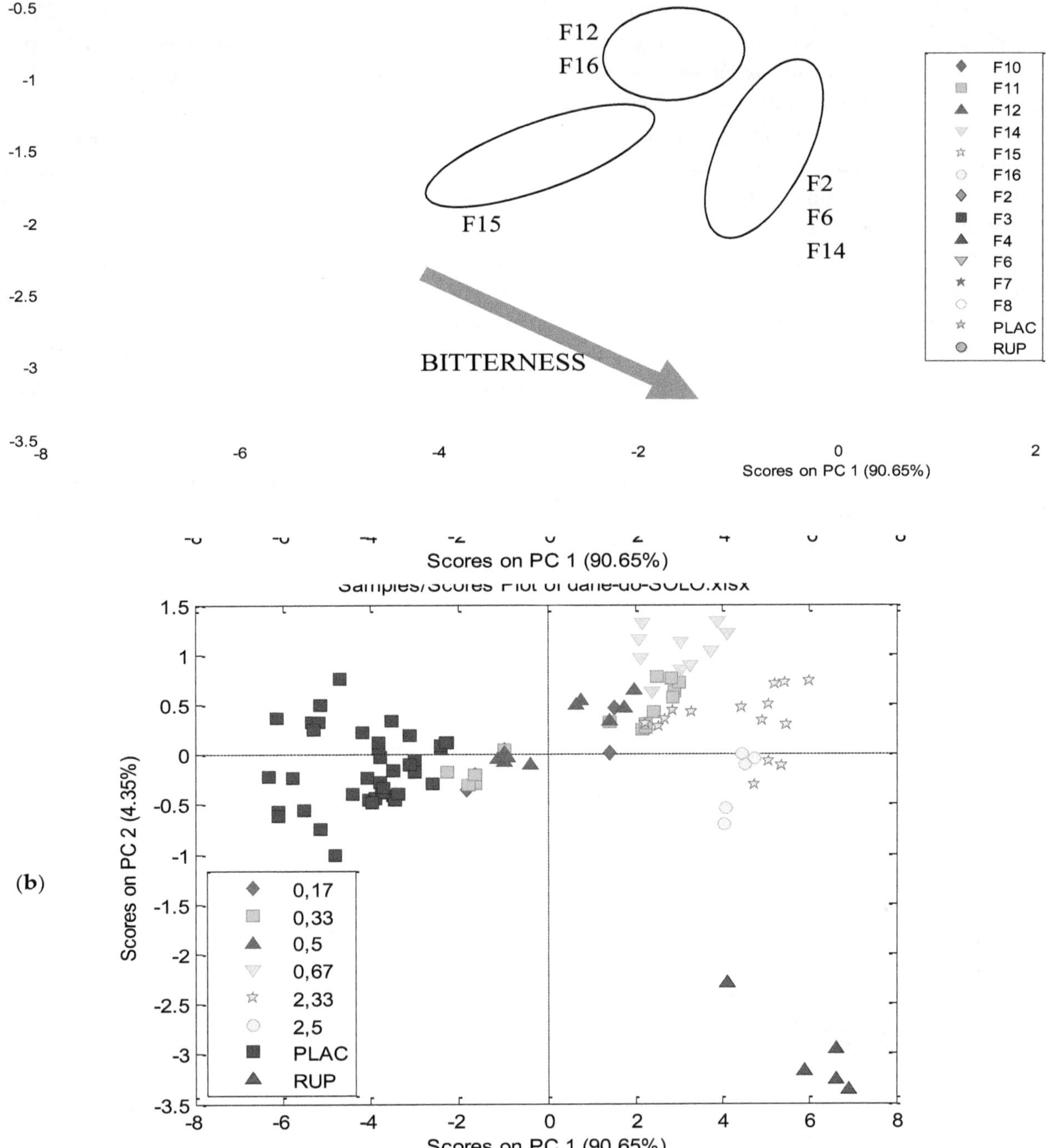

(b)

Figure 8. PC3, PCA score plot of electronic tongue responses for all studied formulations (F2-F16), respective placebos (PLAC) and pure RUP. On both plots the same object are presented, therefore they are in the same configuration, but the symbols are given according to: (**a**) formulation type; (**b**) mean values of bitterness score calculated from Table 5.

3.2.5. Electronic Tongue—Prediction of Dissolution Study

Signals of electrodes forming sensor array of electronic tongue were recorded during 10 min of formulation release. These outputs are related to RUP release, because the sensors are sensitive towards this API; however, they are also strongly influenced by increasing concentration of excipients, which are also released, due to cross-sensitivity of sensors. Therefore, to extract information of RUP release from sensor responses, a supervised data analysis technique was applied. First, we attempted to construct a Partial Least Squares (PLS) model. PLS regression is a chemometric procedure combining PCA and multiple regression. This approach leads to the possibility of the prediction of dependent variables from independent variables (measurement data). It is performed by transforming the obtained results into so-called latent components enabling the calculation of the dependent variables [62]. We applied this data analysis technique for various applications of the electronic tongue system [63–65]. In this paper, electronic tongue signals in appropriate time points were used for PLS modeling. All obtained data were divided into the training and test set. Target matrix was constructed based on %RUP release values that were determined by a standard dissolution test. For establishing a PLS model, a training set of data was applied aiming to find a correlation between the sensor array signals in an appropriate time point and % of RUP released in a respective formulation in a respective time point. When model was ready, the electronic tongue system was capable of predicting of amount of RUP that was released from the respective formulation based on electrodes' signals. The values of the RUP release were obtained for all studied formulations for a few time points. The resulting dissolution curves for independent test set data are presented in Figure 9. It must be underlined that what is predicted by electronic tongue system values are estimates, they do not provide accurate values of RUP release. The most evident example of that fact are negative values of RUP release for F3 minitablets. However, the outputs of PLS model show general tendencies discerning the studied formulations according to release dynamics. Two groups of dissolution curves can be observed. According to electronic tongue signals, four kinds of ODMT: F2, F6, F10, and F14, released RUP very fast, whereas all other formulations were characterized by much slower dynamics of its release. This finding correlates well with the standard dissolution test (Figure 5).

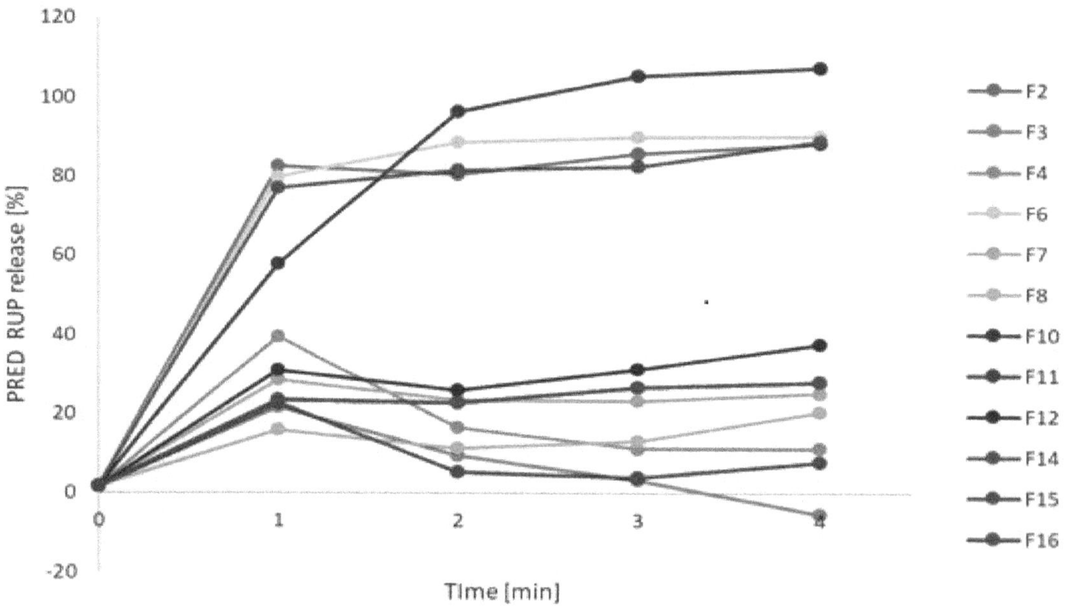

Figure 9. Electronic tongue prediction of RUP release (the results for independent test set).

4. Conclusions

Minitablets are getting increasingly significant among modern solid oral drug dosage forms, enabling the application of medicinal substances for patients of all ages by dose multiplying. Due to their small size they are easy to administer and swallow. Minitablets in orodispersible form improve patient compliance in relation to rapid disintegration in the oral cavity within seconds in the presence of the saliva without requirement of drinking water. Orodispersible minitablets (ODMT) with rupatadine fumarate were successfully prepared by direct compression of commercially available ready to use blends and ethylcellulose microparticles. Designed ODMT were characterized by beneficial physicochemical parameters. The presented study also indicates that MP made of etyhylcellulose with rupatadine fumarare might be efficiently utilized in preparation of ODMT by direct compression technique. The evaluation of taste masking level undertaken by three alternative approaches (e-tongue assessment, volunteers, and the drug release) established that designed ODMT are efficient taste–masking carriers of rupatadine fumarate and are supposed to be a promising alternative for traditional tablets.

Author Contributions: Conceptualization, K.W. (Katarzyna Wasilewska) and K.W. (Katarzyna Winnicka); methodology, K.W. (Katarzyna Wasilewska), P.C.-S., J.L., S.S., A.B., and K.W. (Katarzyna Winnicka); software, P.C.-S. and J.L.; validation, K.W. (Katarzyna Wasilewska), P.C.-S., and J.L.; formal analysis, K.W. (Katarzyna Winnicka); investigation, K.W. (Katarzyna Wasilewska), P.C.-S., J.L., S.S., and A.B.; resources, K.W. (Katarzyna Wasilewska) and K.W. (Katarzyna Winnicka); data curation, K.W. (Katarzyna Wasilewska); writing–original draft preparation, K.W. (Katarzyna Wasilewska), P.C.-S., J.L., and K.W. (Katarzyna Winnicka); writing–review and editing, K.W. (Katarzyna Wasilewska) and K.W. (Katarzyna Winnicka); visualization, K.W. (Katarzyna Wasilewska); supervision, K.W. (Katarzyna Winnicka); project administration, K.W. (Katarzyna Wasilewska) and K.W. (Katarzyna Winnicka); funding acquisition, K.W. (Katarzyna Wasilewska) and K.W. (Katarzyna Winnicka). All authors have read and agreed to the published version of the manuscript.

Acknowledgments: We are thankful to the following companies: Colorcon Inc., Harleysville, PA, USA; FMC BioPolymer, Newark, NJ, USA; Merck, Darmstadt, Germany; Shin-Etsu Chemical Co., Ltd., Tokyo, Japan; Fuji Chemical Industry Co., Ltd., Toyama, Japan; Roquette, Lestrem, France for kindly donating materials.

References

1. Gore, R.; Chugh, P.K.; Tripathi, C.D.; Lhamo, Y.; Gautam, S. Paediatric off-label and unlicensed drug use and its implications. *Curr. Clin. Pharmacol.* **2017**, *12*, 18–25. [CrossRef]
2. McIntyre, J.; Conroy, S.; Avery, A.; Corns, H.; Choonara, I. Unlicensed and of label prescribing of drugs in general practice. *Arch. Dis. Child.* **2000**, *83*, 498–501. [CrossRef] [PubMed]
3. Batchelor, H.K.; Marriott, J.F. Formulations for children: Problems and solutions. *Br. J. Clin. Pharmacol.* **2015**, *79*, 405–418. [CrossRef] [PubMed]
4. Lopez, F.L.; Ernest, T.B.; Tuleu, C.; Gul, M.O. Formulation approaches to paediatric oral drug delivery: Benefits and limitations of current platforms. *Expert Opin. Drug Deliv.* **2015**, *12*, 1727–1740. [CrossRef] [PubMed]
5. Spomer, N.; Klingmann, V.; Stoltenberg, I.; Lerch, C.; Meissner, T.; Breitkreutz, J. Acceptance of uncoated mini-tablets in young children: Results from a prospective exploratory cross-over study. *Arch. Dis. Child.* **2012**, *97*, 283–286. [CrossRef] [PubMed]
6. Klingmann, V.; Spomer, N.; Lerch, C.; Stoltenberg, I.; Frömke, C.; Bosse, H.M.; Breitkreutz, J.; Meissner, T. Favorable acceptance of mini-tablets compared with syrup: A randomized controlled trial in infants and preschool children. *J. Pediatr.* **2013**, *163*, 1728–1732. [CrossRef]
7. Klingmann, V.; Seitz, A.; Meissner, T.; Breitkreutz, J.; Moeltner, A.; Bosse, H.M. Acceptability of uncoated mini-tablets in neonates-a randomized controlled trial. *J. Pediatr.* **2015**, *167*, 893–896. [CrossRef]
8. Kluk, A.; Sznitowska, M.; Brandt, A.; Sznurkowska, K.; Plata-Nazar, K.; Mysliwiec, M.; Kaminska, B.; Kotłowska, H. Can preschool-aged children swallow several minitablets at a time? Results from a clinical pilot study. *Int. J. Pharm.* **2015**, *485*, 1–6. [CrossRef]
9. Kumar, K.P.; Teotia, D. A comprehensieve review on pharmaceutical minitablets. *J. Drug Deliv. Ther.* **2018**, *8*, 382–390.
10. Aleksovski, A.; Dreu, R.; Gašperlin, M.; Planinšek, O. Mini-tablets: A contemporary system for oral drug delivery in targeted patient group. *Expert Opin. Drug Deliv.* **2015**, *12*, 65–84. [CrossRef]
11. Guidance for Industry. Orally Disintegrating Tablets. Available online: https://www.fda.gov/media/70877/download (accessed on 20 February 2020).
12. Sharma, S.; Lewis, S. Taste masking technologies: A review. *Int. J. Pharm. Sci.* **2010**, *2*, 1–8.
13. Pandey, S.; Kumar, S.; Prajapati, S.K.; Madhar, N.M. An overview on taste physiology and masking of bitter drugs. *Int. J. Pharm. Bio. Sci.* **2010**, *1*, 1–11.
14. Jyothi, N.V.N.; Sakarkar, S.N.; Kumar, G.Y.; Prasanna, M. Microencapsulation techniques, factors influencing encapsulation efficiency: A review. *J. Microencapsul.* **2010**, *27*, 187–197. [CrossRef] [PubMed]
15. Faisal, W.; Farag, F.; Abdellatif, A.A.H.; Abbas, A. Taste masking approaches for medicines. *Curr. Drug Deliv.* **2018**, *15*, 167–185. [CrossRef] [PubMed]

16. Liu, W.; Chen, X.D.; Selomuyla, C. On the spray drying of uniform functional microparticles. *Particuology* **2015**, *22*, 1–12. [CrossRef]
17. Wasilewska, K.; Szekalska, M.; Ciosek-Skibinska, P.; Lenik, J.; Basa, A.; Jacyna, J.; Markuszewski, M.; Winnicka, K. Ethylcellulose in organic solution or aqueous dispersion form in designing taste-masked microparticles by the spray drying technique with a model bitter drug: Rupatadine fumarate. *Polymers* **2019**, *11*, 17. [CrossRef]
18. Bowles, B.J.; Dziemidowicz, K.; Lopez, F.L.; Orlu, M.; Tuleu, C.; Edwards, A.; Ernest, T.B. Co-processed excipients for dispersible tablets—Part 1: Manufacturability. *AAPS PharmSciTech* **2018**, *19*, 2598–2609. [CrossRef]
19. Prosolv® ODT. Available online: https://www.jrspharma.com/pharma_en/products-services/excipients/hfe/prosolv-odt-g2.php (accessed on 20 February 2020).
20. Parteck® ODT. Available online: http://www.phexcom.cn/uploadfiles/2011126103726995.pdf (accessed on 20 February 2020).
21. Fmelt®. Available online: http://www.fujichemical.co.jp/english/newsletter/newsletter_pharma_0802.html (accessed on 20 February 2020).
22. SmartEx® QD-50. Available online: http://www.metolose.jp/en/pharmaceutical/smartexr.html (accessed on 20 February 2020).
23. Pearlitol® Flash. Available online: https://www.roquette.com/pharma-and-nutraceuticals-coprocessed-mannitol-starch (accessed on 20 February 2020).
24. Ludiflash®. Available online: https://pharmaceutical.basf.com/global/en/drug-formulation/products/ludiflash.html (accessed on 20 February 2020).
25. Council of Europe. *The European Pharmacopoeia*, 9th ed.; Council of Europe: Strasburg, France, 2016.
26. Choudekar, R.L.; Mahajan, M.P.; Sawant, S.D. Validated RP-HPLC method for the estimation of rupatadine fumarate in bulk and tablet dosage form. *Pharma Chem.* **2012**, *4*, 1047–1053.
27. Redasani, V.K.; Kothawade, A.R.; Surana, S.J. Stability indicating RP-HPLC method for simultaneous estimation of rupatadine fumarate and montelukast sodium in bulk and tablet dosage form. *J. Anal. Chem.* **2014**, *69*, 384–389. [CrossRef]
28. Rele, R.V.; Mali, R.N. New validated RP-HPLC method for quantification of rupatadine fumarate impurities in solid dosage form supported by forced degradation studies. *Der Pharm. Lett.* **2016**, *8*, 66–72.
29. Stoltenberg, I.; Breitkreutz, J. Orally disintegrating mini-tablets (ODMTs)—A novel solid oral dosage form for paediatric use. *Eur. J. Pharm. Biopharm.* **2011**, *78*, 462–469. [CrossRef]
30. FDA; CDER. Guidance for Industry—Orally Disintegrating Tablets. 2008. Available online: https://www.fda.gov/downloads/Drugs/Guidances/ucm070578.pdf (accessed on 20 January 2020).
31. Amelian, A.; Szekalska, M.; Ciosek, P.; Basa, A.; Winnicka, K. Characterization and taste masking evaluation of microparticles with cetirizine dihydrochloride and methacrylate-based copolymer obtained by spray dryling. *Acta Pharm.* **2017**, *67*, 113–124. [CrossRef] [PubMed]
32. Łabańska, M.; Ciosek-Skibińska, P.; Wróblewski, W. Critical evaluation of laboratory potentiometric electronic tongues for pharmaceutical analysis—An overview. *Sensors* **2019**, *19*, 5376. [CrossRef] [PubMed]
33. Shamizadeh, S.; Brockow, K.; Ring, J. Rupatadine: Efficacy and safety of a non-sedating antihistamine with PAF-antagonist effects. *Allergo J. Int.* **2014**, *23*, 87–95. [CrossRef]
34. Mullol, J.; Gonzalez-Nunez, V.; Bachert, C. Rupatadine: Global safety evaluation in allergic rhinitis and urticaria. *Expert Opin. Drug Saf.* **2016**, *15*, 1439–1448.
35. Rao Sudhakara, M.; Dwarakanatha Reddy, D.; Murthy, P.S.N. Rupatadine: Pharmacological profile and its use in the treatment of allergic rhinitis. *Indian J. Otolaryngol. Head Neck Surg.* **2009**, *61*, 320–332. [CrossRef]
36. Picado, C.S. Rupatadine: Pharmacological profile and its use in the treatment of allergic disorders. *Expert Opin. Pharmacoter.* **2006**, *7*, 1989–2001. [CrossRef]
37. Merlos, M.; Giral, M.; Balsa, D.; Ferrando, R.; Queralt, M.; Puigdemont, A.; García-Rafanell, J.; Forn, J. Rupatadine, a new potent, orally active dual antagonist of histamine and platelet-activating factor (PAF). *J. Pharmacol. Exp. Ther.* **1997**, *280*, 114–121.
38. Chuch, M.K. Efficacy and tolerability of rupatadine at four times the recommended dose against histamine- and platelet-activating factor-induced flare responses and ex vivo platelet aggregation in healthy males. *Br. J. Dermatol.* **2010**, *163*, 1330–1332.
39. Izquierdo, I.; Valero, A.; García, O.; Pérez, I.; Mullol, J.; Van Cauwenberge, P. Clinical efficacy of rupatadine in allergic rhinitis under ARIA criteria: Pooled analysis. *Allergy Clin. Immunol. Int.* **2005**, *1*, 271–277.

40. Rupafin®. Available online: https://www.drugs.com/uk/rupafin-10mg-tablets-leaflet.html (accessed on 20 February 2020).
41. FDA Inactive Ingredients Database. Available online: https://search.fda.gov/search?utf8=%E2%9C%93&affiliate=fda1&query=ethylcellulose&commit=Search (accessed on 20 February 2020).
42. WHO. Available online: https://apps.who.int/iris/bitstream/handle/10665/42601/WHO_TRS_913.pdf (accessed on 20 February 2020).
43. Rowe, R.C.; Sheskey, P.J.; Quinn, M.E. *Handbook of Pharmaceutical Excipients*, 6th ed.; Pharmaceutical Press: London, UK; Chicago, IL, USA; Washington, DC, USA, 2009; pp. 262–267.
44. Ethylcellulose. Available online: https://pubchem.ncbi.nlm.nih.gov/compound/24832091#section=ProbableRoutes-of-Human-Exposure (accessed on 20 April 2020).
45. Wasilewska, K.; Winnicka, K. Ethylcellulose—A pharmaceutical excipient with multidirectional application in drug dosage forms development. *Materials* **2019**, *12*, E3386. [CrossRef] [PubMed]
46. Safety & Toxicity of Excipients for Paediatrics, STEP Database. Available online: http://www.eupfi.org/step-database-info/ (accessed on 26 May 2020).
47. Canadian List of Acceptable Non-Medicinal Ingredients. Available online: https://www.canada.ca/en/health-canada/services/drugs-health-products/natural-non-prescription/applications-submissions/product-licensing/compendium-monographs.html. (accessed on 26 May 2020).
48. Surelease®. Available online: https://www.colorcon.com/products-formulation/all-products/filmcoatings/sustained-release/surelease (accessed on 20 February 2020).
49. Aquacoat® ECD. Available online: http://www.fmcbiopolymer.com/Pharmaceutical/Products/Aquacoat.aspx (accessed on 20 February 2020).
50. Müller, K.; Fingueroa, C.; Martinez, C.; Madel, M.; Obreque, E.; Peña-Neira, A.; Morales-Bozo, I.; Toledo, H.; Lopez-Solis, R.O. Measurement of saliva volume in the mouth of members of a trained sensory panel using a beetroot (Beta vulgaris) extract. *Food Qual. Prefer.* **2010**, *21*, 569–574. [CrossRef]
51. Ali, J.; Zgair, A.; Hameed, G.D.S.; Garnet, M.C.; Roberts, C.J.; Vurley, J.C.; Gershkovich, P. Application of biorelevant saliva-based dissolution for optimization of orally disintegrating formulations of felodipin. *Int. J. Pharm.* **2019**, *30*, 228–236. [CrossRef]
52. Brniak, W.; Jachowicz, R.; Pelka, P. The practical approach to the evaluation of methods used to determinate the disintegration time of orally disintegrating tablets (ODTs). *Saudi Pharm. J.* **2015**, *23*, 437–443. [CrossRef]
53. Rupatadine Fumarate. Available online: https://www.drugbank.ca/salts/DBSALT001922 (accessed on 20 February 2020).
54. Henríquez, L.C.; Redondo, G.M.; Zúñiga, R.V.; Berrocal, G.C. Identification of rupatadine fumarate polymorphic crystalline forms in pharmaceutical raw materials. *AJST* **2018**, *9*, 7482–7487.
55. Henríquez, L.C.; Zúñiga, R.V.; Redondo, G.M.; Berrocal, G.C.; Vargas, G.H. Determination of the impact caused by direct compression on the crystalline state of rupatadine fumarate 10 mg tablets. *Int. J. Pharm. Technol. Biotechnol.* **2019**, *6*, 1–12.
56. Mohamed-Ahmed, A.H.; Soto, J.; Ernest, T.; Tuleu, C. Non-human tools for the evaluation of bitter taste in the design and development of medicines: A systematic review. *Drug Discov. Today* **2016**, *21*, 1170–1180. [CrossRef] [PubMed]
57. Pein, M.; Preis, M.; Eckert, C.; Kiene, F.E. Taste-masking assessment of solid oral dosage forms—A critical review. *Int. J. Pharm.* **2014**, *465*, 239–254. [CrossRef] [PubMed]
58. Clapham, D.; Kirsanov, D.; Legin, A.; Rudnitskaya, A.; Saunders, K. Assessing taste without using humans: Rat brief access aversion model and electronic tongue. *Int. J. Pharm.* **2012**, *435*, 137–139. [CrossRef]
59. Legin, A.; Rudnitskaya, A.; Clapham, D.; Seleznev, B.; Lord, K.; Vlasov, Y. Electronic tongue for pharmaceutical analytics: Quantification of tastes and masking effects. *Anal. Bioanal. Chem.* **2004**, *380*, 36–45. [CrossRef]
60. Wesoły, M.; Cal, K.; Ciosek, P.; Wróblewski, W. Influence of dissolution-modifying excipients in various pharmaceutical formulations on electronic tongue results. *Talanta* **2017**, *162*, 203–209. [CrossRef] [PubMed]
61. Wesoły, M.; Zabadaj, M.; Amelian, A.; Winnicka, K.; Wróblewski, W.; Ciosek, P. Tasting cetirizine-based microspheres with an electronic tongue. *Sens. Actuators B* **2017**, *238*, 1190–1198. [CrossRef]
62. Krishnan, A.; Williams, L.J.; McIntosh, A.R.; Abdi, H. Partial Least Squares (PLS) methods for neuroimaging: A tutorial and review. *NeuroImage* **2011**, *56*, 455–475. [CrossRef] [PubMed]

63. Wesoły, M.; Ciosek-Skibińska, P. Comparison of performance of various data analysis techniques applied for the classification of pharmaceutical samples by electronic tongue. *Sens. Actuators B* **2018**, *267*, 570–580. [CrossRef]
64. Zabadaj, M.; Szuplewska, A.; Kalinowska, D.; Chudy, M.; Ciosek-Skibińska, P. Studying pharmacodynamic effects in cell cultures by chemical fingerprinting—SIA electronic tongue versus 2D fluorescence soft sensor. *Sens. Actuators B* **2018**, *272*, 264–273. [CrossRef]
65. Zabadaj, M.; Ufnalska, I.; Chreptowicz, K.; Mierzejewska, J.; Wróblewski, W.; Ciosek-Skibińska, P. Performance of hybrid electronic tongue and HPLC coupled with chemometric analysis for the monitoring of yeast biotransformations. *Chemometr. Intell. Lab.* **2017**, *167*, 69–77. [CrossRef]

4

CO-Releasing Materials: An Emphasis on Therapeutic Implications, as Release and Subsequent Cytotoxicity are the Part of Therapy

Muhammad Faizan [1], Niaz Muhammad [2], Kifayat Ullah Khan Niazi [3], Yongxia Hu [1], Yanyan Wang [1], Ya Wu [1], Huaming Sun [1], Ruixia Liu [4], Wensheng Dong [1], Weiqiang Zhang [1,*] and Ziwei Gao [1,*]

1. Key Laboratory of Applied Surface and Colloid Chemistry MOE, School of Chemistry and Chemical Engineering, Shaanxi Normal University, Xi'an 710062, China; faizanattari@snnu.edu.cn (M.F.); huyongxia@snnu.edu.cn (Y.H.); yyw@snnu.edu.cn (Y.W.); wuya@snnu.edu.cn (Y.W.); hmsun@snnu.edu.cn (H.S.); wsdong@snnu.edu.cn (W.D.)
2. Department of Biochemistry, College of Life Sciences, Shaanxi Normal University, Xi'an 710062, China; niazpk@hotmail.com
3. School of Materials Science and Engineering, Xi'an Jiaotong University, Xi'an 710049, China; niazikifayat@stu.xjtu.edu.cn
4. Institute of Process Engineering, Chinese Academy of Science, Beijing 100190, China; rxliu@ipe.ac.cn

* Correspondence: zwq@snnu.edu.cn (W.Z.); zwgao@snnu.edu.cn (Z.G.);

Abstract: The CO-releasing materials (CORMats) are used as substances for producing CO molecules for therapeutic purposes. Carbon monoxide (CO) imparts toxic effects to biological organisms at higher concentration. If this characteristic is utilized in a controlled manner, it can act as a cell-signaling agent for important pathological and pharmacokinetic functions; hence offering many new applications and treatments. Recently, research on therapeutic applications using the CO treatment has gained much attention due to its nontoxic nature, and its injection into the human body using several conjugate systems. Mainly, there are two types of CO insertion techniques into the human body, i.e., direct and indirect CO insertion. Indirect CO insertion offers an advantage of avoiding toxicity as compared to direct CO insertion. For the indirect CO inhalation method, developers are facing certain problems, such as its inability to achieve the specific cellular targets and how to control the dosage of CO. To address these issues, researchers have adopted alternative strategies regarded as CO-releasing molecules (CORMs). CO is covalently attached with metal carbonyl complexes (MCCs), which generate various CORMs such as CORM-1, CORM-2, CORM-3, ALF492, CORM-A1 and ALF186. When these molecules are inserted into the human body, CO is released from these compounds at a controlled rate under certain conditions or/and triggers. Such reactions are helpful in achieving cellular level targets with a controlled release of the CO amount. However on the other hand, CORMs also produce a metal residue (termed as i-CORMs) upon degradation that can initiate harmful toxic activity inside the body. To improve the performance of the CO precursor with the restricted development of i-CORMs, several new CORMats have been developed such as micellization, peptide, vitamins, MOFs, polymerization, nanoparticles, protein, metallodendrimer, nanosheet and nanodiamond, etc. In this review article, we shall describe modern ways of CO administration; focusing primarily on exclusive features of CORM's tissue accumulations and their toxicities. This report also elaborates on the kinetic profile of the CO gas. The comprehension of developmental phases of CORMats shall be useful for exploring the ideal CO therapeutic drugs in the future of medical sciences.

Keywords: CO administration; therapeutic agent; pharmaceutical drugs; heme oxygenase; CO-releasing materials; CO-releasing molecules; organometallic complexes; pharmacokinetic functions; pathological role; CO kinetic profile; cellular targets

1. Introduction

Carbon monoxide (CO) is considered harmful due to its toxic behavior since the last century. It has a tasteless, odorless and colorless nature. Its colorless nature allows CO to remain undetectable even at high concentrations and toxic levels, thus marked as the "silent killer" [1,2]. This poisonous CO behavior is exerted due to the formation of carboxy hemoglobin (COHb) along with oxygen present in the mainstream blood circulation. Haldane and Douglas scientifically explored it the first time through dissociation curves of CO-hemoglobin using a constant percentage of CO along with a variable percentage of oxygen at an atmospheric pressure [3,4]. The ubiquitous enzyme, heme oxygenase (HO) has been investigated in most of the biological species. In the middle of the 19th century, two scientists Tenhunen and Schmidt discovered the intracellular CO production by heme oxygenase with an enzyme being the heme catalyst [5,6]. HO is categorized under two isoforms: HO-1 (HMOX1; gene name), with its capability to remain inducible in all cell functions; and HO-2 (HMOX2; gene name), that is constitutively expressed and substantially contained in vasculature and testes [7,8]. HO-1 is identified as an element exclusively found in spleen and liver [9]; however it might be influenced by varying intensity in most biological tissues. Both HO-1 and HO-2 indicate the rate-determining step, drag-out biliverdin from the heme conversion with the CO release and Iron product associated with a tetra pyrrole ring. Biliverdin using biliverdin reductase transforms into bilirubin while generating ferritin quickly from the Iron segregate (Figure 1) [10]. The released amount of CO attaches with the Iron containing objects due to its higher diffusion rate and tendency. It tends to make itself bonded with blood in the circulatory system; and ultimately it is exhaled through lungs. CO causes a common sagginess by bringing affliction for the mammalians, completely dependent on oxygen for the blood transport system and mitochondrial respiration. Collectively, endogenously generated CO is featured in the physiological role. Generally, a low dose of CO gas endures tremendous benefits and can achieve remarkable therapeutic targets.

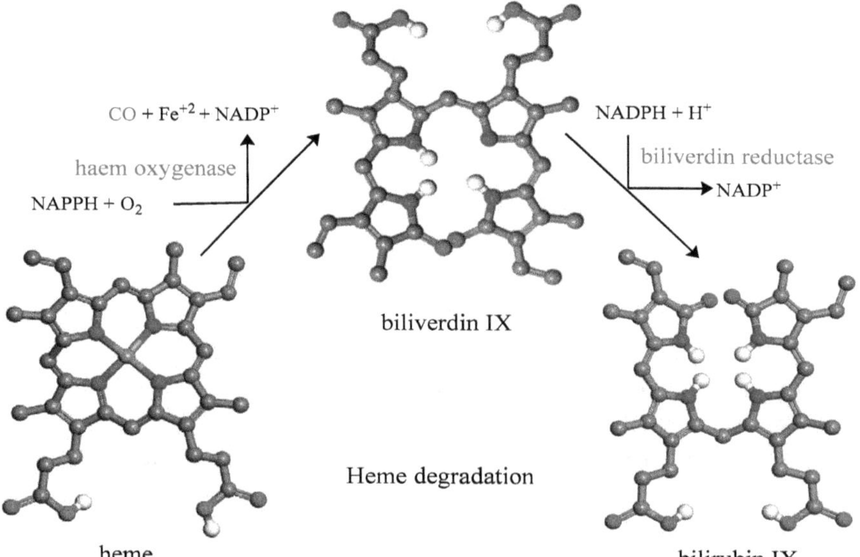

Figure 1. The intracellular carbon monoxide (CO) production by heme oxygenase (HO) in the mammalian system justifies its biological role.

CO is endogenously produced by either specific enzymes or through gas transmission into a biological system, both types exhibit the physiology and pathophysiology functions through inter- and intra- cellular interactions. The endogenously produced CO also raises their potential as a therapeutic agent. The scientists and researchers are availing this opportunity and spending their time and energies for developing modern drug techniques [11]. Their aim is to explore the modern work with the novelty of this great strategy.

1.1. CO Biological Scope

The CO gas is known for its leading role as a molecular messenger in the physiological process for the nervous system [12] and also for following some important therapeutic treatments [2,13]. It has the potential for anti-inflammatory [14], anti-proliferative [15], anti-atherogenic [16], anti-allodynia [17], anti-nociceptive [18], anti-hyperalgesia [17], and anti-apoptotic [19] effects. It is vital for vasodilatory phenomena reducing intraocular pressure [20], immunosuppressive administrated medications [21] and also has the capability to develop the pathological cellular process (Figure 2) [22]. CO also has many advantages for different biological organs: Organ transplantation [2], protection [23] and preservation; heart [24–26]; kidney [23,27–29]; liver [30,31]; lungs [32,33]; pancreatic islet [34] and the small intestine [35]. It is helpful to de-escalate the Ischemia/Reperfusion Injury (IRI) [36], mitigate the myocardial infarction and allograft rejection [37], stimulate the cytoprotective [38], and is also involved in anti-microbial [39] and anti-hypertensive activities [40]. It has a modulated utility for heme-dependent proteins like mitochondrial cytochromes and NADPH [28,41]. Moreover, the intercellular CO production by heme oxygenase has proved itself as a valuable reagent [42]. The pharmaceutical dose through endogenous CO enrichment or exogenous direct transformation is flourishing and will be attracted as a therapeutic interest lately.

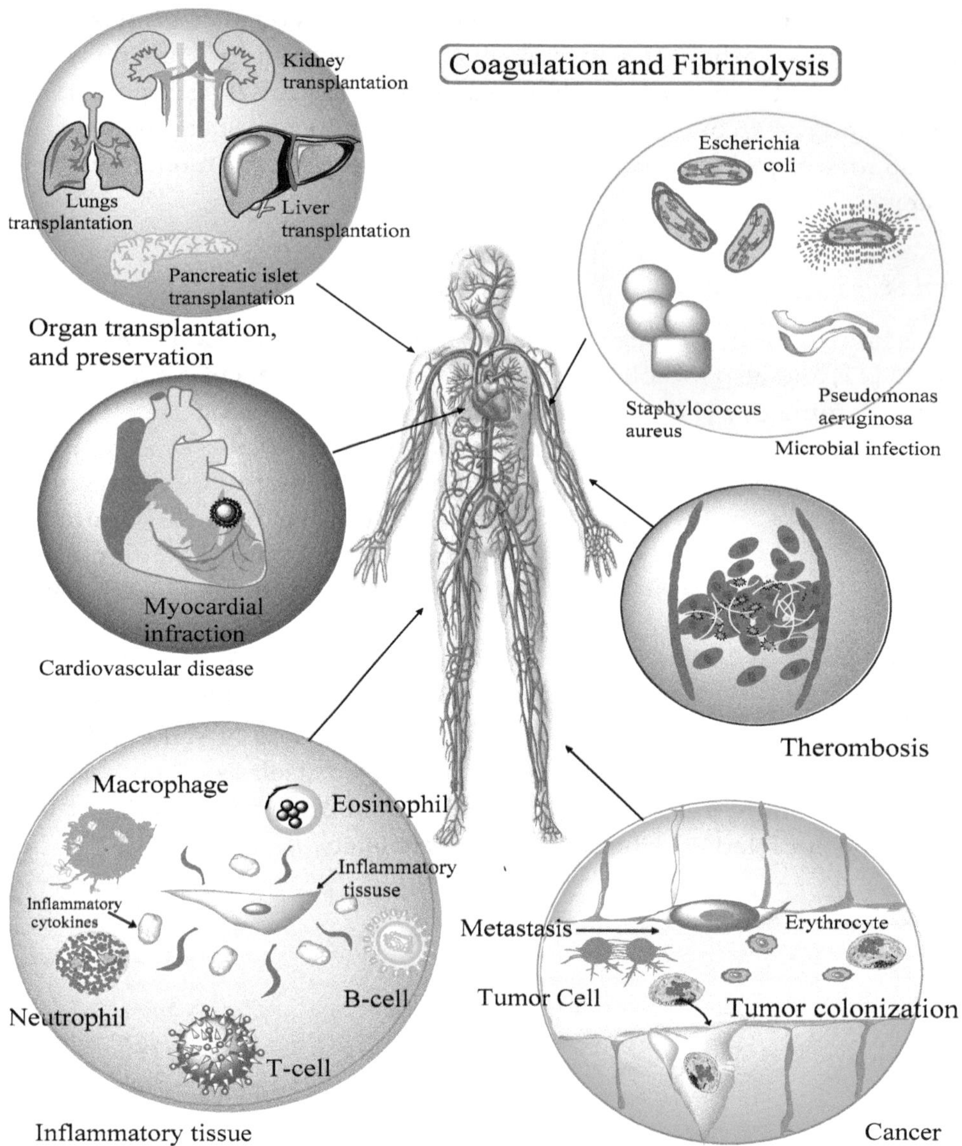

Figure 2. The coagulation and fibrinolysis scope of CO-releasing materials (CORMats).

1.2. CO Therapeutic Ways

Mainly, there are two ways to insert the CO molecules as a therapeutic agent inside the human body, i.e., direct and indirect CO insertion. The direct inhalation has not been preferred, owing to its rise in the COHb level above 10% and lack of tissue selectivity (Figure 3). Moreover, it provides a direct interaction of the CO and lungs only while detainment of CO is also observed in this method. These limitations don't allow CO to approach other biological organisms for therapy. To overcome these problems, researchers have developed an alternate strategy called "Exogenous Endeavor" for obtaining the required therapeutic actions. In the early 19th century, researchers also recognized the toxic gas NO as the nitro drug having therapeutic impacts. The nitric medications are well demonstrated as nitric oxide-releasing molecules (NORMs), and that established their well reputation afterward CORMs cogitation [43].

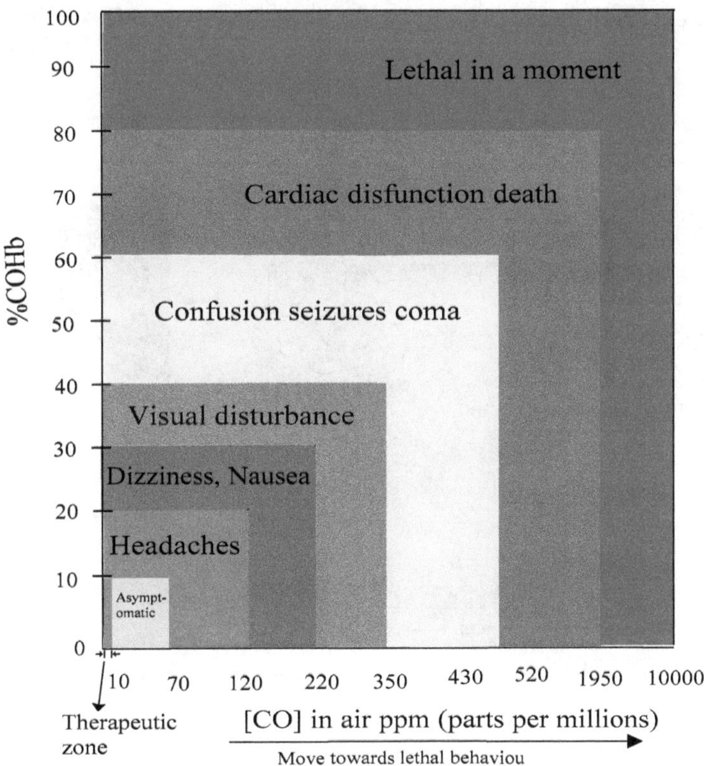

Figure 3. The carboxy hemoglobin (COHb) percentage is increasing in the direct CO inhalation beyond the therapeutic zone (~10%) during the mainstream blood circulation. (This information is based on data reported in reference [44,45]).

1.3. Why Exogenous Endeavor is Required?

The CO-releasing fragment is basically an exogenous endeavor that has opened up the paths for therapeutic treatments (Figure 4). The exogenous stakeholder CO, makes space for searching the affected sites, reaches at the diseased tissue site and makes conflict/collusion with the selected tissues for the destruction of damaged organs or/and diseased cells. If required, the CO-releasing rate can be regulated and modified according to specs. To disintegrate CORMs and CORMats into CO and metal residue, numerous activators are being administratively applied for controlling the CO liberation rate that has already been experienced in Photo-CORMs and Photo-CORMats through Ultra Violet (UV), Visible and NIR light with on/off switching facility [11,46–50]. The photon energy also has a utility to extract CO from its parent organometallic ligand. The main advantage of CO's exogenous interactions with the mammalian organism is that it reduces the CO moiety to be directly induced into blood streams for maintaining the COHb under allowable serum levels (up to 10%). Without an endogenous CO administration, it is quite challenging to get productive outcomes.

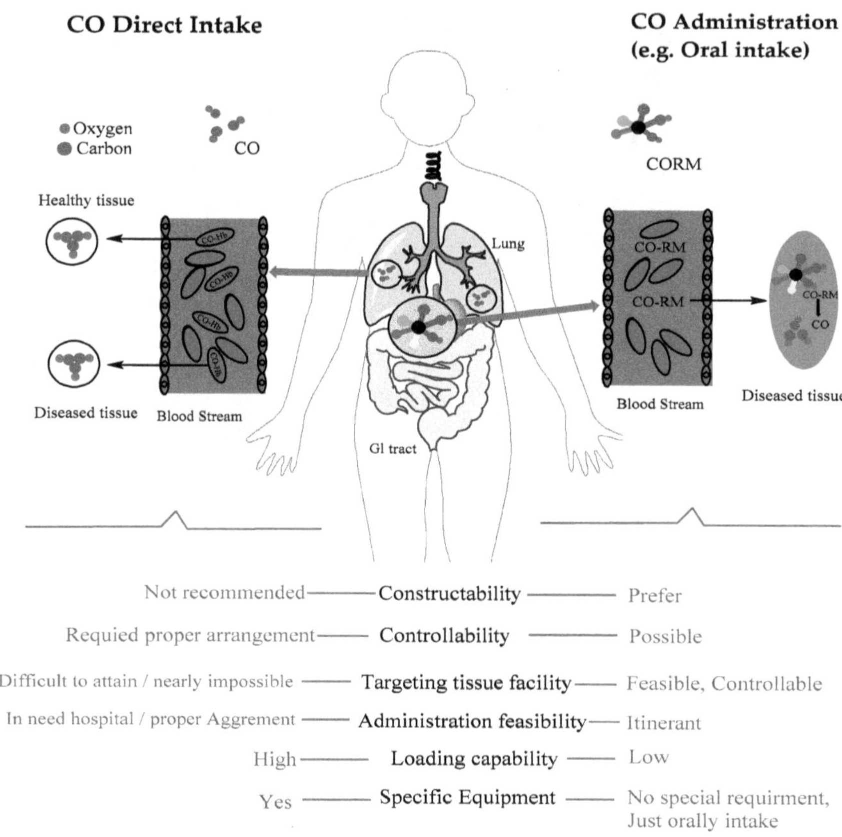

Figure 4. The feasibility analysis of the CO direct and indirect inhalation shows their different biological observance inside a human body.

1.4. *Clinical Translations*

In spite of its hazardous nature, a controlled CO direct inhalation has some therapeutic benefits as well. A clinical trial of controlled CO dosage was conducted on healthy volunteers for temporary paralysis of intestines known as Post-Operative Ileus (POI), and usually every patient is engaged in this POI after surgery of the abdomen. This clinical study revealed that serious POI complications could be significantly reduced if the CO dose (~250 ppm) is inhaled before and after the colon surgery (ClinicalTrials.gov identifier: NCT01050712). Another CO clinical translation test also shows a transplantation protection when the CO–saturated medium is provided for harvesting islets as it protects the cell from chronic pancreatitis (ClinicalTrials.gov identifier: NCT02567240).

This valuable intensive information about the CO therapeutic analysis plays a vital role for all the researchers' attention. Although there are few unfavorable emblems associated with releasing CO moiety, but recent outcomes of therapeutic potential helps to promote CO as preclinical stems [13]. This novel idea was initiated through clinical and pre-clinical trials for either the direct inhaled therapy [13] or oral intake of CO-releasing substances including CORMs or CORMats, which is a modern result of the professional chemistry enterprise [51].

1.5. *Challenges and Demanding Features of CORMs and CORMats*

Although CORMs and CORMats have a tremendous therapeutic utility but it also possesses some sort of following limitations for releasing the embedded CO.

- Availability, solubility and stability of reagents under ambient conditions.
- Feasibility to release the captured CO from in situ CORM.
- Controllability to release CO kinetics up to a desired level.
- Prone to toxicity which arises due to the transition metal foundation of metal-ligand fragments.

The abovementioned fundamentals have been discussed as a prescribed domain while exploring the CO discharge. Considering the CO gas as a therapy treatment based on CORMs and CORMats are easier to control by the transportation of gas molecules rather than the direct CO gas intake. Moreover, the rapid diffusion of these small molecules limits their ability to concentrate in specific tissues. Many challenges also arise during movability of the CO gas molecules by these strategies. Both the carbonyl transition metal and all its degradation products are biologically toxic in nature. Hence, it is difficult to manage the CO discharge with respective biological tissues. Particularly, the release of the CO molecules from CORMs also participates in depositing heavy metal ions inside the human body, which could be harmful for biological organisms.

1.6. Triggers

There are different ways to disintegrate CORMs/CORMats for the release of CO moiety by means of; peculiar physiological conditions [52], trigger by temperature [53], activation by an enzyme [54], pH alteration and increase in reactive oxygen species (ROS) concentration, accessibility to distinct wavelength of light [55,56], either using thermal degradation or ligand exchange/substitution or both [53] and prototypically activation through oxidation mechanism [11,57,58]. In order to deliver the CO molecules at a specified therapeutic rate, it is necessary to characterize the CORMs and CORMats entities, as quantification of such mechanisms might be contingent with its physical conditions like O_2, temperature, assay solution and light conditions.

1.7. CO Identifier

The authorized CO identification method consists of the following techniques: Electrochemical assays [59,60], laser infrared absorption [61] and gas chromatography [62]. Moreover, a colorimetric CO sensor facility is an alternative platform, especially for observing the CO behavior in living cellular tissues or/and organs [63,64]. The vibrational spectroscopy technique (such as IR, infrared and Raman) is one of the quickest ways to monitor the CO attached with transition metal through carbonylation at distinctive bond ranges. To date, the plethora method "Myoglobin Assay" famous as "*Gold Standard*" has been in operation for in vitro interrogation of the CO release from CORMs and CORMats. The "Myoglobin assay" is also a worthy and standard method for observing the behavior of the CO release kinetics in a biological environment and monitors the performed activity of CO (Equation (1)).

$$\text{Mb} + \text{CO} \rightarrow \text{Mb-CO} \quad (1)$$

Recently, It has been observed that binuclear Rhodium compounds, i.e., *cis*-$[Rh_2(C_6H_4PPh_2)_2(O_2CCH_3)_2](HAc)_2]$ can detect CO with a substantial selectivity and superior sensitivity [65]. The gas-phase IR spectroscopy is the most reliable and high-resolution technique for analyzing the CO release activity. For directly sensing the CO, various gas chromatography (GC) detectors have been introduced to date including the gas chromatography-mass spectrometer (GC-MS) [66], reduction gas detector (GC-RGD) [67] and thermal conductivity detector (GC-TCD). The fluorescent probe has the ability to recognize the CO-release entity even at a low concentration as compared with the myoglobin assay, but it is unable to operate in a short interval kinetic measurement (for that at least one hour interaction is required) [68,69].

1.8. The Development Phases of CORMs Motifs

1.8.1. Metal Carbonyl Complexes (MCCs)

To construct the bonding relation between the CO and low valent metal ions for producing carbonyl complexes (M-CO), the M-CO bonds must undergo an inert ambiance along with reducing conditions, which are mostly feasible in organic solvents. Irrespective of a metal physical state, the CO gas can react and develop the volatile metal carbonyl complexes (MCCs) for example, $Ni(CO)_4$ and $Fe(CO)_5$ [70]. MCC acts as a core entity for organometallic transition chemistry. The general representation for MCCs is $[M_m(CO)_xL_y]^{z\pm}[Q^{\pm}]^z$ [53], in which, M, L are the basic entity known as transition metal (B, Cr, Mn, Fe, Co, Mo, Ru, Rh, W, Re, Ir) [71], and ancillary ligand might be the C, O, P, N, S or halide ligand. Furthermore, Q and z represent the counter ion and overall complex charges. If no counter ion is available, then z will be zero. Moreover, m, y, z are calibrated as stoichiometric coefficients and x and m values should be ≥ 1 [53]. Modern and classic complexes can be distinguished by two determining factors: Low oxidation state (OS) or either very low oxidation state (LOS) and total valance electron occupied in the outer coordination sphere. For 4th, 9th, and 10th groups, the compounds were observed to have $16e^-$ configuration and the rest of the complexes were generally observed having $18e^-$ configuration. Each of these commodities must comply with the chemical, biological and physical characteristics of MCCs. Furthermore, it needs to be precisely selected in the configuration of pharmaceutical CORMs [71].

It is important to note that CORM and CORMats are stable in the aqueous medium, and it is also feasible to store it under ambient environmental conditions like the majority of other pharmaceutical drugs. Their circulation must be ensured, as it needs contact both with the diseased and damaged tissues. Moreover, the potent and non-toxic metabolites may be left behind after the CO removal. This is exactly what is required and regarded as therapeutic features. It sets the basic pattern, in the line of action for the development of such challenge-able MCCs. Mostly, during administration MCCs incorporates with the organic solvent and results in traditional oxygen-free atmosphere. These medical conditions might be different from a variety of other biological surroundings, considering that most reactants and their resulting complexes are uncertain under ambient conditions, i.e., oxygen and humidity [71]. Hypothetically, this biological activity of MCCs remains toxic in nature like $Ni(CO)_4$, and $(MeCp)Mn(CO)_3$ (MMT) as an anti-knock gasoline additive [72]. Hence, the common MCCs chemistry can act as a simple guideline for the development of pharmaceutical CORMs. Currently, this research is focused on novel strategies for establishing MCCs-CORM's activity and specifically for therapeutic purposes.

The above discussion suggested that MCCs when triggered as CORM's, become a competitor for the CO availability during its decomposition. In organometallic complexes the releasing strategy is as follows: A new incoming ligand (L') can push itself to a metal center resulting in a new bond, which establishes and influences on the coordination number. The elevated coordination number then promotes it to elongate the M-CO bonds, and eventually it then breaks. Consequently, the CO is liberated by this method and the new L'-M bond is constructed. This information provides the foundations of the CORMs concept. The chemistry of MCCs provides per se different strategies and has an adverse impact on the CO release (Scheme 1) [53].

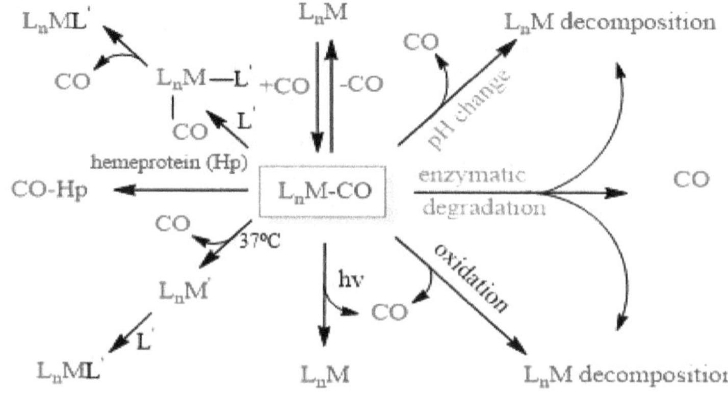

Scheme 1. CO releases from the ligand-metal CO framework (L_nM-CO).

1.8.2. Proposed Strategies for CORMs Development

CORMs based on metal-to-ligand charge transfers (MLCT) morphology. These CORMs are the elementary motifs with organometallic ingredients; corresponding to a series of MCCs occupied at the transition metal core. Other exclusive features are mentioned below:

- Structural variance of unique chemistry;
- Expected divergence with different oxidation states;
- Covalently bound with the metal center;
- Assisting alterations for the attached carbonyl ligands;
- The dynamics of co-ligands binding;
- Tendency of the outer coordination sphere.

As abovementioned, the spectroscopic nature of MCCs confirms the identification and recognition of significant trace elements like ruthenium [73,74], manganese [49,74–78], iron [37,79], cobalt [80,81], tungsten [82], osmium [83], molybdenum [82] and rhenium [84]. The developed organometallic carbonyl complexes CORMs are CORM-1, CORM-2, CORM-3, CORM-401, ALF492, CORM-A1, B_{12}-ReCORM-2, Re-CORM-1, CORMA-1-PLA and ALF186.

Along with organometallic complexes, the miscellaneous compounds can be nominated as the CORMs family. In this scenario, numerous nonmetallic compounds [85] have been accomplished by entertaining the CO release such as silica-carboxylates [86], borano-carbonates [87], borano-carbamates [88], xanthene carboxylic acid (XCA) [89], unsaturated cyclic diketones (DKs) [90], methylene chloride (MC) [91,92], meso-carboxy BODIPYs [46], hydroxy-flavones [93] (Scheme 2). Furthermore, 1,2-disubstituted ferrocenes belongs to an aldehyde family, unfavorably elicits the toxicity and its slow release mechanism restricts the researchers from developing another nonmetallic CORMs (NCORMs). The main drawbacks of NCORM are potentially a low CO content releasing, and always producing organic molecules along with the CO moiety. Anyhow, NCORM clinical traits have shown their utility to communicate with biological activity [94].

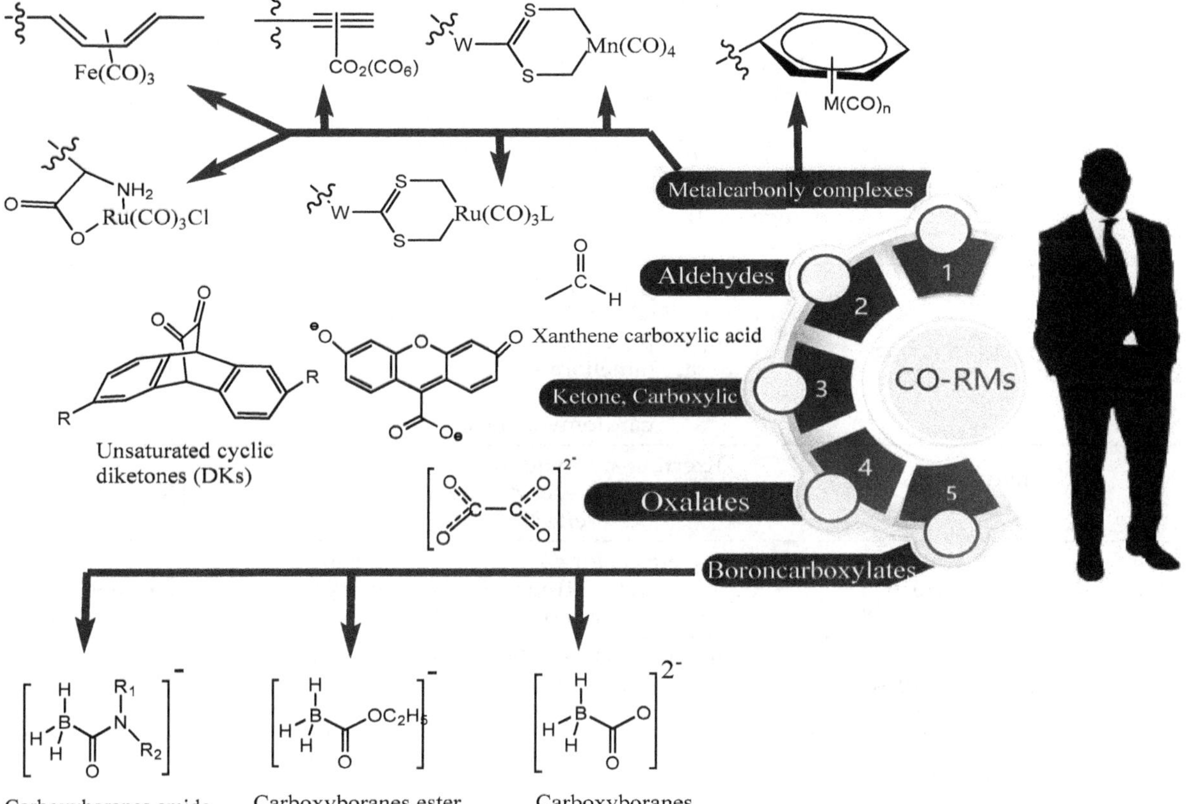

Scheme 2. Various CO-releasing molecules (CORMs) formulation associates with different functional capabilities.

1.9. CORM's Therapeutic Scope

Strategically, the synthesis route of CORMs development is not the only objective. The main theme of this CORM's innovation is to obtain the therapeutic advantage eventually. The biological significance of CORM is associated with their bacterial performance in cells lines, (i.e., standard myoglobin assay). The important biological roles of CORMs are listed below (Table 1).

Table 1. Nonmetallic and organometallics CO-releasing molecules (CORM's) fragments exhibited therapeutics activities.

List	CORMs	Therapeutic Implications	Refs
1	CORM-1	Increase coronary perfusion pressures; attenuates the L-NAME-mediated; restore unstable blood pressure and modulates vessel contractility ex-vivo in animals.	[95]
2	CORM-2	Attenuates inflammatory response in lungs and liver; induces vasorelaxation; protects against IRI; activates K^+/Ca^{+2} channels; possible for pulmonary hypertension.	[95,96]
3	CORM-3	Improves the liver & kidney functions during transplantation; Vasorelaxation induction; prevents sepsis & cardiac graft rejection; helps in bacterial infections; support rheumatoid arthritis; RBF improvement in the treatment of cynomolgus for monkeys.	[23,28,71,97–99]
4	CORM-401	Improves insulin-sensitivity and metabolic switch induces in adipocytes.	[100]
5	ALF492	In severe malaria, fully protects with artesunate combination.	[101]
6	CORM-A1	Induces the vasorelaxation; Increases RBF and reduced vascular; gives resistance in the kidney of mice; good cerebroprotective agent for epileptic seizures treatments.	[102]
7	Re-CORM-1	Anti-oxidative characteristic and protects against IRI from the affected neonatal rat of cardiomyocytes.	[103]
8	B_{12}-ReCORM-2	Protects against IRI (neonatal rat cardio-myocyte); hindrance cell mortality up to 80%; support the cardiac repairing and cardiac disease (ameliorates degenerative); anti-oxidative agent; augments and direct cardiomyogenesis.	[104,105]
9	3-hydroxyflavon CORMs	Exerting anti-oxidative activity; anti-inflammatory services and anti-cancer effects.	[46,55,89]
10	ALF 186	Protective effects for gastric ulcers and neuro protective, while IRI-induced apoptosis of retinal ganglion cells (RGC).	[106–109]
11	CORMA-1-PLA	Prevents fibroblasts and internalized into 3T3 cells during metabolic and hypoxia depletion conditions.	[110]
12	α-DK-CORMs	Absorbs in acute myeloid leukemia (AML) KG-1 cells and releases CO In-vivo upon 470nm irradiation.	[111]

1.10. Solubility

For making CORM acceptable as a pharmaceutical drug in the mammalian biological system, solubility is one of the most prominent factors where the researcher can evaluate the proficiency of the product. Solubility estimates how much CORMs and CORMats are convenient for the practical demonstration. CORM-2 is soluble in DMSO, olive oil and PEG [95,112], while CORM-3 contributes to the water compatibility with a weak acidic nature (pH = 3) [26,37]. Specifically, CORM-A1 possesses the water solubility and stability but it breaks-down immediately after liberating the CO under acidic condition (pH = 11) [87]. CORM-ALF186 can afford the disintegration in the water system and is unstable at an aerobic condition [113] and ALF062 is soluble in methanol and DMSO, while it remains unstable in the air [98,113]. Furthermore, CORM-1 has the compatibility with DMSO and ethanol [114].

Although the CORMs motif is good for releasing the CO moiety, but the tissue selectivity and targeting sites dilemma has reduced its overall biological performance and hence lost its therapeutic significance. Most importantly, the toxicity of organometallic complexes is handled very poorly, so to reduce the toxicity and increase its reactivity, it requires an exploration of all the alternative strategies. Therefore, the researchers have moved from CORMs to CORMats.

2. Research on New CO Transport Materials

As discussed, the MCCs are the admissible and professional class of (soluble) CORMs; however, it has been imperative to examine their probable shortcomings. In fact, a small number of organometallic compounds can be manipulated for pharmaceutical agents predominantly caused by the side-reaction of metals with biological chemical compounds, (e.g., nucleophilic or even electrophilic side chains of proteins) together with the toxicity of several heavy metals. Water-soluble CORMs are approaching the entire body organism and it could accelerate the toxicity against healthy tissues. The spatial and acceptable releasing rate of it into biological tissues/cells is still the utmost challenge. Furthermore, the CO-releasing activity inevitably accumulates a metal and co-ligand fragment, probably takes part in the biological activity as well. This residue (i-CORMs) can be managed through the insoluble framework. On the basis of abovementioned issues and challenges, new and compatible CO transport materials and strategies are emerging in order to get rid of the CO lethal gas dilemma and to convert it into a valuable clinical agent. CORM-1 [115], CORM-2 [116,117], CORM-3 [118] and CORM-A1 [87] have been tested in various disease models to observe their therapeutic effects and to obtain its surprisingly outcomes in typical clinical conditions [2,119]. CORM-3 has good cure-ability for inflammatory disorders like rheumatoid arthritis, osteoarthritis and collagen-induced arthritis (CIA) [97,120,121]. CORM-A1 provides ameliorated course in experimental auto-immune uveoretinitis (EAU) [122], while CORM-2 attenuates the tumor proliferation [123] and a considerable enhancement the coagulation and slow-down of the fibrinolytic bleeding [117,124] and improves survival in the liver injury affected by cecal ligation and perforation (CLP) [116,125]. CORM-3, CORM-2 and ALF-062 corroborates with antimicrobial functions [98,126–131]. The CO is encouraging the proliferation of endothelial cells, progenitor cells and regulatory T-cells [34,132,133]. There is still more interrogation required for further improvement to employ practical knowledge. So, the development of the solid CO precursor in tandem with peculiar trigger for releasing the enclosed CO gas commodity is an imperative research motive. To date, due to the unavailability of a safe delivery system for CORM; none of those prescribed formulations could have been employed in humans as a direct dose for respective damaged tissues or disease. Although a few scientific proposals have been presented in that scenario for making CORMs as a clinically viable project, but none of them exhibits the secure transportation material system for the patient's right choice. All that discussion pursued that the nanoscale and macromolecular carrier system could be exploited to obtain a selected tissue enrichment and proposed mechanism strategy for CORMs delivery (Scheme 3) [134,135].

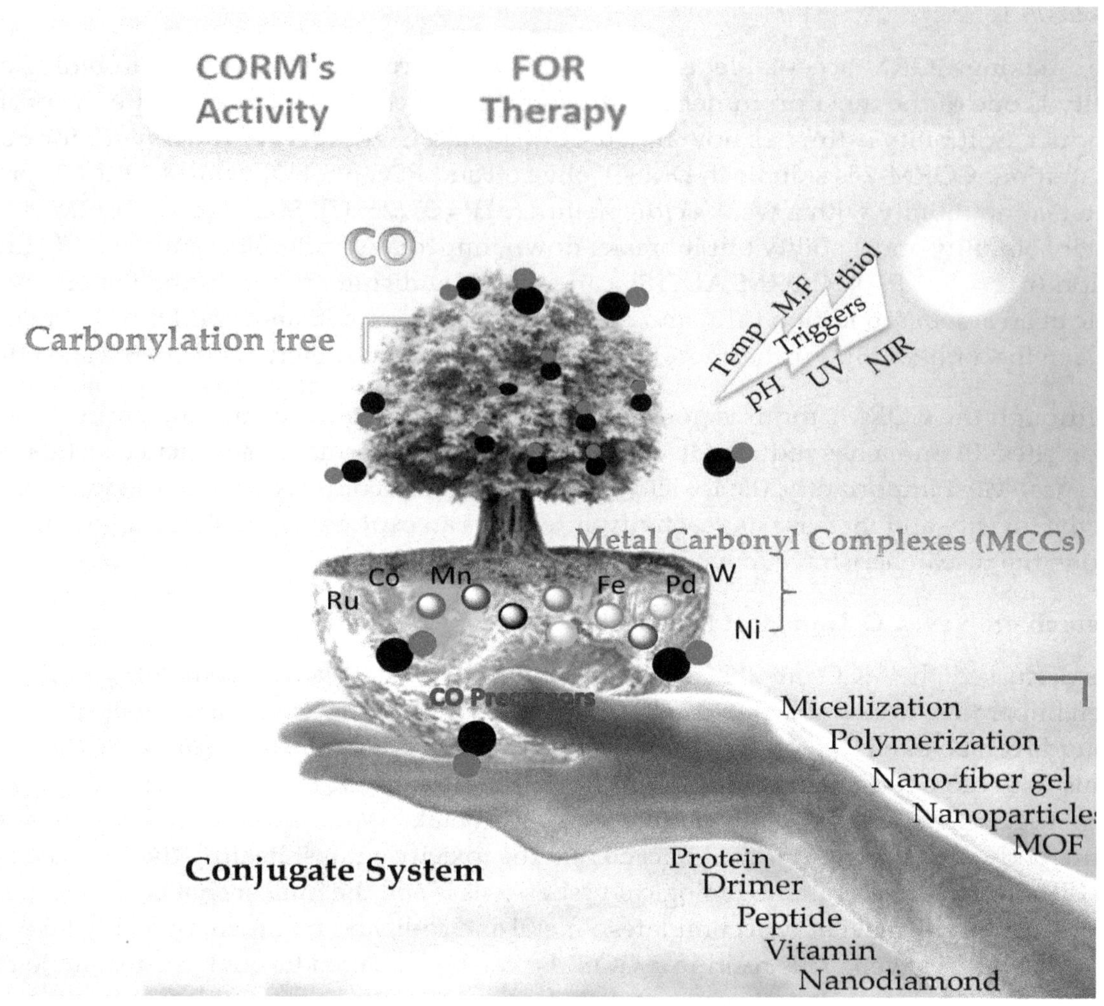

Scheme 3. Various organometallics MCCs incorporate with numerous conjugate systems to produce carbonylation complexes, i.e., CORMats for therapeutic CO release upon trigging.

The clinical trials on CORMs proved that CORMs exhibited the important biological applications, but after CORMs, the degradation metal residue (i-CORMs) also caused toxicity unfortunately [136]. The prohibited i-CORMs activity containment is a big challenge for the researchers. To reduce toxicity and capture the i-CORMs toxic moiety, scientists have explored a strategy known as CORMats. In this strategy, firstly, CO is entrapped inside the CORMats through specific administration, and then upon certain conditions the captured CO is escaped out. Several scaffolds and conjugated formulations have been introduced in this scope and it is still under investigation by compatible conjugate CORM's such as Ruthenium-MCC (Ru-MCC) and Manganese-MCCs (Mn-MCC) by different nano-transporting services such as Iron MOFs [137,138], peptide [139–144], micellization [55,59,145], protein [121,146–149], vitamins [150–153], co-polymer systems [47,154–156], nanofiber gel [142], inorganic hybrid scaffolds [157–160] and metallodendrimers [161] (Figure 5). The intrinsic toxicity control of i-CORMats is the top priority for each developed system.

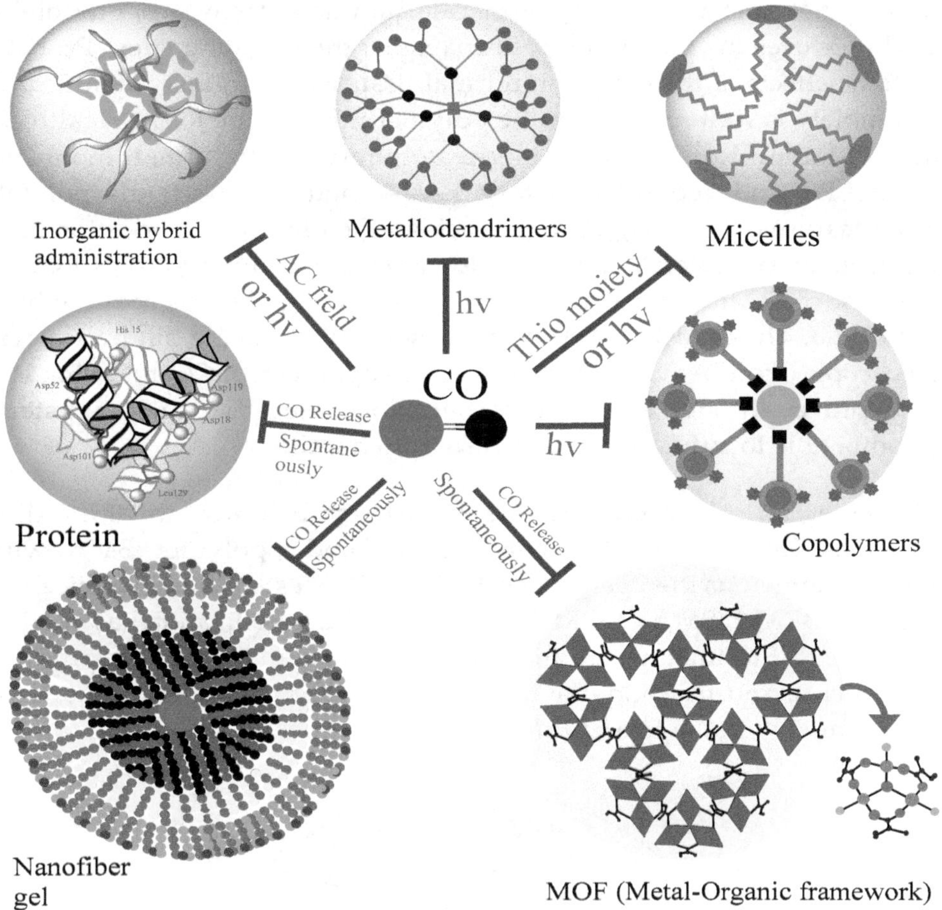

Figure 5. The CO-releasing administration with different conjugate and encapsulate strategies.

2.1. Micellization

Hubbell et al. engineered the micellization technique as the CO-producer with reduced diffusion; creditably targeted to the distal tissue draining sites [59]. Micelles were synthesized by the tri-block copolymer composed of poly(ornithine acrylamide) block and poly(ethylene glycol) block (hydrophilic nature) hosted by $[Ru(CO)_3Cl$-(ornithinate)] moieties with poly(n-butylacrylamide) block (hydrophobic nature). The CO-releasing micelles consists of a triblock copolymers (Figure 6): A hydrophilic poly(ethylene glycol) (PEG) fragment that stabilizes the micelles; a poly-OrnRu fragment that releases CO. A hydrophobic poly(n-butylacrylamide) fragment drives to construct the micelles forms.

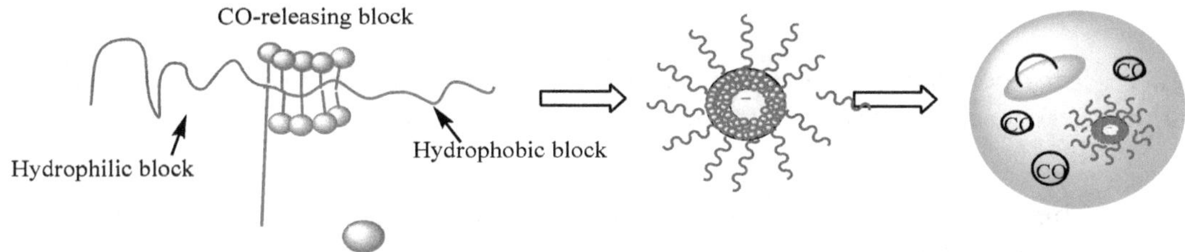

Figure 6. Triblock copolymer assembles for releasing the CO at biological sites.

The micelles polymer can be used as a pharmaceutically acceptable carrier to solubilize the poorly soluble drugs and produces the therapeutic effect against the targeting sites. Probably it promotes the reduction in toxic effects of the drugs on normal tissues and organs. Significantly, the toxicity of the $Ru(CO)_3Cl$ moiety is well-reduced in the polymer micelle due to the stealth characteristic of the PEG fragment. Moreover, the micelles moderately respond to human monocytes against the lipopolysaccharide (LPS) -induced inflammatory disease model. Importantly, poly(ethylene glycol) attenuates the toxic feature of $[Ru(CO)_3Cl(\text{amino acidate})]$ moieties. The addition of cysteine allows the release of CO from an occupied area with a slower rate as compared to $[Ru(CO)_3Cl(\text{glycinate})]$ (CORM-3). The release of CO from micelles was tested in a myoglobin assay and it has been found to be slower than CORM-3. The diffusion of the Orn-Ru substrate is facing hindrance in the cells due to the micelles stereoscopic effect. Anyhow, the mechanism approach of CO-releasing is not obvious. It has been evidently proved through experiments that thiol compounds such as cysteine, glutathione and protein are compatible to induce the CO release from micelles.

Hiroshi Maeda et al. incorporated the tricarbonyldichlororuthenium dimer (CORM-2: $[RuCl(\mu\text{-}Cl)(CO)_3]_2$) as water-soluble styrene-maleic acid and copolymer (SMA) while gaining the optimum half-life and numerous therapeutic effects [145]. They established the micellization structure for encapsulating the CORM-2 (SMA/CORM-2) (Figure 7). The micellization has good water solubility and it is compatible with the aqueous environment. The sustain CO kinetic profile performs well in vivo bioactivity such as murine model of inflammatory colitis. The half-life of this complex was almost 35-folds compared with the free CORM-2.

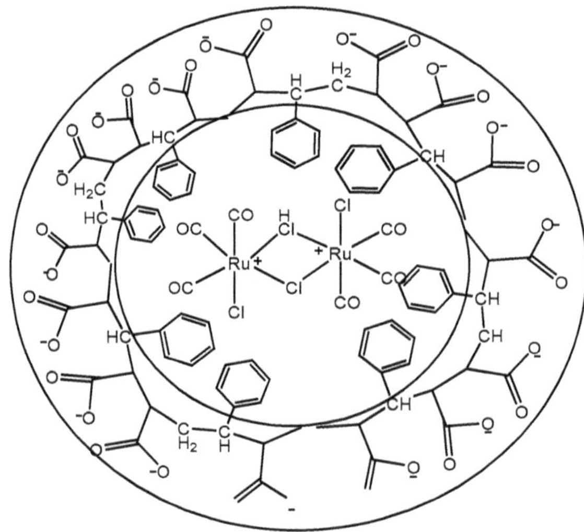

Figure 7. Tricarbonylchlororuthenium (II) dimer (CORM-2) synthesized with water-soluble styrene-maleic acid copolymer (SMA) for micellization CORMats.

In spite of the ligand exchange CO-release mechanism, photo light is able to disintegrate the CORMats moiety as the CO donor. Robert Igarashi and Yi Liao explored the micelle-based photo-CORMs synthesized by the cyclic α-diketones (α-DK) encapsulation [55]. These CORMs require visible photo light for releasing the embedded CO. This research demonstrates the therapeutic potential of CORMs. The photo-activated micelle CORMs strategy has been explained in Figure 8. During the study of these micelle CORMats on the cell proliferation, it has been found that no difference was monitored in the viability of cells in response to the micelles of DKs.

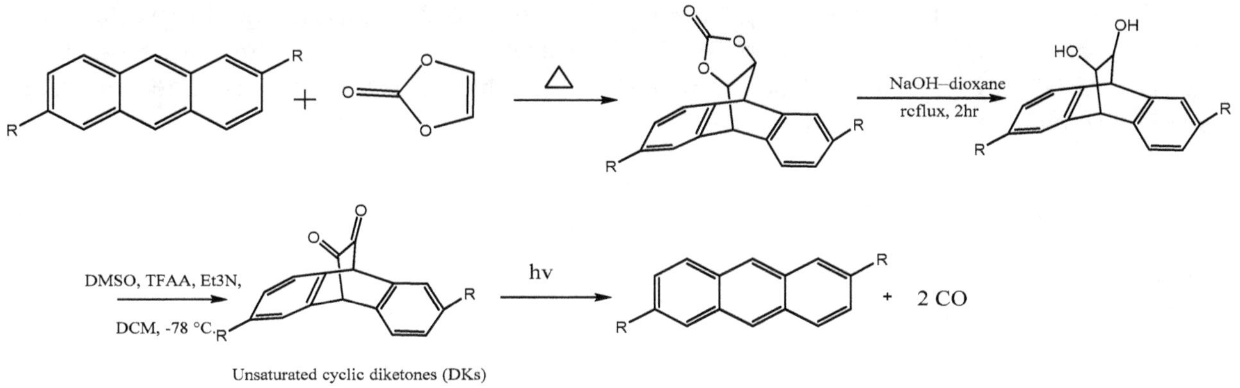

Figure 8. Synthesis route of unsaturated α-diketones (α-DKs) has been activated by photons energy.

2.2. Peptide

John reported a self-assembled amphiphilic peptide (PA) that was used to produce the CO [142]. Thereby, a covalent combination of a hydrophobic alkyl chain and a hydrophilic short sequence peptide endures the self-assembled peptide chain material. Amphiphilic peptides can spontaneously release CO and are prone to toxicity themselves. In that perspective they first designed the amphiphilic peptide PA1; which contains a β-aspartate residue to generate the NH_2-CH-RCOOH unit closely resembling the CORM-3 fragment. Next, PA1 and $[Ru(CO)_3Cl_2]_2$ were synthesized in the presence of sodium methoxide at room temperature to synthesize the CO-releasing peptide PA2 (Figure 9). The CO kinetic release curve proved that peptide P2 was synthesized in an aqueous solution like the first-order rate constant of CORM-3. The half-life of the CO released from both sources is quite identical. The half-life of CO released from CORM-3 is 2.14 ± 0.17 min, while the half-life of the CO released peptide P2 is 2.16 ± 0.05 min. In order to increase the half-life of CO released from P2, the incorporation of nanofiber gel PA2 and a strong gel PA was made. The half-life of the CO released from this nanofiber gel was significantly increased (~17.8 min) compared to PA2 and CORM-3 in an aqueous solution.

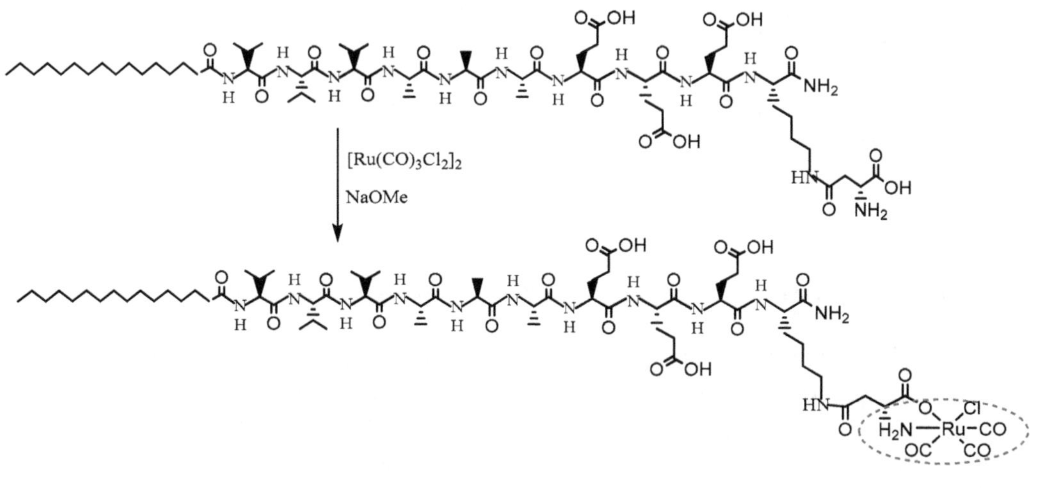

Figure 9. Synthesis of PA2 having CO-moiety for spontaneous release CO.

Rather than encapsulating a mere CO segment inside the transport materials, the CORMs entity incorporates with different functional groups of parent CORM's ligand commodity. In that scenario, peptide is linked with the Manganese-based Photo-CORM $[Mn(CO)_3]^+$ ligand tpm (tris(pyrazolyl)methane) using a Pd-catalyzed based Songashira cross-coupling mechanism and click reaction at N-terminal (azide-) and side-chain (iodoarene-) functionalization [140].

Ulrich Schatzschneider exposed the peptide linkage for the CORMats development [144]. They introduced the Mo-carbonyl $[Mo(CO)_4(bpy^{CH3,CHO})]$ associated with aldehyde functional groups at the peripheral position. The bioactive β-target peptide ligand 2,20-bipyridine (bpy) attached with molybdenum-carbonyl by *N*-terminal bonds of aminoxy acetic through catalyst-free and bio-orthogonal oxime ligation (Figure 10). The photo-activated CORMats gets activated upon 468 nm photons lights irradiations.

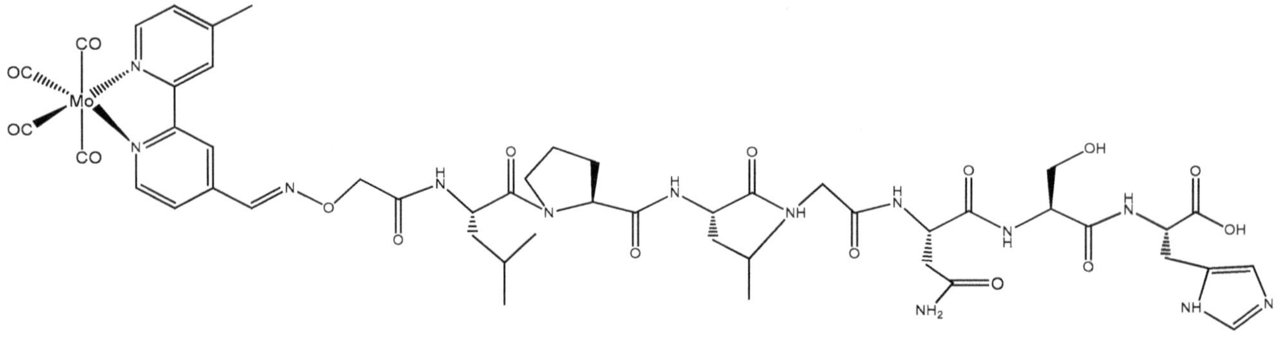

Figure 10. [$Mo(CO)_4(bpy_{CH3,CHO})$] complex has been constructed through bio-orthogonal peptide conjugate.

Radacki and Ulrich Schatzschneider jointly synthesized the Manganese carbonyl complexes [$Mn(bpea^{NHCH2C6H4CHO})(CO)_3]PF_6$ [139]. The peptides ligand 2,2-bis(pyrazolyl)ethylamine (bpea) is bearing aminoxy, azide and N-terminal alkyne residues (Figure 11). The researchers applied the transforming growth factor β-recognizing (TGF-β) peptide sequence for developing the photo-activated delivery agent. This peptide conjugation could be utilized for further development of new CORMats.

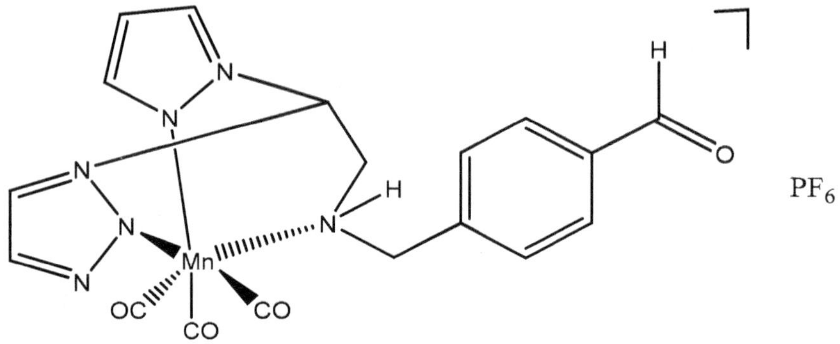

Figure 11. The synthesis route of [$Mn(bpea_{NHCH2C6H4CHO})(CO)_3]PF_6$ for Photo-CORMats.

The JJ Kodanko group successfully synthesized the ionic water-soluble compound [$Fe^{II}(CO)(N4Py)$] by a method of continuous CO bubbling through a ligand N4Py and one equivalent of $Fe^{II}(ClO_4)_2$ under the action of the organic solvent acetone $(ClO_4)_2$ (Figure 12A) [141]. A myoglobin experiment shows that the compound is stable under dark conditions and its releasing half-life is more than one day. When it was irradiated with 365 nm ultraviolet light, the CO can be quickly released. According to MTT experimental studies, [$Fe^{II}(CO)(N4Py)](ClO_4)_2$ exhibited the effective cytotoxicity against human prostate cancer cell line (PC-3) under light-induced conditions. When the concentration reaches 10 μM the cell survival rate was monitored as 63% of the control group. In order to further investigate the CO release behavior, the carbonyl segment with acetonitrile was replaced. The UV-vis analysis found that the substitution process is very slow [Fe^{II}-(MeCN)(N4Py)]$^{2+}$ and the concentration of acetonitrile was a quick step to replace CO. Moreover, it was also found that the N4Py ligand can be modified with a peptide (Ac-Ala-Gly-OBn) to obtain a peptide-conjugated photo-induced release molecule (Figure 12B). Biological experiments have showed that the peptide chain conjugation might be evaluated for the improvement of cell-specific itself or tissue-specific CO transport properties.

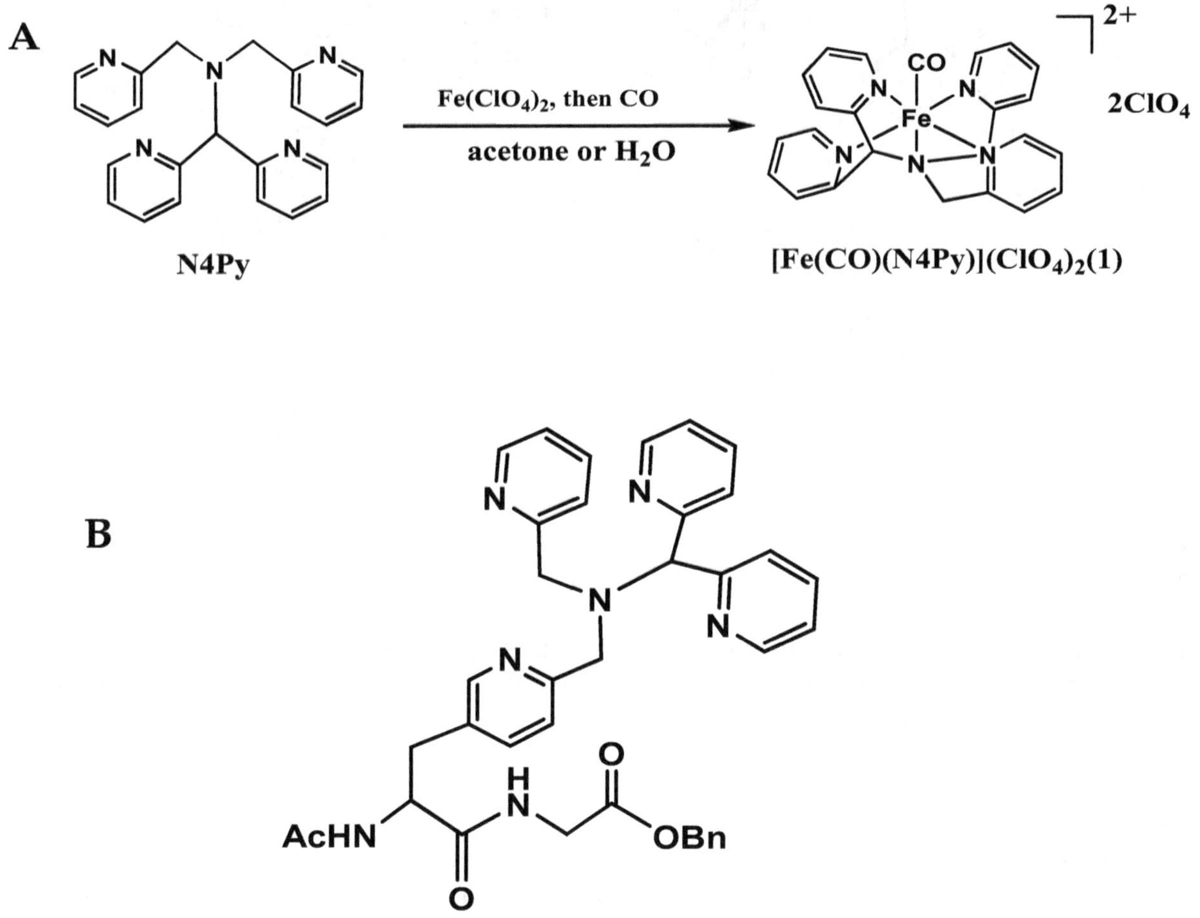

A

N4Py

$Fe(ClO_4)_2$, then CO

acetone or H_2O

$[Fe(CO)(N4Py)](ClO_4)_2(1)$

$2ClO_4$

B

AcHN

OBn

Figure 12. The ionic water-soluble Iron complexes $[Fe^{II}(CO)(N4Py)]$ (**A**) could be modified into Photo-CORMats by the replacement of the N4Py ligand with peptide china Ac-Ala-Gly-OBn (**B**) for the improvement of the cell-specific itself or tissue-specific therapeutic properties.

In the development of Photo-CORMats, metal-coligand plays a vital role in the photoexcitation at a prescribed wavelength. This allows the photons energy to penetrate and push the CO molecules to pull out these molecules from the metal-ligand fragment. In other words, these wavelengths are providing extra energy that enables the CO molecules excitation from its parent location. The CORM-2 and CORM-3 are hydrolytically active. Synthetically, these CORMs could be transformed into the photo-activated reagent. Leone Spiccia and Ulrich Schatzschneider described the ruthenium (II) dicarbonyl complexes functionalized with 2-(2-pyridyl)pyrimidine-4-carboxylic acid (CppH) (Figure 13A) [143]. They were able to successfully construct the monomeric PNA backbone with ruthenium (II) di-carbonyl complexes to produce ruthenium (II) dicarbonyl dichloride-based PNA-like monomer $[RuCl_2(Cpp\text{-}L\text{-}PNA)CO_2]$ (where PNA= peptide nucleic acid) (Figure 13B).

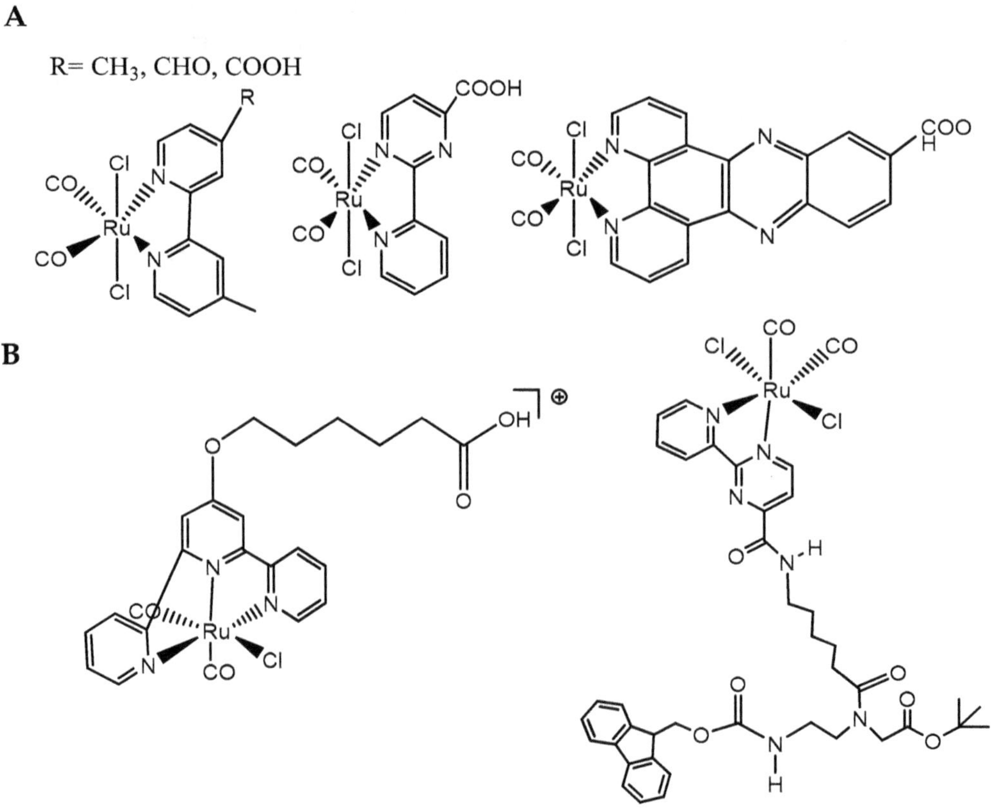

Figure 13. The hydrolytically activated Ruthenium dicarbonyl complexes CORM-2 and CORM-3 could be transformed into Photo-CORMats by peptide ligands through different functionalization: (**A**) Polypyridyl ligand of 2-(2-pyridyl)pyrimidine-4-carboxylic acide (CppH); (**B**) monomeric PNA backbone.

2.3. Proteins

G. J. Bernardes et al. disclosed that CORMs was compatible with the protein complexes transportation (Figure 14) [121]. They presented that the $Ru^{II}(CO)_2$-protein complexes using the reaction between CORM-3 and histidine fragment at the protein surface, the spontaneous CO is released to deliver in cells and mice. They also discussed that plasma protein acts as a CO carrier for in vivo by the CORM-3 formulation. Therapeutically, the controlled CO release favors in downregulation of the cytokines interleukin, i.e., IL-6 and IL-10.

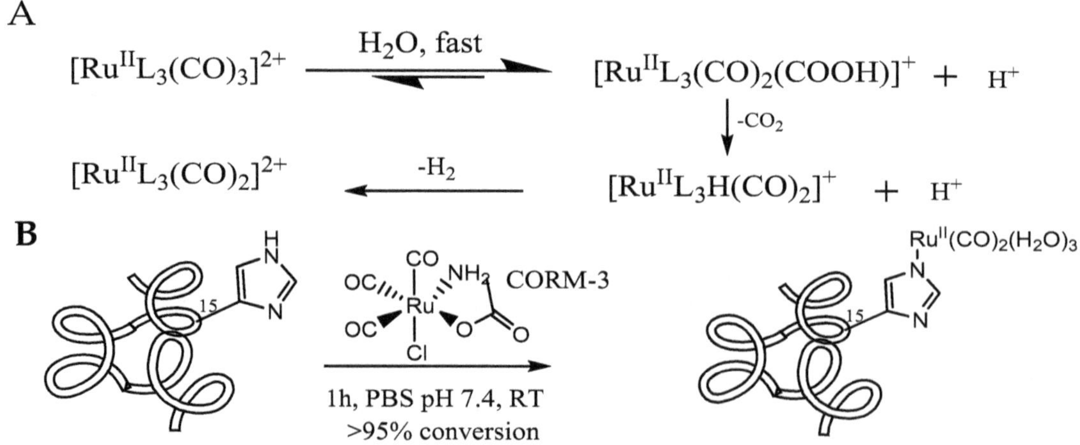

Figure 14. The reactivity of the *fac*-$[RuL_3(CO)_3]^{2+}$ complex (**A**) and CORM-3 react with single-His protein (**B**).

Another Ruthenium (II) carbonyl reagent *cis*-$[Ru(CO)_2(H_2O)_4]^{2+}$ has been reported for the spontaneous CO release in live cells using histidine (His) metalloprotein and retained at IL-8 (Figure 15a) [148]. The *cis*-$[Ru(CO)_2]^{2+}$ carbonyl segment could be produced by aqua dirutheniumcarbonyl *cis*-$[Ru(CO)_2(H_2O)_4]^{2+}$ (Figure 15b). It was also explained that metalloproteins can be modified as organometallic pro-drugs rather than catalysis. Such artificial metallohydrolase performance can be compared with the human carbonic anhydrase (CA)-II.

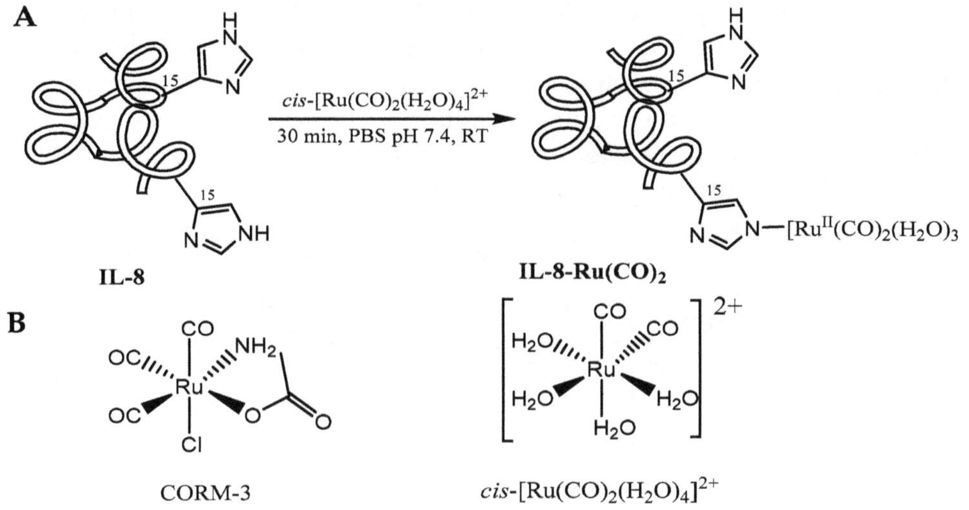

Figure 15. The spontaneous CO release by metalloprotein: (**A**) The carbonyl reagent *cis*-$[Ru(CO)_2(H_2O)_4]^{2+}$ spontaneous CO release in live cells using histidine (His) metalloprotein and retained at IL-8; (**B**) the *cis*-$[Ru(CO)_2]^{2+}$ carbonyl segment can be produced by the aqua carbonyl *cis*-$[Ru^{II}(CO)_2(H_2O)_4]^{2+}$.

In spite of the CORMs fragment incorporation with protein, Takafumi Ueno et al. explored the cages of protein for CO releasing [149]. They administrated the ferritin (Fr) cage of protein for capturing the CORM-3 moiety (Figure 16). Furthermore, it was observed that the half-life of the CO release could be enhanced; which indicates a good sign for ideal drug development. When they interrogated their performance at the biological sites, they described that the nuclear factor kappa B (NF-κB) becomes 10-times higher than the parent CORM-3. The CORM-3 protein cage is quite a unique way of CORM's engineering.

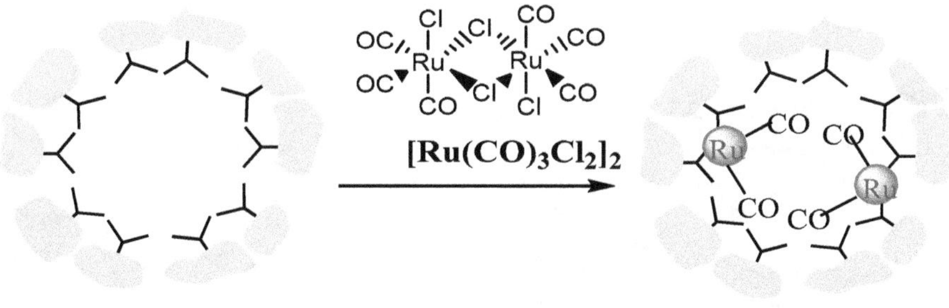

Figure 16. The recombinant L-chain apoferritin (apo-rHLFr) of Ru carbonyl complexes.

Additionally, Takafumi Ueno et al. explored the immobilization of the crosslinked hen egg white lysozyme CL-HEWL crystal deposit on MCCs for therapeutic purposes [146]. The scientist disclosed that NF-κB is remarkably high in order to respond to the pathological signals. The extra scaffold Ruthenium carbonyl moiety (Ru·CL-HEWL), was used to induce the NF-κB activation and immobilized Ruthenium carbonyl [*cis*-$Ru(CO)_2X_4]^{2-}$ moieties inside the protein cage (Ru·CL-HEWL). Optimist approaches of this transport service bear the potential of the artificial extracellular scaffold.

NF-κB can be regulated by the protein fragment. Susumu Kitagawa et al. disclosed the crystalline assembly of protein with CORM-2 in polyhedra crystals (PhC) [147]. They introduced the ruthenium carbonyls immobilized on hexahistidine. The activation of NF-κB was significantly improved up to six folds. This therapeutic research will lead to further investigation on the extracellular scaffold.

2.4. Vitamins

Anna Yu. Bogdanovab et al. presented the cyanocobalamin (B_{12}) as a biocompatible B_{12}-$Re^{II}(CO)_2$ scaffold for CORMats (Figure 17) [150]. They incorporated the *cis-trans*-$[Re^{II}(CO)_2Br_2]^0$ core having $17e^-$ dicarbonyl complexes. This research also elaborated that ReCORM-1 is compatible with B_{12} for pharmaceutical applications, and the obtained cobalamin conjugates are also feasible with aqueous aerobic media. Interestingly, after CO releasing, metal degradation is not involved in toxicity due to the exclusive configuration and metal oxidation of ReO_4^- generation.

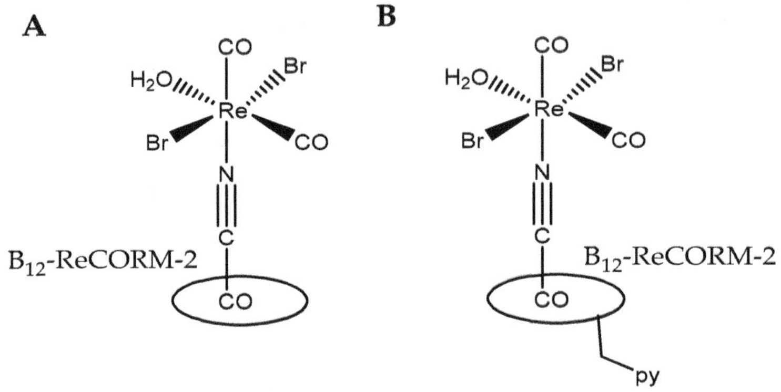

Figure 17. B_{12}-$Re^{II}(CO)_2$ CORMats conjugate: (**A**) B_{12}-ReCORM-2; (**B**) B_{12}-ReCORM-4.

The most promising anticancer drug agent is a macromolecular conjugate. The HO-1 and transcription factor Nrf2 are the prime parameters to provide resistance against inflammation and oxidative stress disease. In this analogy, biliverdin is the enzymatic activity of HO-1, while CO directs the therapeutic exploitation. Roberta Foresti et al. found that hybrid molecules were simultaneously involved in the CO liberation and Nrf2 activation [151]. The newly developed CORMats termed as hybrid-CORMats (HY-CORMats) is shown in Figure 18.

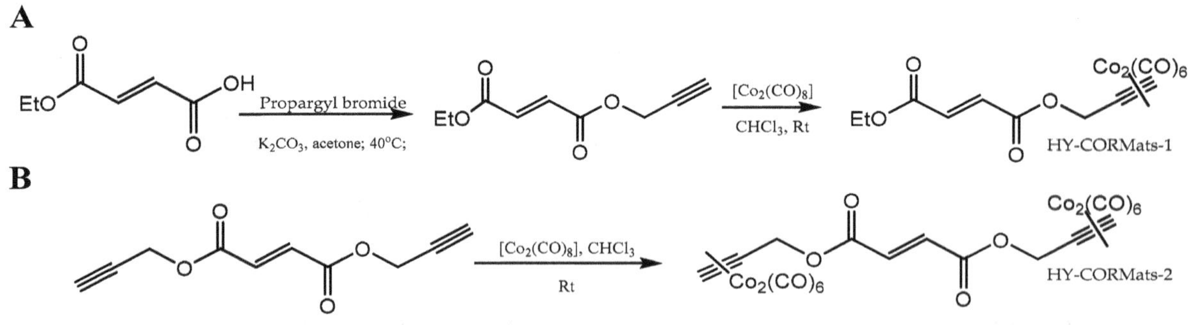

Figure 18. Synthesis route of hybrid CORMats: (**A**) HY-CORMats-1; (**B**) HY-CORMats-2.

After synthesizing the HY-CORMats, researchers further interrogated the biological activities and described the HO-1 expression along with the nuclear accumulation of Nrf2 and showed viability in different cell types (Scheme 4).

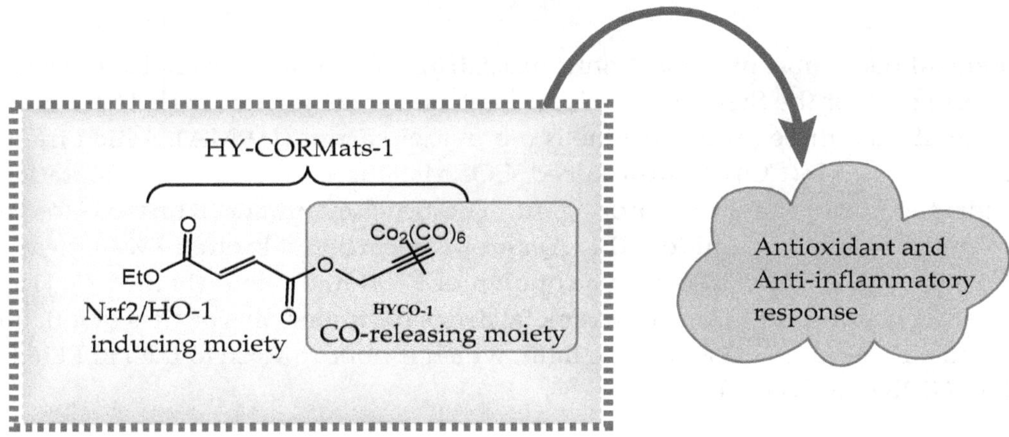

Scheme 4. The hybrid CORMats (HY-CORMats-1) has a CO moiety for various anti-inflammatory, antioxidant actions and induced nuclear accumulation of Nrf2.

A. Pamplona's group coordinated the galactose with a central metal to synthesize a polyhydric-containing water-soluble CORMats [$RuCl_2$-thiogalacto-pyranoside$(CO)_3$] (ALF492) through Sulphur bond (Figure 19) [152]. The Sulphur bond coordination of the galactose ligand with the central metal increases the water solubility and biocompatibility. This compound also exhibited the appropriate drug-like properties. The presence of the galactose ligand increases the specificity of liver glycoprotein. A myoglobin study was used to monitor the CO release kinetic profile. The target selectivity of ALF492 can be well administrated. Significantly, when ALF492 is mixed with the antimalarial drug artesunate, ALF492 responds to the effective adjuvant treatment for cerebral malaria. Collectively, this marks the outstanding potential of ALF492 in the treatment of falciparum malaria.

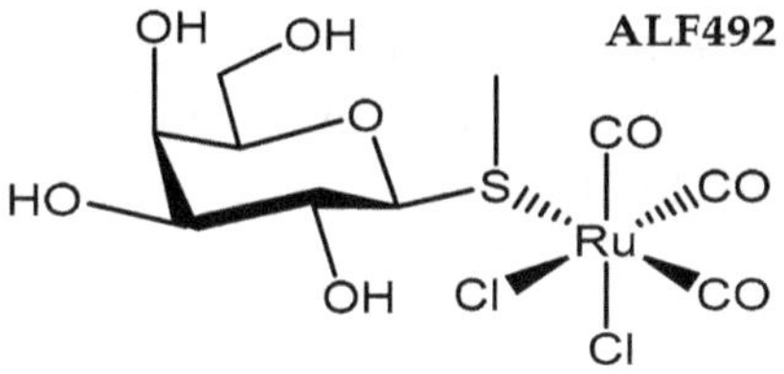

ALF492

Figure 19. Galactose chelated three carbonyl ruthenium complexes.

The CC Romao group synthesized the molybdenum-based water-soluble release molecule $Mo(CO)_3(CNCR'R''CO_2H)_3$ (R'=R''=H, ALF795) (R'=R''=CH_3, ALF794) (Figure 20) [153]. Myoglobin experiments have shown that compounds were stable and did not decompose in an aerobic aqueous solution for at least 1 hr. ALF794 is less toxic and suitable for drug-like properties. It can deliver CO to acetamido phenol-induced liver in mice with acute liver failure. After 5 min, intravenous injection, the ratio of ALF794 in liver/blood and liver/kidney were reported at 5.27 and 12.58, respectively and ALF795 liver/blood and liver/kidney ratios were observed at 0.33 and 0.50, respectively.

ALF795: R'=R''=H,

ALF794: R'=R''=CH_3

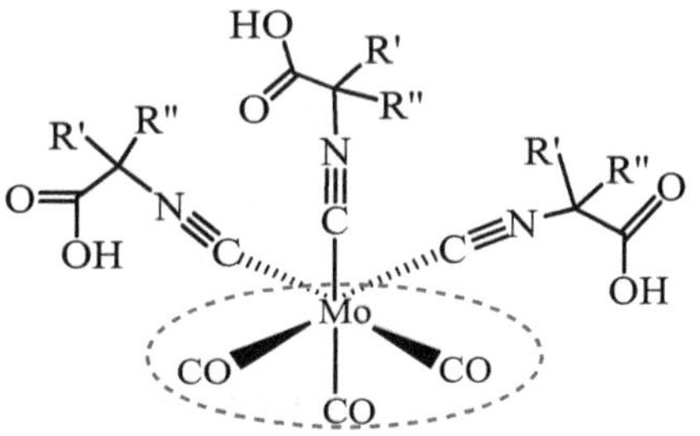

Figure 20. β-isocyanate coordinated molybdenum carbonyl complexes.

2.5. Polymers

The aforementioned most promising anticancer drug agent is a macromolecular conjugate. Ruth Duncan et al. reported for the first time a polymer-anticancer conjugate [154]. These macromolecular drugs consist of at least three (3) parts: One is a polymer carrier (HPMA), which transports metal organic drugs such as $Mn(CO)_3$ light-induced CORMs; the second is a biodegradable polymer drug connector; the third is an anti-tumor agent. The Bruckmann and Kunz groups reported that N-(2-hydroxypropyl)methacrylamide (HPMA) and pentacarbonyl bromide were heated under the re-flux of a dry acetone solution to obtain a copolymer P1 at high yield (Figure 21) [155]. Inducing CORMs can passively transport CO to release metal drugs for tumor cells or sites of inflammation. The polymer conjugate P1 releases CO at 365 nm light, which is not cytotoxic to the HCT116 human colon cancer and HepG2 liver cancer cells.

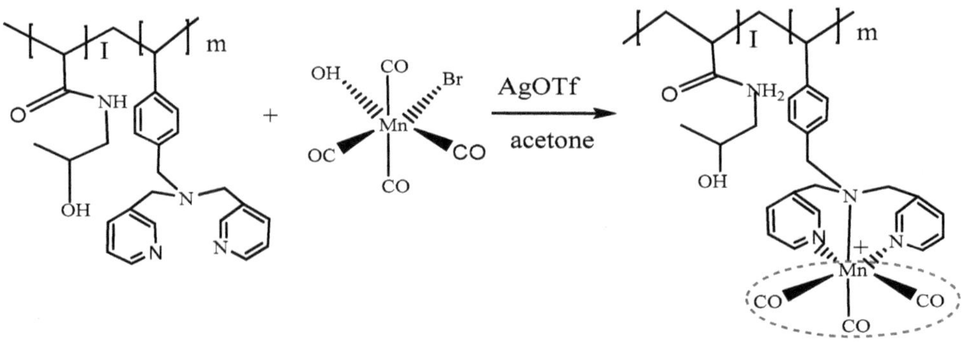

Figure 21. The copolymer P1 synthesized for releasing CO segment.

HPMA-copolymer has a great nature of water solubility. Bernhard Spingler et al. discovered the copolymer materials [156]. The bis(2-pyridylmethyl)benzylamine ligand was prepared from picolyl chloride and benzylamine, then this ligand coordinated with $Re(CO)_3$ moiety to construct the HPMA-co-bis(2-pyridylmethyl)-4-vinylbenzylamine copolymers (Figure 22). HPMA-copolymer characteristics such as the average molecular weight can be modified according to the requirement by replacing the radical starter and co-monomers. For instance, the molecular weight 52KDa is the appropriate choice for remarkably enhancing the permeability and retention (EPR) effect. The established copolymer system with the $Re(CO)_3$ fragment has an ability to diagnose the used 99mTc. Moreover, the identical behavior in IR spectra and X-ray crystallography have shown their resemblance in the binding sites of $Re(CO)_3$-labelled copolymer and bis(2-pyridylmethyl)-amine-derived complexes (solid-state structures (SSS) of $\cdot CH_2Cl_2$ and$\cdot CH_2Cl_2 \cdot H_2O$). HPMA-morphology can be efficient for targeting the tumor sites for the EPR effect.

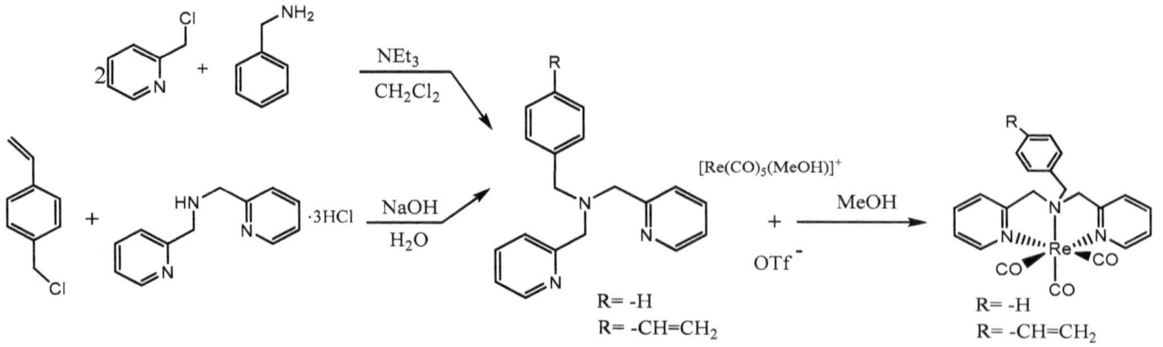

Figure 22. The copolymers HPMA-co-bis(2-pyridylmethyl)-4-vinyl-benzylamine construct through $Re(CO)_3$ moiety.

Not only solvent exchange triggers complexes have been reported but photons energy has also been explored in this research area. Pierri et al. have shown that the water-soluble photo-CORM can be controlled through NIR photons energy. They utilized the amphiphilic polymer for encapsulating the Photo-CORM *trans*-Mn(bpy)(PPh_3)(CO_2)$_2$ (Figure 23) [47]. Since CO has a strong ligand field (L.F), so its absorption bands lies in higher energy zone almost closer to the UV-region [162]. Usually Photo-CORMats belongs to the MCCs family and having CO photolysis-lability from the excited states of LF associated metal-centered [163]. Although the higher MLCT transitions obviate the ligand re-configuration, during the MLCT exhibition, the photolysis might be affected due to π-back-bonding of metal-to-CO configuration [164]. The energy gaps were found between the MLCT and LF excited states. The lower excitation states of MCLT have reduced the ligand lability as compared to LF states [163]. Thus, it is difficult to construct the Photo-induced-CO-release upon NIR or longer visible wavelengths. Up-conversion nanoparticles (UCNPs), (i.e., lanthanide ion doped) have a utility of uncaging from NIR photolysis wavelengths. UCNPs are already claimed as photodynamic therapy [165,166]. Those research analysts firstly developed the polymer matrix UNCPs@PL-PEG (an amphiphilic phospholipid-functionalized poly(ethylene glycol) then used NIR photons energy as a trigger to release the CO segment for biological purposes. PL-PEG shows a remarkable characteristic of water solubility and it has also provided space for incoming other soluble photo-organic CORMs. These organic compounds might be helpful for searching the special physiological targets.

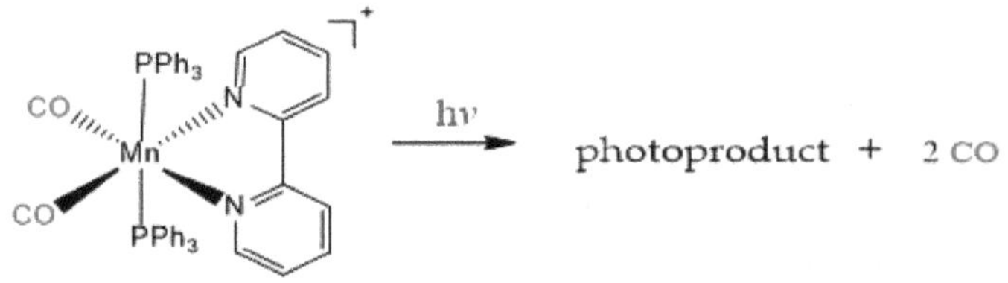

Figure 23. NIR-responsive amphiphilic polymer conjugates (PhotoCORMats).

2.6. Metal Organic Frameworks (MOFs-CORMats)

Metzler-Nolte et al. synthesized the hybrid material metal-organic framework as a class of porous coordinated polymer to encapsulate the CO segment. [138]. They established the bio-compatibility with MOFs; NH_2-MIL-88B (Fe) and MIL-88B (Fe) by capturing the CO at susceptible Fe^{II} and Fe^{III} coordinative unsaturated metal sites (CUSs). Unfavorably, it requires higher activation temperature [167] ($\geq$ 550 K). An adventuring feature of MOF has a breathing effect while providing accommodation for CO at the adjacent site; probably having a controlled CO release, potential through the opening/closing gesture of porous MOF.

Instead, it encapsulates the mere CO segment. The research can also accommodate the CORM's fragment inside MOFs. A new class of Manganese carbonyl complex Photo-CORMs has been explored from Zr(IV) based MOF. MnBr(bpydc)($CO)_3$ (bpydc=5,5′-dicarboxylate-2,2′-bipyridine) embedded into Zr(IV) MOFs [137]. This photo-activated commodity has been evaluated into cellular substrates along with the biocompatible polymer matrix, claimed to be controlled and efficient light-induced CO-release. After the successful CO release from CORMats, the inability in containment of metal degradation growth, this leads to scientists being reluctant for the employment of genuine medication. The CO has played its own role effectively; how other body organisms responds remains questionable.

2.7. Porous Structure Materials

Porous structure materials have already been in use for encapsulation of the CORMs commodity for the usage of the CO release. Maldonado, Elisa Barea et al. shared the amazing research work about the organometallic community by embedding the anion porous framework with the exhibition of the cation exchange strategy (Figure 24) [50]. This innovation invigorates under physiological condition while it is triggered by visible light. At first, they developed the air-stable, nontoxic, photoactive and water-soluble cation species CORM [Mn(tacn)($CO)_3$]$^+$ (ALF472$^+$) then encapsulates into anionic porous matrixes belonging to the inorganic framework. Anionic silica matrix exerts the good administration by reducing the CO release kinetics and providing the control-able rate. The ALF472@hybrid silica-SO_3 material might support the on/off switch delivery management, probably experiencing the command and control on the released CO. For ensuring the safety of the CORMats, the process metal degradation fragment was examined for ALF472@MCM-41-SO_3 up to 72 h and no significant appearance was reported. This silica framework is providing an 80% CORMs metal fragment containment. In phototherapies, the CO supplied is a provocative feature in the controlled manner, such as many inflammatory skin issues and topical skin cancer treatment.

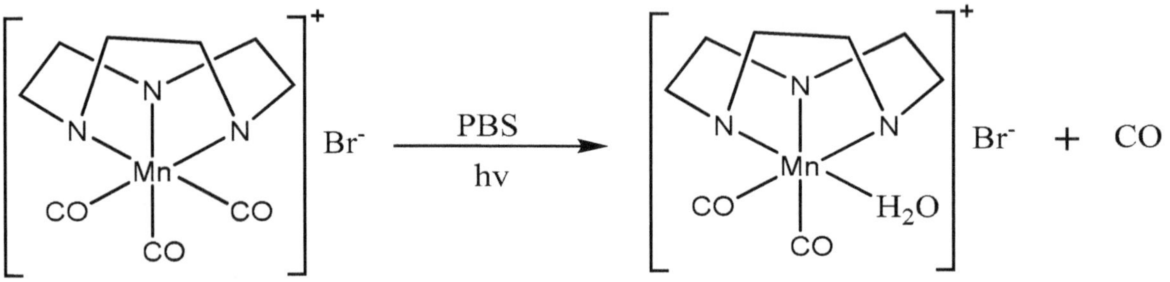

Figure 24. Photo-activated ALF472 CORM $[Mn(tacn)(CO)_3]Br$ simulated under physiological parameter.

Although many of the CORMats have been explored for therapeutic purposes, but the lack of biocompatibility and inconvenient features like solubility and toxicity from organometallic compounds, it could not be used as a drug agent. To overcome this dilemma, CORM-1 has been embedded into the nonporous fibers structure poly(L-lactide-co-D/L-lactide). The bioavailability and water accessibility were confidently achieved by photo-activated electro-spinning [111]. Specifically, there was no toxicity observed during the mouse fibroblast 3T3 cells culture. This feature might be promoting the CORMats into viable drug materials in the future.

2.8. Nanaoparticles

Among the CO-carrying support system, nanoparticles are intensely focused because nanoparticles can passively target the malignant cells and actively involve with the targeted tumor cells. Ulrich Schatzschneider et al. open the gateway for the nanoparticles carriers of Silicium dioxide as photoactivatable CORMats [157]. These research analysts, first time synthesized the 3-azidopropane-functionalized SiO_2 nanoparticles, followed by $[Mn(CO)_3(tpm\text{-}L1)]$ in a dimethylamide solution at room temperature. Manganese-based Photo-CORM $[Mn(CO)_3(tpm)]^+$ whose tpm ligand is linked with Silicium dioxide nanoparticles by CuAAC "click" reaction through construction of the Azido group by emulsion copolymerization of (3-azidopropyl)triethoxysilane and trimethoxymethylsilane at the surface. In this mechanism nanoparticles were functionalized with manganese tricarbonyl as light-induced CORMats (Figure 25). SiO_2 nanoparticles are stable in nature with an amazing bio-compatibly and easy to modify at the surface. It means that various target molecules could be incorporated at the surface to achieve the drug delivery objectives. Eventually, it will increase the drug delivery capacity at specific sites. So therefore, reduce the systemic risk. To reduce the side effects of chemotherapy, SiO_2 nanoparticles provide the most valuable platform for tumor drug delivery.

In the nanoparticle carrier strategy, Urara Hasegawa et al. introduced the CO-releasing polymeric nanoparticles (CONPs) through phenylboronic acid-catechol complexation of catechol-bearing

CO-donor $Ru(CO)_3Cl$(L-DOPA) and phenylboronic acid-containing framboidal nanoparticles. It has been testified in a biological organism and gives feedback to cysteine, and subdues the pro-inflammatory mediator's IL-6 [168].

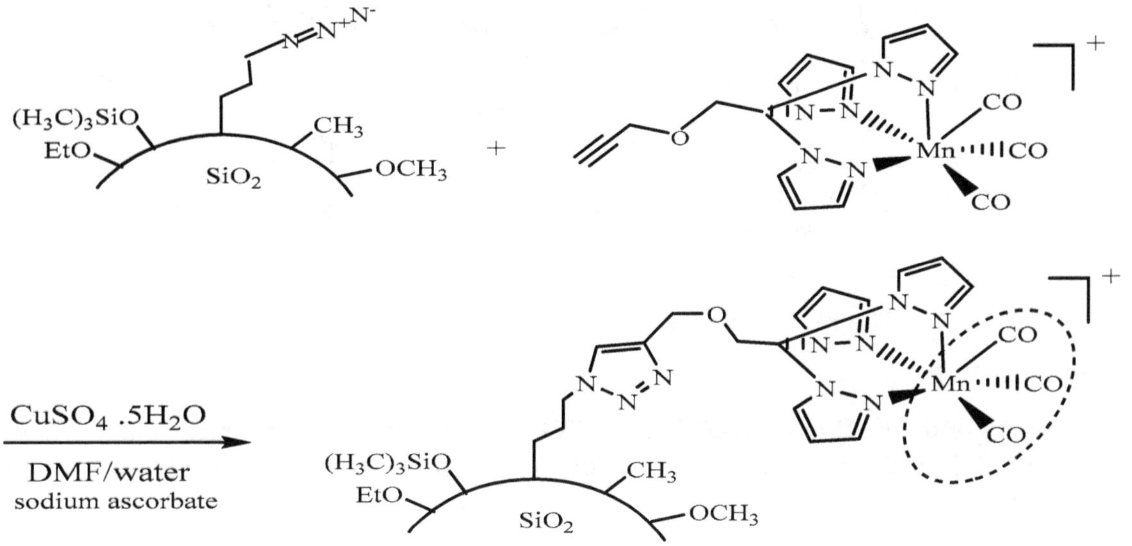

Figure 25. The mechanism of Manganese tricarbonyl functionalized with silica nanoparticles.

2.9. Nanosheets

The encapsulation of CORM's commodity shows promising features. X. Chen et al. worked out to cage the Manganese-carbonyl CORM inside the small MnCO-graphene oxide (PEG-BPY[$MnBr(CO)_3$]-GO) nanosheet, recruited as a drug carrier trigger by NIR light energy with on-demand CO release for photochemical CORMats [48]. They successfully constructed the novel combinations of the CO-release mechanism but triggered facility provided inconvenience for therapeutic purposes. However, we also need to pay attention to its complete management system, as in some cases big trouble may be faced for its state of being clinically applied or not. Merely an advantage for the CO releasing behavior is not enough, as it will always be difficult to handle it and nearly impossible for remote area patients, thus it raises a concern for being a practically viable medicine or not. Moreover, there might be no concern to what happens to metal degradation and leftover residue, which actually needs to be addressed properly too. Apart from this, how can we provide this medication to the patient using NIR trigging, so its mobility will remain the utmost challenge. In reality, the novel production in terms of its laboratory scale is quite different from its practical application as a cure agent.

2.10. Metallodendrimers

Metallodendrimers has a monodisperse nature with facile preparation. This exclusive feature is demonstrated by Smith et al. to entrepreneur the Photo-CORMats (Figure 26) [161]. For this purpose, Photo-CORM $Mn(CO)_3$ moiety scaffolds with polypyridyl dendritic. The general representation of polypyridyl dendritic is [DAB-PPI-{$MnBr(bpy^{CH3,CH=N})(CO)_3$}n] (whereas DAB=1,4-diaminobutane, PPI=poly(propyleneimine), bpy=bipyridyl). Photo-activated metallodendritic CORMats has been observed to liberate CO molecules upon 410 nm visible light photons penetration.

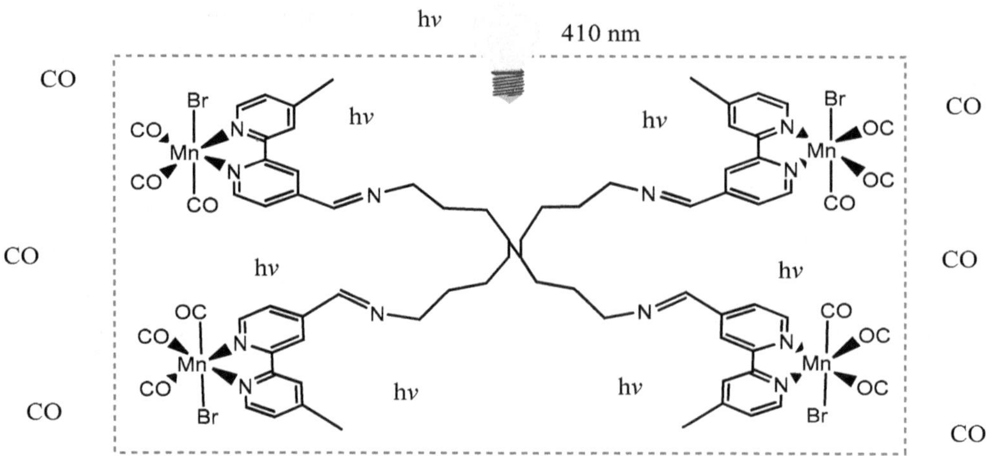

Figure 26. Metallodendrimers photoactivated CORMats.

2.11. Nanodiamond (ND)

The tpm ligand of Photo-CORM $[Mn(CO)_3(tpm)]^+$ peptide material and nanoparticle $[Mn(CO)_3(tpm\text{-}L1)]$ could further be constructed to explore the azide-modified nanodiamond (ND) by CuAAC (copper-catalyzed 1,3-dipolar azide–alkyne cycloaddition) "click" formation as Manganese-MCCs Photo-CORMats (Figure 27) [159]. Dordelmann, G. et al. introduced the first-time CuAAC coupling to attach the CO-liberating agent with ND as a biocompatible supporter. Photoactivatable CORM $[Mn(CO)_3(tpm)]^+$ retained at the ND's surface for CO biological services and therapeutic purposes and were evaluated through standard myoglobin assay.

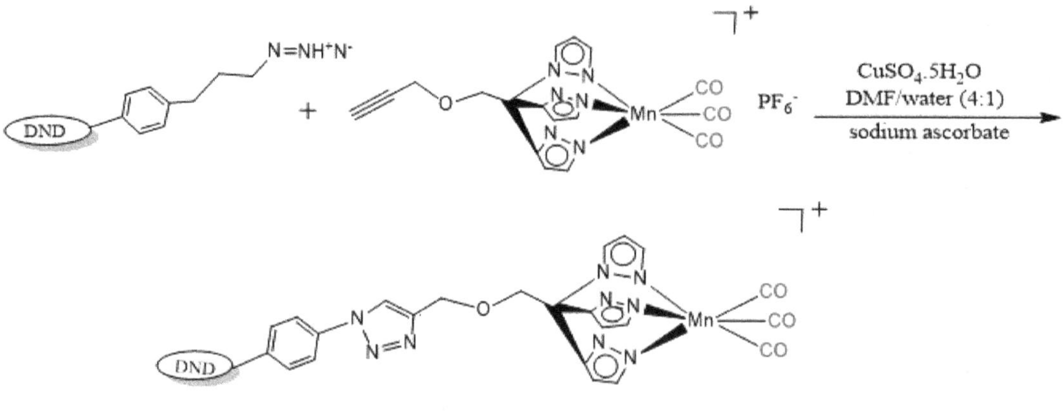

Figure 27. The $[Mn(CO)_3(tpm)]^+$-functionalized nanodiamond (ND) immobilized on azidemodified ND'surface through CuAAC "click" reaction.

Different CORMats are compatible with special cellular environments and are free to perform their therapeutic activities. Certain conditions restrict CORMats activities; definitely it would directly affect the therapeutic performance. CORMats therapeutic potential relies on the material's nature such as solubility, compatibility and activation mechanism. Another advantage of CORMats is to modify the CORMats assembly according to respective disease cells, which could be more helpful in searching the selective targets. For cancer treatment, the redirected T-cells, i.e., chimeric antigen receptor (CAR) T-cell might be providing a governing principle for cancer therapy [169]. CAR-Tcell is easier to find its own therapeutic targets from the peculiar receptor configuration. This exclusive feature facilitates gene-therapy. Similarly, this morphology can be applied to the CORMats development for special tissue selectivity. Numerous CORMats with their biological significance are described in Table 2.

Table 2. Conjugate strategies for therapeutic CO release.

Sr. #	CORMats	Therapeutic Implications	Refs
1	Micellization	Bioactive in a murine model of inflammatory colitis; potential for curing the ROS affected inflammatory disease; In response to human monocytes and attenuates the LPS-induced inflammatory.	[55,59,145]
2	Proteins	Regulation the cytokines IL-6 and IL-10; artificial metallohydrolase performance and elevated NF-κB factor (10 folds).	[121,146–149]
3	Vitamins	Shows HO-1 expression; inducing nuclear accumulation of Nrf2; antimalarial drug artesunate and acute liver failure.	[150–153]
4	Polymers	HCT116 human colon cancer and HepG2 liver cancer cells; enhance the EPR effect and targeting the tumor sites; achieve special and selective physiological targets.	[47,154–156]
5	Porous structure materials	Inflammatory skin issues and topical skin cancer treatment. Surprisingly, no toxicity was found in mouse fibroblast 3T3 cells.	[50,111].
6	Nanoparticles	Cysteine and subdues feedback to pro-inflammatory mediator's IL-6; cardiovascular therapy and relax the rat aorta muscle rings.	[157,168]
7	Peptide	Human prostate cancer cell line (PC-3) and supported cardiomyocyte viability.	[139–144]
8	Nano-sheets	Controllable CO release (e.g. GO-MnCORMats) suitable for inflammatory diseases after LPS stimulation and responsive intracellular CO release.	[48]
9	Nano-diamond	Nano-diamond precursor compatible with photons, hopefully, could be modified for special cell targeting.	[159]
10	MOFs	Inflammatory bowel disease and expected pharmacological applications by downsizing the MOF crystals to the nanoscale.	[137,138]
11	Metallodendrimers	Potential for inflammatory disease and cancer cells.	[161]

Briefly if the above intensive research discussion is summarized; it is evident that Ru-MCCs and Mn-MCCs are the right choices for nano-medicine due to bio-compatibility and tremendous prescribed feasibility analysis especially Ru-MCCs due to its lessened toxicity. Scrolling down from micellization to nanodiamond, all CO-prescriptions have CO liberation capability, but none of them could be claimed as safe therapeutic management and can't be directly applied for exogenous CO-prodrug. During the CORMats administration, rather than focus on the exploration of new advanced materials, the researchers might be considering already existing pharmaceutical materials. A pharmaceutical drug like substance such as crystalline smectite clay; is one of the promising biocompatible and pharmaceutical composites, which could be transformed into CORMats after proper formulation and careful administration. There are two types of strategies that have been introduced for the CORMats production. One is exploiting from the already developed CORMs with biocompatible materials as CO carriers. Another analogy is captured from the CO moiety in the vicinity of material specific akin to MOFs [138]. Already developed CO incorporating strategies are generalized in Table 3.

Table 3. Summarize the CO-releasing substrate along with their association.

Strategies	CO-Release Mechanism	Molecules/Materials
CO-releasing molecules (CORMs)	organometallics	CORM-1, CORM-2, CORM-3, ALF492, CORM-A1, B_{12}-ReCORM-2, Re-CORM-1, CORMA-1-PLA and ALF186.
	nonmetallic	Silica-carboxylates, boranocarbonates, boranocarbamates, xanthene carboxylic acid (XCA), hydroxy-flavones, 1,2-disubstituted ferrocenes, methylene chloride, meso-carboxy BODIPYs, unsaturated cyclic and diketones (DKs).
CO-releasing materials (CORMats)	conjugated systems	Micellization, peptide, vitamins, proteins, polymers, metal organic framework, nanoparticles, nano-sheets, porous structure materials, metallodendrimer and nano-diamond.

3. CO-Releasing Kinetic Profile

CORMs and CORMats must have a CO utility to deliver in response to the biological system soon after trigger. The specified trigger plays a decisive role for therapeutic applications. Their kinetics is highly dependent on the trigger facility at which they are applied for. The CO discharging rate was exclusively committed for searching the affected sites of selected targets. The half-life ($t_{1/2}$) of CORMs/CORMats ($t_{1/2}$ is defined in time duration as half of the introduced CORMs/CORMats amount will be dis-integrated) is the key parameter for examining the CORMs/CORMats stability and sustainability. The fast CO-releasing rate is difficult to attain predetermined clinical objectives.

Just an illustration [170], the half-life ($t_{1/2}$) of CORM-3 is 3.6 min only when anticipated with the human plasma. At that moment, CORM-3 dissolves in plasma configuration and suddenly reacting with albumin, supplies CO_2 and $Ru(CO)_2$ segment; and also makes an alliance with protein in vivo circulation, where CO serves slowly and nonspecifically [171]. Non-technical CO release is unable to deliver the necessary pharmaceutical features. Likewise slow and fast CO release molecules would be engineered to accommodate the distinct clinical trials (Figure 28).

The half-life of CORM-1 and CORM-2 is about 1 min in PBS (*phosphate buffered saline*) at 37 temperature with pH~7.4 [37,172]. Such types of half-lives are considered very short intervals. The CORMs and CORMats deliberation must be regulated along with integral body fluids in order to communicate with victim organs and/or tissues before CORMs/CORMats (as CO-producer) consume entire CO quantity [173]. To improve the sustainability of CO carriers, the half-life ($t_{1/2}$) should be extended for few minutes, but somehow few seconds and milliseconds extension will be more beneficial. A different designated strategy has promoted the transient CO releases. These mechanisms will be observed through ion-channel kinetic studies [174]. The extended pharmacokinetic qualities containing nanomaterials (NPs) and macromolecular models could be exploited for the management of CO transporters or CO carriers.

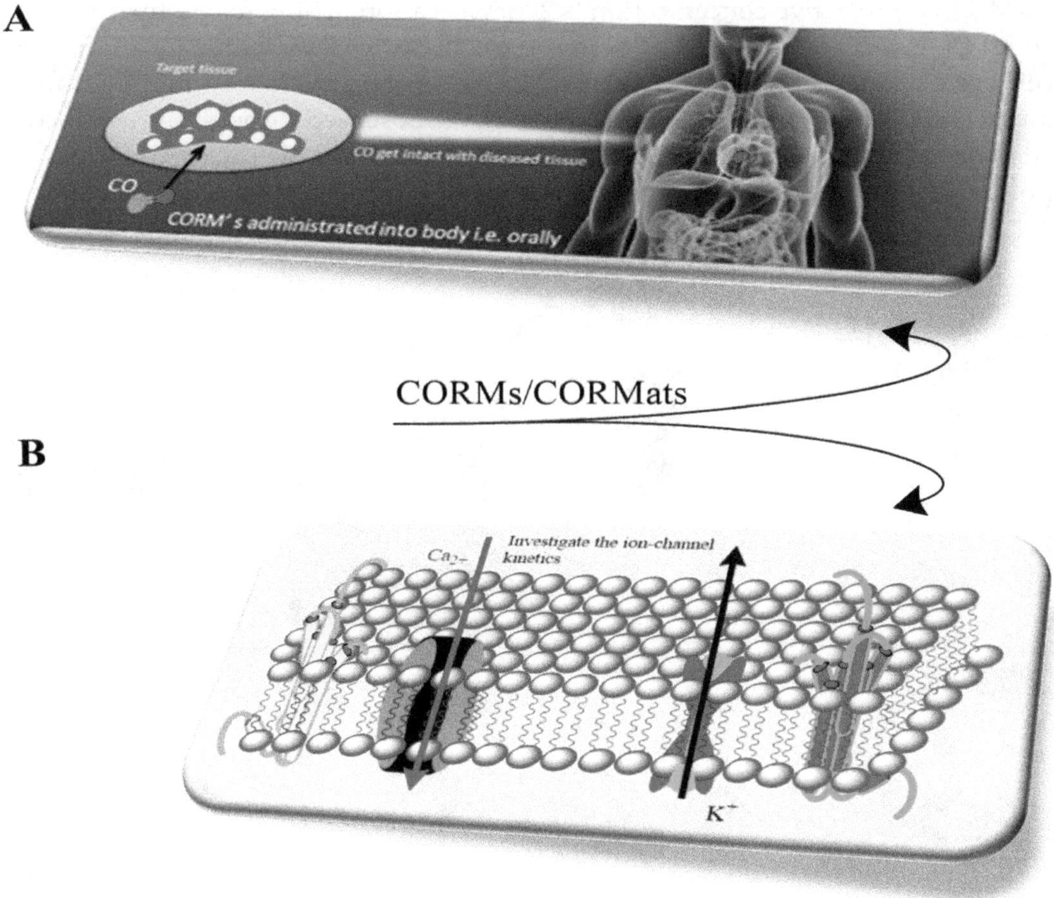

Figure 28. The CO-releasing rate profile reflects the different characteristics: (**a**) Slow CO release has therapeutic significance; (**b**) fast CO release demonstrates the path of ion-channel kinetics.

4. CORMs/CORMats Cytotoxicity and Tissue Accumulation

In addition to CORMs and CORMats pharmaceutical advantages, it delivers some adverse effects too because of their toxicological profile or even proliferation of toxic metal residues (i-CORMs/i-CORMats) resulting soon after CORMs/CORMats launch the CO into the biological environment [95,175–177]. Subsequently, a particular deficiency of CORMs/CORMats is usually observed after the CO excretion; their CO-missing analogues tend to prevail in situ administration. Therefore the transition-heavy metal core usually harbors cofactors and is involved in some uncontrolled reactions/activities with neighboring tissues/cells, thereby contributing serious cellular impairment (Figure 29).

Wang et al. studied the in vivo toxicity, cytotoxicity, metabolism and bio-distribution of two carbonyl metal CORMs series including $Ru(CO)_3ClnL$ and $M(CO)_5L$ (M= Cr, Mo, W) [178]. The cytotoxic effect was monitored on murine macrophages through MTT colorimetric assay with respect to IC_{50} and LD_{50} values; the severely damaged kidney and liver were observed to picture both morphological and functional aspects. The cell culture RAW264.7 was incubated with CORMs/CORMats while examining cytotoxicity and demonstrates their bactericidal activity against a variety of microbes, including *Staphylococcus aureus, Escherichia coli, and Pseudomonas aeruginosa* [126,127]. In this study, they found the uneven distribution of metal complexes in organs and tissues that subsequent damage through metal ions oxidation such as Ruthenium complexes. It was oxidized from Ru^{II} to Ru^{III} by P450 enzymes. This toxicity issue was elucidated by Winburn et al., they also performed the CORM's toxicological profile [179]. CORM-2 and its depleted form i-CORM-2 were studied and compared in two kidney cell lines (MDCK and HeK lines) and primary rat cardiomyocytes. This study explained that the CORM-2 cytoprotective concentration (<20mM) is approaching to cytotoxic value (>100 mM). Moreover, both CORM-2 and i-CORM-2 exerted the cellular toxicity by means of the abnormal cell cytology, cell cycle arrest, reduced cell viability, increased apoptosis and inhibited mitochondrial enzyme activity [136]. These particular consequences were observed through the metal-core mediated toxicity. Different studies have also been explored that intensifying the polarity of CORMs/CORMats would be possibly limiting their penetration over the cellular membrane, and thus attenuating their toxicity [136].

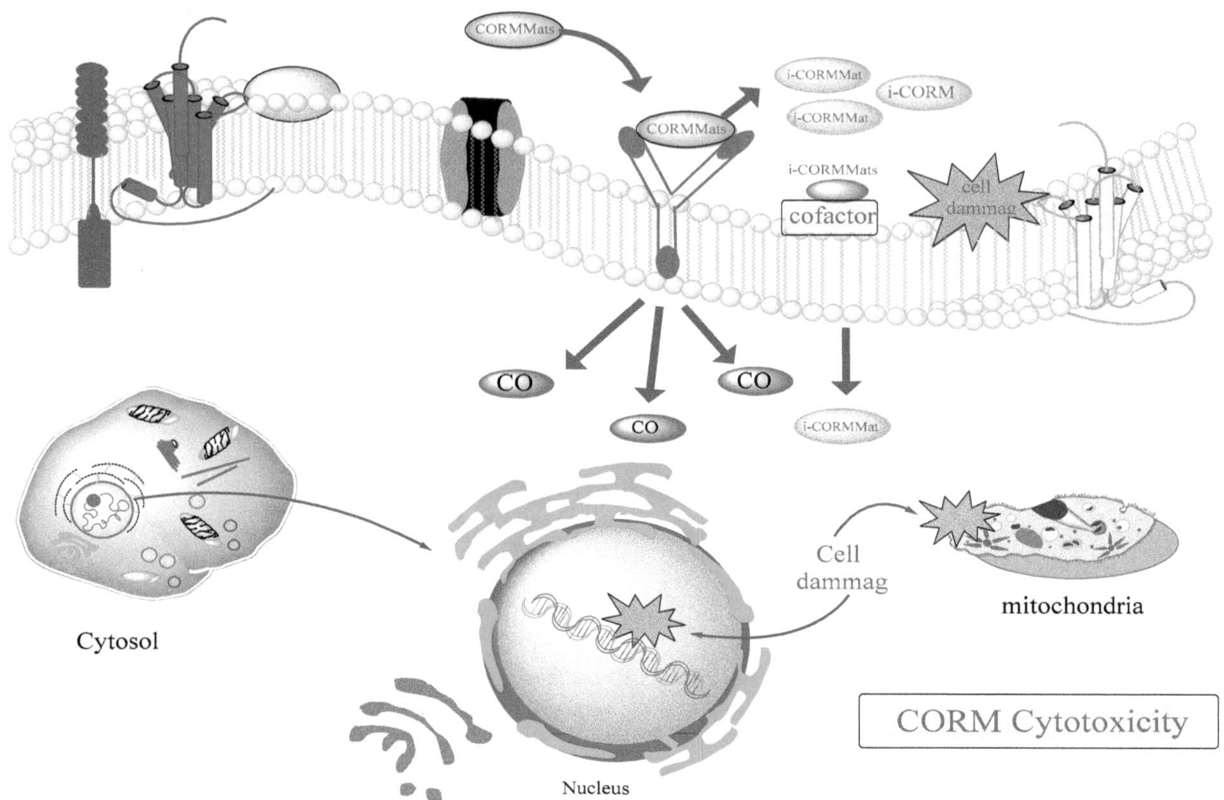

Figure 29. The CORMs/CORMats integration exhibited the cytotoxicity of metal residue (i-CORMs/CORMats).

5. Concluding Remarks

CO is generally infamous for its toxicity, but a controlled dose of CO shows useful biological impacts. The CO's detail analysis exhibits endogenous production by heme oxygenase and explores the therapeutic scope. This scientific study not only confirms the endogenous generation of CO, which has important potential in pathological tissues but also guarantees exogenously released CO's therapeutic impacts. Therefore, the challenges for the pharmaceutical drug chemists have always been and are continuing still, for the development of a risk-free and more convenient strategy to deliver therapeutic CO dosage. The CO administration with biological system suggests their therapeutic potential. This CO administration relies on MCCs for CO liberation. Thus, CORMats were developed by MCCs with different conjugate/scaffold systems. The CORMats have been covalently assembled with different nanomaterial including polymers, silica nanoparticles, proteins cages, vitamins, metallodendrimer, micelles, nanodiamond and nanofiber gel (peptide amphiphilic) or even incorporated with magnetic nanoparticles (maghemite), tablets, non-woven, or either MOFs for following features: To enhance sustainability and stability; to approach the special cellular tissues/organs; to reduce the toxicity; to attain the EPR- effect; or to permit special triggers facilities. CORM has the capability to deliver the CO to tissues and cells in vivo, in-fact constitute the most appropriate scheme to accomplish the therapeutic outcomes. This proof-of-concept refers to the medicinal chemists to endeavor modern

CORMats furnished with ADME (CORMats characteristics: Administration, Distribution, Metabolism, Excretion), prerequisite for the clinical utility. As a prodrug, these developed mechanisms are highly dependent on in vivo performance. It has been worth mentioning that many pharmaceutical materials were also claimed to be non-toxic such as smectite clay that might be transformed into CORMats for promising therapeutic benefits. Probably crystalline smectite clays are the best choice for the CORMats development due to its con-comitant administration. Additionally, their layered structure exfoliations and cation exchange capacity (CEC) have been encouraging for developing the new class of CORMats. Furthermore, it is mandatory to investigate the metal residues (remaining fragments) after CO liberation, if any side effect of newly developed materials is reported should try to minimize it by modern carrier designs. The aim of the controlled CO delivery management was sponsored by tissue selection and distribution. The CORMats activation with different triggers did not permit to develop "universal" CORMats for every disease model. The method of CORMs/CORMats trigger or even CO activation is used to disintegrate the MCCs through photo, thermal, enzyme, pH, oxidation and solvent trigger CORMs/CORMats bearing ligand exchange strategies. These CORMs/CORMats strategies are promising candidates of the therapeutic potential and deserve exclusive attention for thorough therapeutic investigations.

The toxicity of the CO precursor is still a big challenge for the researchers. The CORMs/CORMats toxicity was in-action during and after the CO release with depleted metal residues abbreviated as i-CORMs/CORMats. The fast CO release helps to study the ion-channel path, while the slow release favors tissue targets. It is mandatory that CORMs/i-CORMs and CORMats/i-CORMats (before/after CO release) should not be participating in any toxic activity. Otherwise it will not be possible to prescribe for patients; as the safety of human organs is the utmost priority.

The above discussion confirms that CORMs and CORMats are accountable for the CO-produce being the active ingredient. It should be noted that CORMats did not technically modify specific receptors but only provided a transport and discharge services for the CO gas. Therefore, the therapeutic impacts of CORMats under physiological conditions to employ CO preferentially and professionally against damaged biological tissues/organism must prevail and ensure the quick release of loaded CO upon trigger.

Author Contributions: Conceptualization, W.Z. and Y.W. (Yanyan Wang); Methodology, Y.W. (Yanyan Wang), M.F., Y.H. and W.Z.; Writing —Original Draft Preparation, M.F., H.S., Y.H., N.M., K.N. and Y.W. (Yanyan Wang); Writing —Review and Editing, Y.H., N.M., Y.W. (Ya Wu), W.D., R.L., K.N., W.Z. and M.F.; Supervision, Z.G. and W.Z.; Project Administration, W.Z. and Z.G.

Acknowledgments: This work was performed within the "211 Project" of Ministry of Education (MOE) China at the Key Laboratory of Applied Surface and Colloid Chemistry with the support of China Scholarship Council program at Shaanxi Normal University, Xi'an, China.

References

1. Pitto-Barry, A.; Lupan, A.; Ellingford, C.; Attia, A.A.A.; Barry, N.P.E. New Class of Hybrid Materials for Detection, Capture, and "On-Demand" Release of Carbon Monoxide. *ACS Appl. Mater. Interfaces* **2018**, *10*, 13693–13701. [CrossRef] [PubMed]
2. Motterlini, R.; Otterbein, L.E. The therapeutic potential of carbon monoxide. *Nat. Rev. Drug Discov.* **2010**, *9*, 728–743. [CrossRef] [PubMed]
3. Haldane, J.B.S. Carbon monoxide as a tissue poison. *Biochem. J.* **1927**, *21*, 1068–1075. [CrossRef] [PubMed]
4. Douglas, C.G.; Haldane, J.S.; Haldane, J.B.S. The laws of combination of haemoglobin with carbon monoxide and oxygen. *J. Physiol.* **1912**, *44*, 275–304. [CrossRef]
5. Tenhunen, R.; Marver, H.S.; Schmid, R. Microsomal heme oxygenase. Characterization of the enzyme. *J. Biol. Chem.* **1969**, *244*, 6388–6394.
6. Tenhunen, R.; Marver, H.S.; Schmid, R. The enzymatic conversion of heme to bilirubin by microsomal heme oxygenase. *Proc. Natl. Acad. Sci. USA* **1968**, *61*, 748–755. [CrossRef]
7. Kocer, G.; Nasircilar Ulker, S.; Senturk, U.K. The contribution of carbon monoxide to vascular tonus. *Microcirculation* **2018**, *25*, e12495. [CrossRef]

8. Peng, J.; Hu, T.; Li, J.; Du, J.; Zhu, K.; Cheng, B.; Li, K. Shepherd's Purse Polyphenols Exert Its Anti-Inflammatory and Antioxidative Effects Associated with Suppressing MAPK and NF-kappaB Pathways and Heme Oxygenase-1 Activation. *Oxidative Med. Cell. Longev.* **2019**, *2019*, 7202695. [CrossRef]
9. Dercho, R.A.; Nakatsu, K.; Wong, R.J.; Stevenson, D.K.; Vreman, H.J. Determination of in vivo carbon monoxide production in laboratory animals via exhaled air. *J. Pharmacol. Toxicol. Methods* **2006**, *54*, 288–295. [CrossRef]
10. Heinemann, S.H.; Hoshi, T.; Westerhausen, M.; Schiller, A. Carbon monoxide—Physiology, detection and controlled release. *Chem. Commun.* **2014**, *50*, 3644–3660. [CrossRef]
11. Yang, S.; Chen, M.; Zhou, L.; Zhang, G.; Gao, Z.; Zhang, W. Photo-activated CO-releasing molecules (PhotoCORMs) of robust sawhorse scaffolds [μ^2-OOCR^1, η^1-NH_2CHR^2(C=O] OCH_3, Ru(I)$_2CO_4$]. *Dalton Trans.* **2016**, *45*, 3727–3733. [CrossRef]
12. Stupfel, M.; Bouley, G. Physiological and biochemical effects on rats and mice exposed to small concentrations of carbon monoxide for long periods. *Ann. N. Y. Acad. Sci.* **1970**, *174*, 342–368. [CrossRef]
13. Ling, K.; Men, F.; Wang, W.C.; Zhou, Y.Q.; Zhang, H.W.; Ye, D.W. Carbon Monoxide and Its Controlled Release: Therapeutic Application, Detection, and Development of Carbon Monoxide Releasing Molecules (CORMs). *J. Med. Chem.* **2018**, *61*, 2611–2635. [CrossRef] [PubMed]
14. Otterbein, L.E. Carbon monoxide: Innovative anti-inflammatory properties of an age-old gas molecule. *Antioxid. Redox Signal.* **2002**, *4*, 309–319. [CrossRef]
15. Otterbein, L.E.; Soares, M.P.; Yamashita, K.; Bach, F.H. Heme oxygenase-1: Unleashing the protective properties of heme. *Trends Immunol.* **2003**, *24*, 449–455. [CrossRef]
16. Zamani, M.; Aleyasin, A.; Fakhrzadeh, H.; Kiavar, M.; Raoufzadeh, S.; Larijani, B.; Mahmoodi, E. Heme Oxigenase 2 Gene Polymorphisms as Genetic Risk Factor in Atherosclerosis in Iranian Patients. *Iran. Red Crescent Med. J.* **2010**, *12*, 559–563.
17. Joshi, H.P.; Kim, S.B.; Kim, S.; Kumar, H.; Jo, M.J.; Choi, H.; Kim, J.; Kyung, J.W.; Sohn, S.; Kim, K.T.; et al. Nanocarrier-mediated Delivery of CORM-2 Enhances Anti-allodynic and Anti-hyperalgesic Effects of CORM-2. *Mol. Neurobiol.* **2019**, *56*. [CrossRef]
18. Motterlini, R.; Haas, B.; Foresti, R. Emerging concepts on the anti-inflammatory actions of carbon monoxide-releasing molecules (CO-RMs). *Med. Gas Res.* **2012**, *2*, 28. [CrossRef]
19. Al-Huseini, L.M.; Aw Yeang, H.X.; Hamdam, J.M.; Sethu, S.; Alhumeed, N.; Wong, W.; Sathish, J.G. Heme oxygenase-1 regulates dendritic cell function through modulation of p38 MAPK-CREB/ATF1 signaling. *J. Biol. Chem.* **2014**, *289*, 16442–16451. [CrossRef]
20. Stagni, E.; Privitera, M.G.; Bucolo, C.; Leggio, G.M.; Motterlini, R.; Drago, F. A water-soluble carbon monoxide-releasing molecule (CORM-3) lowers intraocular pressure in rabbits. *Br. J. Ophthalmol.* **2009**, *93*, 254–257. [CrossRef]
21. Allanson, M.; Reeve, V.E. Ultraviolet A (320-400 nm) modulation of ultraviolet B (290-320 nm)-induced immune suppression is mediated by carbon monoxide. *J. Investig. Dermatol.* **2005**, *124*, 644–650. [CrossRef] [PubMed]
22. Mazzola, S.; Forni, M.; Albertini, M.; Bacci, M.L.; Zannoni, A.; Gentilini, F.; Lavitrano, M.; Bach, F.H.; Otterbein, L.E.; Clement, M.G. Carbon monoxide pretreatment prevents respiratory derangement and ameliorates hyperacute endotoxic shock in pigs. *FASEB J.* **2005**, *19*, 2045–2047. [CrossRef]
23. Bagul, A.; Hosgood, S.A.; Kaushik, M.; Nicholson, M.L. Carbon monoxide protects against ischemia-reperfusion injury in an experimental model of controlled nonheartbeating donor kidney. *Transplantation* **2008**, *85*, 576–581. [CrossRef] [PubMed]
24. Sato, K.; Balla, J.; Otterbein, L.; Smith, R.N.; Brouard, S.; Lin, Y.; Csizmadia, E.; Sevigny, J.; Robson, S.C.; Vercellotti, G.; et al. Carbon monoxide generated by heme oxygenase-1 suppresses the rejection of mouse-to-rat cardiac transplants. *J. Immunol.* **2001**, *166*, 4185–4194. [CrossRef]
25. Chen, B.; Guo, L.; Fan, C.; Bolisetty, S.; Joseph, R.; Wright, M.M.; Agarwal, A.; George, J.F. Carbon monoxide rescues heme oxygenase-1-deficient mice from arterial thrombosis in allogeneic aortic transplantation. *Am. J. Pathol.* **2009**, *175*, 422–429. [CrossRef] [PubMed]
26. Clark, J.E.; Naughton, P.; Shurey, S.; Green, C.J.; Johnson, T.R.; Mann, B.E.; Foresti, R.; Motterlini, R. Cardioprotective actions by a water-soluble carbon monoxide-releasing molecule. *Circ. Res.* **2003**, *93*, e2–e8. [CrossRef]

27. Yoshida, J.; Ozaki, K.S.; Nalesnik, M.A.; Ueki, S.; Castillo-Rama, M.; Faleo, G.; Ezzelarab, M.; Nakao, A.; Ekser, B.; Echeverri, G.J.; et al. Ex vivo application of carbon monoxide in UW solution prevents transplant-induced renal ischemia/reperfusion injury in pigs. *Am. J. Transplant.* **2010**, *10*, 763–772. [CrossRef]
28. Sandouka, A.; Fuller, B.J.; Mann, B.E.; Green, C.J.; Foresti, R.; Motterlini, R. Treatment with CO-RMs during cold storage improves renal function at reperfusion. *Kidney Int.* **2006**, *69*, 239–247. [CrossRef]
29. Nakao, A.; Faleo, G.; Shimizu, H.; Nakahira, K.; Kohmoto, J.; Sugimoto, R.; Choi, A.M.; McCurry, K.R.; Takahashi, T.; Murase, N. Ex vivo carbon monoxide prevents cytochrome P450 degradation and ischemia/reperfusion injury of kidney grafts. *Kidney Int.* **2008**, *74*, 1009–1016. [CrossRef] [PubMed]
30. Pizarro, M.D.; Rodriguez, J.V.; Mamprin, M.E.; Fuller, B.J.; Mann, B.E.; Motterlini, R.; Guibert, E.E. Protective effects of a carbon monoxide-releasing molecule (CORM-3) during hepatic cold preservation. *Cryobiology* **2009**, *58*, 248–255. [CrossRef] [PubMed]
31. Kaizu, T.; Ikeda, A.; Nakao, A.; Tsung, A.; Toyokawa, H.; Ueki, S.; Geller, D.A.; Murase, N. Protection of transplant-induced hepatic ischemia/reperfusion injury with carbon monoxide via MEK/ERK1/2 pathway downregulation. *Am. J. Physiol. Gastrointest. Liver Physiol.* **2008**, *294*, G236–G244. [CrossRef]
32. Kohmoto, J.; Nakao, A.; Sugimoto, R.; Wang, Y.; Zhan, J.; Ueda, H.; McCurry, K.R. Carbon monoxide-saturated preservation solution protects lung grafts from ischemia-reperfusion injury. *J. Thorac. Cardiovasc. Surg.* **2008**, *136*, 1067–1075. [CrossRef]
33. Minamoto, K.; Harada, H.; Lama, V.N.; Fedarau, M.A.; Pinsky, D.J. Reciprocal regulation of airway rejection by the inducible gas-forming enzymes heme oxygenase and nitric oxide synthase. *J. Exp. Med.* **2005**, *202*, 283–294. [CrossRef] [PubMed]
34. Lee, S.S.; Gao, W.; Mazzola, S.; Thomas, M.N.; Csizmadia, E.; Otterbein, L.E.; Bach, F.H.; Wang, H. Heme oxygenase-1, carbon monoxide, and bilirubin induce tolerance in recipients toward islet allografts by modulating T regulatory cells. *FASEB J.* **2007**, *21*, 3450–3457. [CrossRef] [PubMed]
35. Nakao, A.; Toyokawa, H.; Tsung, A.; Nalesnik, M.A.; Stolz, D.B.; Kohmoto, J.; Ikeda, A.; Tomiyama, K.; Harada, T.; Takahashi, T.; et al. Ex vivo application of carbon monoxide in University of Wisconsin solution to prevent intestinal cold ischemia/reperfusion injury. *Am. J. Transplant.* **2006**, *6*, 2243–2255. [CrossRef] [PubMed]
36. Bojakowski, K.; Gaciong, Z.; Grochowiecki, T.; Szmidt, J. Carbon monoxide may reduce ischemia reperfusion injury: A case report of complicated kidney transplantation from a carbon monoxide poisoned donor. *Transplant. Proc.* **2007**, *39*, 2928–2929. [CrossRef]
37. Motterlini, R.; Mann, B.E.; Foresti, R. Therapeutic applications of carbon monoxide-releasing molecules. *Expert Opin. Investig. Drugs* **2005**, *14*, 1305–1318. [CrossRef]
38. Ryter, S.W.; Choi, A.M. Cytoprotective and anti-inflammatory actions of carbon monoxide in organ injury and sepsis models. *Novartis Found. Symp.* **2007**, *280*, 165–175.
39. Nobre, L.S.; Jeremias, H.; Romao, C.C.; Saraiva, L.M. Examining the antimicrobial activity and toxicity to animal cells of different types of CO-releasing molecules. *Dalton Trans.* **2016**, *45*, 1455–1466. [CrossRef] [PubMed]
40. Motterlini, R.; Gonzales, A.; Foresti, R.; Clark, J.E.; Green, C.J.; Winslow, R.M. Heme oxygenase-1-derived carbon monoxide contributes to the suppression of acute hypertensive responses in vivo. *Circ. Res.* **1998**, *83*, 568–577. [CrossRef] [PubMed]
41. Taille, C.; El-Benna, J.; Lanone, S.; Boczkowski, J.; Motterlini, R. Mitochondrial respiratory chain and NAD(P)H oxidase are targets for the antiproliferative effect of carbon monoxide in human airway smooth muscle. *J. Biol. Chem.* **2005**, *280*, 25350–25360. [CrossRef]
42. Siow, R.C.; Sato, H.; Mann, G.E. Heme oxygenase-carbon monoxide signalling pathway in atherosclerosis: Anti-atherogenic actions of bilirubin and carbon monoxide? *Cardiovasc. Res.* **1999**, *41*, 385–394. [CrossRef]
43. Crespy, D.; Landfester, K.; Schubert, U.S.; Schiller, A. Potential photoactivated metallopharmaceuticals: From active molecules to supported drugs. *Chem. Commun.* **2010**, *46*, 6651–6662. [CrossRef]
44. Otterbein, L.E. The evolution of carbon monoxide into medicine. *Respir. Care* **2009**, *54*, 925–932. [CrossRef]
45. Omaye, S.T. Metabolic modulation of carbon monoxide toxicity. *Toxicology* **2002**, *180*, 139–150. [CrossRef]
46. Palao, E.; Slanina, T.; Muchová, L.; Šolomek, T.; Vítek, L.; Klán, P. Transition-Metal-Free CO-Releasing BODIPY Derivatives Activatable by Visible to NIR Light as Promising Bioactive Molecules. *J. Am. Chem. Soc.* **2016**, *138*, 126–133. [CrossRef] [PubMed]

47. Pierri, A.E.; Huang, P.J.; Garcia, J.V.; Stanfill, J.G.; Chui, M.; Wu, G.; Zheng, N.; Ford, P.C. A photoCORM nanocarrier for CO release using NIR light. *Chem. Commun.* **2015**, *51*, 2072–2075. [CrossRef] [PubMed]
48. He, Q.; Kiesewetter, D.O.; Qu, Y.; Fu, X.; Fan, J.; Huang, P.; Liu, Y.; Zhu, G.; Liu, Y.; Qian, Z.; et al. NIR-Responsive On-Demand Release of CO from Metal Carbonyl-Caged Graphene Oxide Nanomedicine. *Adv. Mater.* **2015**, *27*, 6741–6746. [CrossRef]
49. Mede, R.; Hoffmann, P.; Klein, M.; Goerls, H.; Schmitt, M.; Neugebauer, U.; Gessner, G.; Heinemann, S.H.; Popp, J.; Westerhausen, M. A Water-Soluble Mn(CO)3-Based and Non-Toxic PhotoCORM for Administration of Carbon Monoxide Inside of Cells. *Z. Anorg. Allg. Chem.* **2017**, *643*, 2057–2062. [CrossRef]
50. Carmona, F.J.; Rojas, S.; Sanchez, P.; Jeremias, H.; Marques, A.R.; Romao, C.C.; Choquesillo-Lazarte, D.; Navarro, J.A.; Maldonado, C.R.; Barea, E. Cation Exchange Strategy for the Encapsulation of a Photoactive CO-Releasing Organometallic Molecule into Anionic Porous Frameworks. *Inorg. Chem.* **2016**, *55*, 6525–6531. [CrossRef]
51. Foresti, R.; Bani-Hani, M.G.; Motterlini, R. Use of carbon monoxide as a therapeutic agent: Promises and challenges. *Intensive Care Med.* **2008**, *34*, 649–658. [CrossRef]
52. Kueh, J.T.B.; Stanley, N.J.; Hewitt, R.J.; Woods, L.M.; Larsen, L.; Harrison, J.C.; Rennison, D.; Brimble, M.A.; Sammut, I.A.; Larsen, D.S. Norborn-2-en-7-ones as physiologically-triggered carbon monoxide-releasing prodrugs. *Chem. Sci.* **2017**, *8*, 5454–5459. [CrossRef]
53. Romão, C.C.; Blättler, W.A.; Seixas, J.D.; Bernardes, G.J.L. Developing drug molecules for therapy with carbon monoxide. *Chem. Soc. Rev.* **2012**, *41*, 3571–3583. [CrossRef] [PubMed]
54. Stamellou, E.; Storz, D.; Botov, S.; Ntasis, E.; Wedel, J.; Sollazzo, S.; Krämer, B.K.; van Son, W.; Seelen, M.; Schmalz, H.G.; et al. Different design of enzyme-triggered CO-releasing molecules (ET-CORMs) reveals quantitative differences in biological activities in terms of toxicity and inflammation. *Redox Biol.* **2014**, *2*, 739–748. [CrossRef] [PubMed]
55. Peng, P.; Wang, C.; Shi, Z.; Johns, V.K.; Ma, L.; Oyer, J.; Copik, A.; Igarashi, R.; Liao, Y. Visible-light activatable organic CO-releasing molecules (PhotoCORMs) that simultaneously generate fluorophores. *Org. Biomol. Chem.* **2013**, *11*, 6671–6674. [CrossRef] [PubMed]
56. Schatzschneider, U. Photoactivated Biological Activity of Transition-Metal Complexes. *Eur. J. Inorg. Chem.* **2010**, *2010*, 1451–1467. [CrossRef]
57. Seixas, J.D.; Mukhopadhyay, A.; Santos-Silva, T.; Otterbein, L.E.; Gallo, D.J.; Rodrigues, S.S.; Guerreiro, B.H.; Gonçalves, A.M.L.; Penacho, N.; Marques, A.R.; et al. Characterization of a versatile organometallic pro-drug (CORM) for experimental CO based therapeutics. *Dalton Trans.* **2013**, *42*, 5985–5998. [CrossRef]
58. Queiroga, C.S.F.; Vercelli, A.; Vieira, H.L.A. Carbon monoxide and the CNS: Challenges and achievements. *Br. J. Pharmacol.* **2015**, *172*, 1533–1545. [CrossRef] [PubMed]
59. Hasegawa, U.; van der Vlies, A.J.; Simeoni, E.; Wandrey, C.; Hubbell, J.A. Carbon monoxide-releasing micelles for immunotherapy. *J. Am. Chem. Soc.* **2010**, *132*, 18273–18280. [CrossRef]
60. Park, S.S.; Kim, J.; Lee, Y. Improved electrochemical microsensor for the real-time simultaneous analysis of endogenous nitric oxide and carbon monoxide generation. *Anal. Chem.* **2012**, *84*, 1792–1796. [CrossRef]
61. Morimoto, Y.; Durante, W.; Lancaster, D.G.; Klattenhoff, J.; Tittel, F.K. Real-time measurements of endogenous CO production from vascular cells using an ultrasensitive laser sensor. *Am. J. Physiol. Heart Circ. Physiol.* **2001**, *280*, H483–H488. [CrossRef]
62. Marks, G.S.; Vreman, H.J.; McLaughlin, B.E.; Brien, J.F.; Nakatsu, K. Measurement of endogenous carbon monoxide formation in biological systems. *Antioxid. Redox Signal.* **2002**, *4*, 271–277. [CrossRef]
63. Barbe, J.M.; Canard, G.; Brandes, S.; Guilard, R. Selective chemisorption of carbon monoxide by organic-inorganic hybrid materials incorporating cobalt(III) corroles as sensing components. *Chemistry* **2007**, *13*, 2118–2129. [CrossRef]
64. McLean, S.; Mann, B.E.; Poole, R.K. Sulfite species enhance carbon monoxide release from CO-releasing molecules: Implications for the deoxymyoglobin assay of activity. *Anal. Biochem.* **2012**, *427*, 36–40. [CrossRef]
65. Esteban, J.; Ros-Lis, J.V.; Martinez-Manez, R.; Marcos, M.D.; Moragues, M.; Soto, J.; Sancenon, F. Sensitive and selective chromogenic sensing of carbon monoxide by using binuclear rhodium complexes. *Angew. Chem.* **2010**, *49*, 4934–4937. [CrossRef]
66. Nandi, C.; Debnath, R.; Debroy, P. Intelligent Control Systems for Carbon Monoxide Detection in IoT Environments. In *Guide to Ambient Intelligence in the IoT Environment: Principles, Technologies and Applications*; Mahmood, Z., Ed.; Springer International Publishing: Cham, Switzerland, 2019; pp. 153–176.

67. Vreman, H.J.; Stevenson, D.K. Heme oxygenase activity as measured by carbon monoxide production. *Anal. Biochem.* **1988**, *168*, 31–38. [CrossRef]
68. Yuan, L.; Lin, W.; Tan, L.; Zheng, K.; Huang, W. Lighting up carbon monoxide: Fluorescent probes for monitoring CO in living cells. *Angew. Chem.* **2013**, *52*, 1628–1630. [CrossRef]
69. Michel, B.W.; Lippert, A.R.; Chang, C.J. A Reaction-Based Fluorescent Probe for Selective Imaging of Carbon Monoxide in Living Cells Using a Palladium-Mediated Carbonylation. *J. Am. Chem. Soc.* **2012**, *134*, 15668–15671. [CrossRef]
70. Bauschlicher, C.W., Jr; Bagus, P.S. The metal–carbonyl bond in $Ni(CO)_4$ and $Fe(CO)_5$: A clear–cut analysis. *J. Chem. Phys.* **1984**, *81*, 5889–5898. [CrossRef]
71. Schatzschneider, U. Novel lead structures and activation mechanisms for CO-releasing molecules (CORMs). *Br. J. Pharmacol.* **2015**, *172*, 1638–1650. [CrossRef]
72. Kitazawa, M.; Wagner, J.R.; Kirby, M.L.; Anantharam, V.; Kanthasamy, A.G. Oxidative stress and mitochondrial-mediated apoptosis in dopaminergic cells exposed to methylcyclopentadienyl manganese tricarbonyl. *J. Pharmacol. Exp. Ther.* **2002**, *302*, 26–35. [CrossRef]
73. Gessner, G.; Sahoo, N.; Swain, S.M.; Hirth, G.; Schonherr, R.; Mede, R.; Westerhausen, M.; Brewitz, H.H.; Heimer, P.; Imhof, D.; et al. CO-independent modification of K(+) channels by tricarbonyldichlororuthenium(II) dimer (CORM-2). *Eur. J. Pharmacol.* **2017**, *815*, 33–41. [CrossRef]
74. Mansour, A.M. Rapid green and blue light-induced CO release from bromazepam Mn(I) and Ru(II) carbonyls: Synthesis, density functional theory and biological activity evaluation. *Appl. Organomet. Chem.* **2017**, *31*, e3564. [CrossRef]
75. Carmona, F.J.; Jimenez-Amezcua, I.; Rojas, S.; Romao, C.C.; Navarro, J.A.R.; Maldonado, C.R.; Barea, E. Aluminum Doped MCM-41 Nanoparticles as Platforms for the Dual Encapsulation of a CO-Releasing Molecule and Cisplatin. *Inorg. Chem.* **2017**, *56*, 10474–10480. [CrossRef]
76. Wareham, L.K.; McLean, S.; Begg, R.; Rana, N.; Ali, S.; Kendall, J.J.; Sanguinetti, G.; Mann, B.E.; Poole, R.K. The Broad-Spectrum Antimicrobial Potential of [Mn(CO)4(S2CNMe(CH2CO2H))], a Water-Soluble CO-Releasing Molecule (CORM-401): Intracellular Accumulation, Transcriptomic and Statistical Analyses, and Membrane Polarization. *Antioxid. Redox Signal.* **2018**, *28*, 1286–1308. [CrossRef] [PubMed]
77. Mansour, A.M.; Shehab, O.R. Reactivity of visible-light induced CO releasing thiourea-based Mn(I) tricarbonyl bromide (CORM-NS1) towards lysozyme. *Inorg. Chim. Acta* **2018**, *480*, 159–165. [CrossRef]
78. Aucott, B.J.; Ward, J.S.; Andrew, S.G.; Milani, J.; Whitwood, A.C.; Lynam, J.M.; Parkin, A.; Fairlamb, I.J.S. Redox-tagged carbon monoxide-releasing molecules (CORMs): Ferrocene-containing [Mn(C-N)(CO)4] complexes as a promising new CORM class. *Inorg. Chem.* **2017**, *56*, 5431–5440. [CrossRef]
79. Kretschmer, R.; Gessner, G.; Goerls, H.; Heinemann, S.H.; Westerhausen, M. Dicarbonyl-bis(cysteamine)iron(II): A light induced carbon monoxide releasing molecule based on iron (CORM-S1). *J. Inorg. Biochem.* **2011**, *105*, 6–9. [CrossRef]
80. Li, J.; Zhang, J.; Zhang, Q.; Bai, Z.; Zhao, Q.; Wang, Z.; Chen, Y.; Liu, B. Synthesis and biological activities of carbonyl cobalt CORMs with selectively inhibiting cyclooxygenase-2. *J. Organomet. Chem.* **2018**, *874*, 49–62. [CrossRef]
81. Gong, Y.; Zhang, T.; Li, M.; Xi, N.; Zheng, Y.; Zhao, Q.; Chen, Y.; Liu, B. Toxicity, bio-distribution and metabolism of CO-releasing molecules based on cobalt. *Free Radic. Biol. Med.* **2016**, *97*, 362–374. [CrossRef]
82. Wong, J.; MacDonald, N.; Mottillo, C.; Hiskic, I.; Butler, I.S.; Friscic, T. *Synthesis of Organometallic C0-Releasing Molecules (CORMs) in the Absence of a Bulk Organic Solvent*; American Chemical Society: Denver, CO, USA, 2015; INOR-785.
83. Finze, M.; Bernhardt, E.; Willner, H.; Lehmann, C.W.; Aubke, F. Homoleptic, sigma-bonded octahedral superelectrophilic metal carbonyl cations of iron(II), ruthenium(II), and osmium(II). Part 2: Syntheses and characterizations of [M(CO)(6)][BF(4)](2) (M = Fe, Ru, Os). *Inorg. Chem.* **2005**, *44*, 4206–4214. [CrossRef]
84. Kottelat, E.; Chabert, V.; Crochet, A.; Fromm, K.M.; Zobi, F. Towards Cardiolite-Inspired Carbon Monoxide Releasing Molecules—Reactivity of d4, d5 Rhenium and d6 Manganese Carbonyl Complexes with Isocyanide Ligands. *Eur. J. Inorg. Chem.* **2015**, *2015*, 5628–5638. [CrossRef]
85. Abeyrathna, N.; Washington, K.; Bashur, C.; Liao, Y. Nonmetallic carbon monoxide releasing molecules (CORMs). *Org. Biomol. Chem.* **2017**, *15*, 8692–8699. [CrossRef]
86. Friis, S.D.; Taaning, R.H.; Lindhardt, A.T.; Skrydstrup, T. Silacarboxylic acids as efficient carbon monoxide releasing molecules: Synthesis and application in palladium-catalyzed carbonylation reactions. *J. Am. Chem. Soc.* **2011**, *133*, 18114–18117. [CrossRef] [PubMed]

87. Motterlini, R.; Sawle, P.; Hammad, J.; Bains, S.; Alberto, R.; Foresti, R.; Green, C.J. CORM-A1: A new pharmacologically active carbon monoxide-releasing molecule. *FASEB J.* **2005**, *19*, 284–286. [CrossRef] [PubMed]
88. Klein, M.; Neugebauer, U.; Schmitt, M.; Popp, J. Elucidation of the CO-Release Kinetics of CORM-A1 by Means of Vibrational Spectroscopy. *Chemphyschem A Eur. J. Chem. Phys. Phys. Chem.* **2016**, *17*, 985–993. [CrossRef]
89. Antony, L.A.; Slanina, T.; Sebej, P.; Solomek, T.; Klan, P. Fluorescein analogue xanthene-9-carboxylic acid: A transition-metal-free CO releasing molecule activated by green light. *Org. Lett.* **2013**, *15*, 4552–4555. [CrossRef]
90. Mondal, R.; Okhrimenko, A.N.; Shah, B.K.; Neckers, D.C. Photodecarbonylation of alpha-diketones: A mechanistic study of reactions leading to acenes. *J. Phys.Chem. B* **2008**, *112*, 11–15. [CrossRef] [PubMed]
91. Martins, P.N.A.; Reuzel-Selke, A.; Jurisch, A.; Atrott, K.; Pascher, A.; Pratschke, J.; Buelow, R.; Neuhaus, P.; Volk, H.D.; Tullius, S.G. Induction of carbon monoxide in the donor reduces graft immunogenicity and chronic graft deterioration. *Transplant. Proc.* **2005**, *37*, 379–381. [CrossRef]
92. Chauveau, C.; Bouchet, D.; Roussel, J.C.; Mathieu, P.; Braudeau, C.; Renaudin, K.; Tesson, L.; Soulillou, J.P.; Iyer, S.; Buelow, R.; et al. Gene Transfer of Heme Oxygenase-1 and Carbon Monoxide Delivery Inhibit Chronic Rejection. *Am. J. Transplant.* **2002**, *2*, 581–592. [CrossRef]
93. Anderson, S.N.; Richards, J.M.; Esquer, H.J.; Benninghoff, A.D.; Arif, A.M.; Berreau, L.M. A Structurally-Tunable 3-Hydroxyflavone Motif for Visible Light-Induced Carbon Monoxide-Releasing Molecules (CORMs). *ChemistryOpen* **2015**, *4*, 590–594. [CrossRef]
94. Petrovski, Ž.; Norton de Matos, M.R.P.; Braga, S.S.; Pereira, C.C.L.; Matos, M.L.; Gonçalves, I.S.; Pillinger, M.; Alves, P.M.; Romão, C.C. Synthesis, characterization and antitumor activity of 1,2-disubstituted ferrocenes and cyclodextrin inclusion complexes. *J. Organomet. Chem.* **2008**, *693*, 675–684. [CrossRef]
95. Motterlini, R.; Clark, J.E.; Foresti, R.; Sarathchandra, P.; Mann, B.E.; Green, C.J. Carbon monoxide-releasing molecules: Characterization of biochemical and vascular activities. *Circ. Res.* **2002**, *90*, E17–E24. [CrossRef]
96. Steiger, C.; Luhmann, T.; Meinel, L. Oral drug delivery of therapeutic gases—Carbon monoxide release for gastrointestinal diseases. *J. Control. Release* **2014**, *189*, 46–53. [CrossRef] [PubMed]
97. Ferrandiz, M.L.; Maicas, N.; Garcia-Arnandis, I.; Terencio, M.C.; Motterlini, R.; Devesa, I.; Joosten, L.A.; van den Berg, W.B.; Alcaraz, M.J. Treatment with a CO-releasing molecule (CORM-3) reduces joint inflammation and erosion in murine collagen-induced arthritis. *Ann. Rheum. Dis.* **2008**, *67*, 1211–1217. [CrossRef]
98. Nobre, L.S.; Seixas, J.D.; Romao, C.C.; Saraiva, L.M. Antimicrobial action of carbon monoxide-releasing compounds. *Antimicrob. Agents Chemother.* **2007**, *51*, 4303–4307. [CrossRef] [PubMed]
99. Bikiel, D.E.; Gonzalez Solveyra, E.; Di Salvo, F.; Milagre, H.M.; Eberlin, M.N.; Correa, R.S.; Ellena, J.; Estrin, D.A.; Doctorovich, F. Tetrachlorocarbonyliridates: Water-soluble carbon monoxide releasing molecules rate-modulated by the sixth ligand. *Inorg. Chem.* **2011**, *50*, 2334–2345. [CrossRef] [PubMed]
100. Braud, L.; Pini, M.; Wilson, J.L.; Czibik, G.; Sawaki, D.; Derumeaux, G.; Foresti, R.; Motterlini, R. A carbon monoxide-releasing molecule (CORM-401) induces a metabolic switch in adipocytes and improves insulin-sensitivity on high fat diet-induced obesity in mice. *Arch. Cardiovasc. Dis. Suppl.* **2018**, *10*, 188. [CrossRef]
101. Wareham, L.K.; Poole, R.K.; Tinajero-Trejo, M. CO-releasing Metal Carbonyl Compounds as Antimicrobial Agents in the Post-antibiotic Era. *J. Biol. Chem.* **2015**, *290*, 18999–19007. [CrossRef]
102. Zhang, W.Q.; Atkin, A.J.; Thatcher, R.J.; Whitwood, A.C.; Fairlamb, I.J.; Lynam, J.M. Diversity and design of metal-based carbon monoxide-releasing molecules (CO-RMs) in aqueous systems: Revealing the essential trends. *Dalton Trans.* **2009**, 4351–4358. [CrossRef] [PubMed]
103. Seixas, J.D.; Santos, M.F.; Mukhopadhyay, A.; Coelho, A.C.; Reis, P.M.; Veiros, L.F.; Marques, A.R.; Penacho, N.; Goncalves, A.M.; Romao, M.J.; et al. A contribution to the rational design of Ru(CO)3Cl2L complexes for in vivo delivery of CO. *Dalton Trans.* **2015**, *44*, 5058–5075. [CrossRef]
104. Suliman, H.B.; Zobi, F.; Piantadosi, C.A. Heme Oxygenase-1/Carbon Monoxide System and Embryonic Stem Cell Differentiation and Maturation into Cardiomyocytes. *Antioxid. Redox Signal.* **2016**, *24*, 345–360. [CrossRef]
105. Musameh, M.D.; Green, C.J.; Mann, B.E.; Fuller, B.J.; Motterlini, R. Improved myocardial function after cold storage with preservation solution supplemented with a carbon monoxide-releasing molecule (CORM-3). *J. Heart Lung Transplant.* **2007**, *26*, 1192–1198. [CrossRef]

106. Ulbrich, F.; Hagmann, C.; Buerkle, H.; Romao, C.C.; Schallner, N.; Goebel, U.; Biermann, J. The Carbon monoxide releasing molecule ALF-186 mediates anti-inflammatory and neuroprotective effects via the soluble guanylate cyclase ß1 in rats' retinal ganglion cells after ischemia and reperfusion injury. *J. Neuroinflamm.* **2017**, *14*, 130. [CrossRef]
107. Zhang, W.Q.; Whitwood, A.C.; Fairlamb, I.J.; Lynam, J.M. Group 6 carbon monoxide-releasing metal complexes with biologically-compatible leaving groups. *Inorg. Chem.* **2010**, *49*, 8941–8952. [CrossRef]
108. Long, L.; Jiang, X.; Wang, X.; Xiao, Z.; Liu, X. Water-soluble diiron hexacarbonyl complex as a CO-RM: Controllable CO-releasing, releasing mechanism and biocompatibility. *Dalton Trans.* **2013**, *42*, 15663–15669. [CrossRef]
109. Zobi, F.; Degonda, A.; Schaub, M.C.; Bogdanova, A.Y. CO releasing properties and cytoprotective effect of cis-trans-[Re(II)(CO)2Br2L2]n complexes. *Inorg. Chem.* **2010**, *49*, 7313–7322. [CrossRef]
110. Schatzschneider, U. PhotoCORMs: Light-triggered release of carbon monoxide from the coordination sphere of transition metal complexes for biological applications. *Inorg. Chim. Acta* **2011**, *374*, 19–23. [CrossRef]
111. Bohlender, C.; Gläser, S.; Klein, M.; Weisser, J.; Thein, S.; Neugebauer, U.; Popp, J.; Wyrwa, R.; Schiller, A. Light-triggered CO release from nanoporous non-wovens. *J. Mater. Chem. B* **2014**, *2*, 1454–1463. [CrossRef]
112. Lomont, J.P.; Nguyen, S.C.; Harris, C.B. Exploring the utility of tandem thermal-photochemical CO delivery with CORM-2. *Organometallics* **2014**, *33*, 6179–6185. [CrossRef]
113. Bannenberg, G.L.; Vieira, H.L. Therapeutic applications of the gaseous mediators carbon monoxide and hydrogen sulfide. *Expert Opin. Ther. Pat.* **2009**, *19*, 663–682. [CrossRef]
114. Motterlini, R.; Mann, B.E.; Johnson, T.R.; Clark, J.E.; Foresti, R.; Green, C.J. Bioactivity and pharmacological actions of carbon monoxide-releasing molecules. *Curr. Pharm. Des.* **2003**, *9*, 2525–2539. [CrossRef]
115. Fiumana, E.; Parfenova, H.; Jaggar, J.H.; Leffler, C.W. Carbon monoxide mediates vasodilator effects of glutamate in isolated pressurized cerebral arterioles of newborn pigs. *Am. J. Physiol. Heart Circ. Physiol.* **2003**, *284*, H1073–H1079. [CrossRef]
116. Cepinskas, G.; Katada, K.; Bihari, A.; Potter, R.F. Carbon monoxide liberated from carbon monoxide-releasing molecule CORM-2 attenuates inflammation in the liver of septic mice. *Am. J. Physiol. Gastrointest. Liver Physiol.* **2008**, *294*, G184–G191. [CrossRef]
117. Nielsen, V.G.; Chawla, N.; Mangla, D.; Gomes, S.B.; Arkebauer, M.R.; Wasko, K.A.; Sadacharam, K.; Vosseller, K. Carbon monoxide-releasing molecule-2 enhances coagulation in rabbit plasma and decreases bleeding time in clopidogrel/aspirin-treated rabbits. *Blood Coagul. Fibrinolysis Int. J. Haemost. Thromb.* **2011**, *22*, 756–759. [CrossRef]
118. Santos-Silva, T.; Mukhopadhyay, A.; Seixas, J.D.; Bernardes, G.J.; Romao, C.C.; Romao, M.J. Towards improved therapeutic CORMs: Understanding the reactivity of CORM-3 with proteins. *Curr. Med. Chem.* **2011**, *18*, 3361–3366. [CrossRef]
119. Maines, M.D. Heme oxygenase: Function, multiplicity, regulatory mechanisms, and clinical applications. *FASEB J.* **1988**, *2*, 2557–2568. [CrossRef]
120. Freitas, A.; Alves-Filho, J.C.; Secco, D.D.; Neto, A.F.; Ferreira, S.H.; Barja-Fidalgo, C.; Cunha, F.Q. Heme oxygenase/carbon monoxide-biliverdin pathway down regulates neutrophil rolling, adhesion and migration in acute inflammation. *Br. J. Pharmacol.* **2006**, *149*, 345–354. [CrossRef]
121. Chaves-Ferreira, M.; Albuquerque, I.S.; Matak-Vinkovic, D.; Coelho, A.C.; Carvalho, S.M.; Saraiva, L.M.; Romao, C.C.; Bernardes, G.J. Spontaneous CO release from Ru(II)(CO)2-protein complexes in aqueous solution, cells, and mice. *Angew. Chem.* **2015**, *54*, 1172–1175. [CrossRef]
122. Chora, A.A.; Fontoura, P.; Cunha, A.; Pais, T.F.; Cardoso, S.; Ho, P.P.; Lee, L.Y.; Sobel, R.A.; Steinman, L.; Soares, M.P. Heme oxygenase-1 and carbon monoxide suppress autoimmune neuroinflammation. *J. Clin. Investig.* **2007**, *117*, 438–447. [CrossRef]
123. Vitek, L.; Gbelcova, H.; Muchova, L.; Vanova, K.; Zelenka, J.; Konickova, R.; Suk, J.; Zadinova, M.; Knejzlik, Z.; Ahmad, S.; et al. Antiproliferative effects of carbon monoxide on pancreatic cancer. *Dig. Liver Dis.* **2014**, *46*, 369–375. [CrossRef]
124. Chlopicki, S.; Lomnicka, M.; Fedorowicz, A.; Grochal, E.; Kramkowski, K.; Mogielnicki, A.; Buczko, W.; Motterlini, R. Inhibition of platelet aggregation by carbon monoxide-releasing molecules (CO-RMs): Comparison with NO donors. *Naunyn Schmiedeberg's Arch. Pharmacol.* **2012**, *385*, 641–650. [CrossRef]
125. Chung, S.W.; Liu, X.; Macias, A.A.; Baron, R.M.; Perrella, M.A. Heme oxygenase-1-derived carbon monoxide enhances the host defense response to microbial sepsis in mice. *J. Clin. Investig.* **2008**, *118*, 239–247. [CrossRef]

126. Desmard, M.; Davidge, K.S.; Bouvet, O.; Morin, D.; Roux, D.; Foresti, R.; Ricard, J.D.; Denamur, E.; Poole, R.K.; Montravers, P.; et al. A carbon monoxide-releasing molecule (CORM-3) exerts bactericidal activity against Pseudomonas aeruginosa and improves survival in an animal model of bacteraemia. *FASEB J.* **2009**, *23*, 1023–1031. [CrossRef]
127. Desmard, M.; Foresti, R.; Morin, D.; Dagouassat, M.; Berdeaux, A.; Denamur, E.; Crook, S.H.; Mann, B.E.; Scapens, D.; Montravers, P.; et al. Differential antibacterial activity against Pseudomonas aeruginosa by carbon monoxide-releasing molecules. *Antioxid. Redox Signal.* **2012**, *16*, 153–163. [CrossRef]
128. Murray, T.S.; Okegbe, C.; Gao, Y.; Kazmierczak, B.I.; Motterlini, R.; Dietrich, L.E.; Bruscia, E.M. The carbon monoxide releasing molecule CORM-2 attenuates Pseudomonas aeruginosa biofilm formation. *PLoS ONE* **2012**, *7*, e35499. [CrossRef]
129. Wegiel, B.; Larsen, R.; Gallo, D.; Chin, B.Y.; Harris, C.; Mannam, P.; Kaczmarek, E.; Lee, P.J.; Zuckerbraun, B.S.; Flavell, R.; et al. Macrophages sense and kill bacteria through carbon monoxide-dependent inflammasome activation. *J. Clin. Investig.* **2014**, *124*, 4926–4940. [CrossRef]
130. Otterbein, L.E.; May, A.; Chin, B.Y. Carbon monoxide increases macrophage bacterial clearance through Toll-like receptor (TLR)4 expression. *Cell. Mol. Biol.* **2005**, *51*, 433–440.
131. Tavares, A.F.; Teixeira, M.; Romao, C.C.; Seixas, J.D.; Nobre, L.S.; Saraiva, L.M. Reactive oxygen species mediate bactericidal killing elicited by carbon monoxide-releasing molecules. *J. Biol. Chem.* **2011**, *286*, 26708–26717. [CrossRef]
132. Hu, C.M.; Lin, H.H.; Chiang, M.T.; Chang, P.F.; Chau, L.Y. Systemic expression of heme oxygenase-1 ameliorates type 1 diabetes in NOD mice. *Diabetes* **2007**, *56*, 1240–1247. [CrossRef]
133. Wegiel, B.; Gallo, D.J.; Raman, K.G.; Karlsson, J.M.; Ozanich, B.; Chin, B.Y.; Tzeng, E.; Ahmad, S.; Ahmed, A.; Baty, C.J.; et al. Nitric oxide-dependent bone marrow progenitor mobilization by carbon monoxide enhances endothelial repair after vascular injury. *Circulation* **2010**, *121*, 537–548. [CrossRef] [PubMed]
134. Nguyen, D.; Boyer, C. Macromolecular and Inorganic Nanomaterials Scaffolds for Carbon Monoxide Delivery: Recent Developments and Future Trends. *ACS Biomater. Sci. Eng.* **2015**, *1*, 895–913. [CrossRef]
135. Kautz, A.C.; Kunz, P.C.; Janiak, C. CO-releasing molecule (CORM) conjugate systems. *Dalton Trans.* **2016**, *45*, 18045–18063. [CrossRef]
136. Schallner, N.; Otterbein, L.E. Friend or foe? Carbon monoxide and the mitochondria. *Front. Physiol.* **2015**, *6*, 17. [CrossRef]
137. Diring, S.; Carné-Sánchez, A.; Zhang, J.; Ikemura, S.; Kim, C.; Inaba, H.; Kitagawa, S.; Furukawa, S. Light responsive metal–organic frameworks as controllable CO-releasing cell culture substrates. *Chem. Sci.* **2017**, *8*, 2381–2386. [CrossRef] [PubMed]
138. Ma, M.; Noei, H.; Mienert, B.; Niesel, J.; Bill, E.; Muhler, M.; Fischer, R.A.; Wang, Y.; Schatzschneider, U.; Metzler-Nolte, N. Iron metal-organic frameworks MIL-88B and NH2-MIL-88B for the loading and delivery of the gasotransmitter carbon monoxide. *Chemistry* **2013**, *19*, 6785–6790. [CrossRef]
139. Pai, S.; Radacki, K.; Schatzschneider, U. Sonogashira, CuAAC, and Oxime Ligations for the Synthesis of MnI Tricarbonyl PhotoCORM Peptide Conjugates. *Eur. J. Inorg. Chem.* **2014**, *2014*, 2886–2895. [CrossRef]
140. Pfeiffer, H.; Rojas, A.; Niesel, J.; Schatzschneider, U. Sonogashira and Click reactions for the N-terminal and side-chain functionalization of peptides with [Mn(CO)3(tpm)]+-based CO releasing molecules (tpm = tris(pyrazolyl)methane). *Dalton Trans.* **2009**, 4292–4298. [CrossRef]
141. Jackson, C.S.; Schmitt, S.; Dou, Q.P.; Kodanko, J.J. Synthesis, characterization, and reactivity of the stable iron carbonyl complex [Fe(CO)(N4Py)](ClO4)2: Photoactivated carbon monoxide release, growth inhibitory activity, and peptide ligation. *Inorg. Chem.* **2011**, *50*, 5336–5338. [CrossRef]
142. Matson, J.B.; Webber, M.J.; Tamboli, V.K.; Weber, B.; Stupp, S.I. A peptide-based material for therapeutic carbon monoxide delivery. *Soft Matter* **2012**, *8*, 6689–6692. [CrossRef]
143. Bischof, C.; Joshi, T.; Dimri, A.; Spiccia, L.; Schatzschneider, U. Synthesis, spectroscopic properties, and photoinduced CO-release studies of functionalized ruthenium(II) polypyridyl complexes: Versatile building blocks for development of CORM-peptide nucleic acid bioconjugates. *Inorg. Chem.* **2013**, *52*, 9297–9308. [CrossRef] [PubMed]
144. Pfeiffer, H.; Sowik, T.; Schatzschneider, U. Bioorthogonal oxime ligation of a Mo(CO)4(N–N) CO-releasing molecule (CORM) to a TGF β-binding peptide. *J. Organomet. Chem.* **2013**, *734*, 17–24. [CrossRef]
145. Yin, H.; Fang, J.; Liao, L.; Nakamura, H.; Maeda, H. Styrene-maleic acid copolymer-encapsulated CORM2, a water-soluble carbon monoxide (CO) donor with a constant CO-releasing property, exhibits therapeutic potential for inflammatory bowel disease. *J. Control. Release* **2014**, *187*, 14–21. [CrossRef] [PubMed]

146. Tabe, H.; Fujita, K.; Abe, S.; Tsujimoto, M.; Kuchimaru, T.; Kizaka-Kondoh, S.; Takano, M.; Kitagawa, S.; Ueno, T. Preparation of a Cross-Linked Porous Protein Crystal Containing Ru Carbonyl Complexes as a CO-Releasing Extracellular Scaffold. *Inorg. Chem.* **2015**, *54*, 215–220. [CrossRef]
147. Tabe, H.; Shimoi, T.; Fujita, K.; Abe, S.; Ijiri, H.; Tsujimoto, M.; Kuchimaru, T.; Kizaka-Kondo, S.; Mori, H.; Kitagawa, S.; et al. Design of a CO-releasing Extracellular Scaffold Using in Vivo Protein Crystals. *Chem. Lett.* **2015**, *44*, 342–344. [CrossRef]
148. Albuquerque, I.S.; Jeremias, H.F.; Chaves-Ferreira, M.; Matak-Vinkovic, D.; Boutureira, O.; Romão, C.C.; Bernardes, G.J.L. An artificial CO-releasing metalloprotein built by histidine-selective metallation. *Chem. Commun.* **2015**, *51*, 3993–3996. [CrossRef]
149. Fujita, K.; Tanaka, Y.; Sho, T.; Ozeki, S.; Abe, S.; Hikage, T.; Kuchimaru, T.; Kizaka-Kondoh, S.; Ueno, T. Intracellular CO release from composite of ferritin and ruthenium carbonyl complexes. *J. Am. Chem. Soc.* **2014**, *136*, 16902–16908. [CrossRef]
150. Zobi, F.; Blacque, O.; Jacobs, R.A.; Schaub, M.C.; Bogdanova, A.Y. 17 e−rhenium dicarbonyl CO-releasing molecules on a cobalamin scaffold for biological application. *Dalton Trans.* **2012**, *41*, 370–378. [CrossRef]
151. Wilson, J.L.; Fayad Kobeissi, S.; Oudir, S.; Haas, B.; Michel, B.; Dubois Rande, J.L.; Ollivier, A.; Martens, T.; Rivard, M.; Motterlini, R.; et al. Design and synthesis of new hybrid molecules that activate the transcription factor Nrf2 and simultaneously release carbon monoxide. *Chemistry* **2014**, *20*, 14698–14704. [CrossRef]
152. Pena, A.C.; Penacho, N.; Mancio-Silva, L.; Neres, R.; Seixas, J.D.; Fernandes, A.C.; Romao, C.C.; Mota, M.M.; Bernardes, G.J.; Pamplona, A. A novel carbon monoxide-releasing molecule fully protects mice from severe malaria. *Antimicrob. Agents Chemother.* **2012**, *56*, 1281–1290. [CrossRef]
153. Marques, A.R.; Kromer, L.; Gallo, D.J.; Penacho, N.; Rodrigues, S.S.; Seixas, J.D.; Bernardes, G.J.L.; Reis, P.M.; Otterbein, S.L.; Ruggieri, R.A.; et al. Generation of Carbon Monoxide Releasing Molecules (CO-RMs) as Drug Candidates for the Treatment of Acute Liver Injury: Targeting of CO-RMs to the Liver. *Organometallics* **2012**, *31*, 5810–5822. [CrossRef]
154. Duncan, R. Polymer conjugates as anticancer nanomedicines. *Nat. Rev. Cancer* **2006**, *6*, 688–701. [CrossRef]
155. Brückmann, N.E.; Wahl, M.; Reiß, G.J.; Kohns, M.; Wätjen, W.; Kunz, P.C. Polymer Conjugates of Photoinducible CO-Releasing Molecules. *Eur. J. Inorg. Chem.* **2011**, *2011*, 4571–4577. [CrossRef]
156. Kunz, P.C.; Brückmann, N.E.; Spingler, B. Towards Polymer Diagnostic Agents—Copolymers of N-(2-Hydroxypropyl)methacrylamide and Bis(2-pyridylmethyl)-4-vinylbenzylamine: Synthesis, Characterisation and Re(CO)3-Labelling. *Eur. J. Inorg. Chem.* **2007**, *2007*, 394–399. [CrossRef]
157. Dördelmann, G.; Pfeiffer, H.; Birkner, A.; Schatzschneider, U. Silicium Dioxide Nanoparticles As Carriers for Photoactivatable CO-Releasing Molecules (PhotoCORMs). *Inorg. Chem.* **2011**, *50*, 4362–4367. [CrossRef]
158. Gonzales, M.A.; Han, H.; Moyes, A.; Radinos, A.; Hobbs, A.J.; Coombs, N.; Oliver, S.R.J.; Mascharak, P.K. Light-triggered carbon monoxide delivery with Al-MCM-41-based nanoparticles bearing a designed manganese carbonyl complex. *J. Mater. Chem. B* **2014**, *2*, 2107–2113. [CrossRef]
159. Dordelmann, G.; Meinhardt, T.; Sowik, T.; Krueger, A.; Schatzschneider, U. CuAAC click functionalization of azide-modified nanodiamond with a photoactivatable CO-releasing molecule (PhotoCORM) based on [Mn(CO)3(tpm)]+. *Chem. Commun.* **2012**, *48*, 11528–11530. [CrossRef]
160. Kunz, P.C.; Meyer, H.; Barthel, J.; Sollazzo, S.; Schmidt, A.M.; Janiak, C. Metal carbonyls supported on iron oxide nanoparticles to trigger the CO-gasotransmitter release by magnetic heating. *Chem. Commun.* **2013**, *49*, 4896–4898. [CrossRef]
161. Govender, P.; Pai, S.; Schatzschneider, U.; Smith, G.S. Next generation PhotoCORMs: Polynuclear tricarbonylmanganese(I)-functionalized polypyridyl metallodendrimers. *Inorg. Chem.* **2013**, *52*, 5470–5478. [CrossRef]
162. Cadranel, A.; Pieslinger, G.E.; Tongying, P.; Kuno, M.K.; Baraldo, L.M.; Hodak, J.H. Spectroscopic signatures of ligand field states in {Ru(II)(imine)} complexes. *Dalton Trans.* **2016**, *45*, 5464–5475. [CrossRef]
163. Gonzales, M.A. Iron, Manganese and Ruthenium Metal Carbonyls as Photoactive Carbon Monoxide Releasing Molecules (photoCORMS): Ligand Design Strategies, Syntheses and Structure Characterizations. Ph.D. Thesis, University of California, Santa Cruz, CA, USA, 2013.
164. Khramov, D.M.; Lynch, V.M.; Bielawski, C.W. N-Heterocyclic Carbene−Transition Metal Complexes: Spectroscopic and Crystallographic Analyses of π-Back-bonding Interactions. *Organometallics* **2007**, *26*, 6042–6049. [CrossRef]

165. Wang, C.; Cheng, L.; Liu, Z. Drug delivery with upconversion nanoparticles for multi-functional targeted cancer cell imaging and therapy. *Biomaterials* **2011**, *32*, 1110–1120. [CrossRef]
166. Zhao, Z.; Han, Y.; Lin, C.; Hu, D.; Wang, F.; Chen, X.; Chen, Z.; Zheng, N. Multifunctional core-shell upconverting nanoparticles for imaging and photodynamic therapy of liver cancer cells. *Chem. Asian J.* **2012**, *7*, 830–837. [CrossRef] [PubMed]
167. Yoon, J.W.; Seo, Y.-K.; Hwang, Y.K.; Chang, J.-S.; Leclerc, H.; Wuttke, S.; Bazin, P.; Vimont, A.; Daturi, M.; Bloch, E.; et al. Controlled Reducibility of a Metal–Organic Framework with Coordinatively Unsaturated Sites for Preferential Gas Sorption. *Angew. Chem. Intl. Ed.* **2010**, *49*, 5949–5952. [CrossRef]
168. van der Vlies, A.J.; Inubushi, R.; Uyama, H.; Hasegawa, U. Polymeric Framboidal Nanoparticles Loaded with a Carbon Monoxide Donor via Phenylboronic Acid-Catechol Complexation. *Bioconjugate Chem.* **2016**, *27*, 1500–1508. [CrossRef]
169. Muhammad, N.; Mao, Q.; Xia, H. CAR T-cells for cancer therapy. *Biotechnol. Genet. Eng. Rev.* **2017**, *33*, 190–226. [CrossRef]
170. Johnson, T.R.; Mann, B.E.; Teasdale, I.P.; Adams, H.; Foresti, R.; Green, C.J.; Motterlini, R. Metal carbonyls as pharmaceuticals? [Ru(CO)3Cl(glycinate)], a CO-releasing molecule with an extensive aqueous solution chemistry. *Dalton Trans.* **2007**, 1500–1508. [CrossRef] [PubMed]
171. Narayan, S.P.; Choi, C.H.; Hao, L.; Calabrese, C.M.; Auyeung, E.; Zhang, C.; Goor, O.J.; Mirkin, C.A. The Sequence-Specific Cellular Uptake of Spherical Nucleic Acid Nanoparticle Conjugates. *Small (Weinh. Bergstr. Ger.)* **2015**, *11*, 4173–4182. [CrossRef]
172. Nguyen, D.; Adnan, N.N.; Oliver, S.; Boyer, C. The Interaction of CORM-2 with Block Copolymers Containing Poly(4-vinylpyridine): Macromolecular Scaffolds for Carbon Monoxide Delivery in Biological Systems. *Macromol. Rapid Comm.* **2016**, *37*, 739–744. [CrossRef] [PubMed]
173. Garcia-Gallego, S.; Bernardes, G.J. Carbon-monoxide-releasing molecules for the delivery of therapeutic CO in vivo. *Angew. Chem.* **2014**, *53*, 9712–9721. [CrossRef] [PubMed]
174. Dallas, M.L.; Scragg, J.L.; Peers, C. Modulation of hTREK-1 by carbon monoxide. *Neuroreport* **2008**, *19*, 345–348. [CrossRef]
175. Lundvig, D.M.; Immenschuh, S.; Wagener, F.A. Heme oxygenase, inflammation, and fibrosis: The good, the bad, and the ugly? *Front. Pharmacol.* **2012**, *3*, 81. [CrossRef]
176. Szeremeta, M.; Petelska, A.D.; Kotynska, J.; Niemcunowicz-Janica, A.; Figaszewski, Z.A. The effect of fatal carbon monoxide poisoning on the surface charge of blood cells. *J. Membr. Biol.* **2013**, *246*, 717–722. [CrossRef]
177. Petelska, A.D.; Kotynska, J.; Figaszewski, Z.A. The effect of fatal carbon monoxide poisoning on the equilibria between cell membranes and the electrolyte solution. *J. Membr. Biol.* **2015**, *248*, 157–161. [CrossRef]
178. Wang, P.; Liu, H.; Zhao, Q.; Chen, Y.; Liu, B.; Zhang, B.; Zheng, Q. Syntheses and evaluation of drug-like properties of CO-releasing molecules containing ruthenium and group 6 metal. *Eur. J. Med. Chem.* **2014**, *74*, 199–215. [CrossRef]
179. Winburn, I.C.; Gunatunga, K.; McKernan, R.D.; Walker, R.J.; Sammut, I.A.; Harrison, J.C. Cell damage following carbon monoxide releasing molecule exposure: Implications for therapeutic applications. *Basic Clin. Pharmacol. Toxicol.* **2012**, *111*, 31–41. [CrossRef]

5

Silicon Nanofluidic Membrane for Electrostatic Control of Drugs and Analytes Elution

Nicola Di Trani [1,2], Antonia Silvestri [1,3], Yu Wang [1], Danilo Demarchi [3], Xuewu Liu [1] and Alessandro Grattoni [1,4,5,*]

1 Department of Nanomedicine, Houston Methodist Research Institute, Houston, TX 77030, USA; nditrani@houstonmethodist.org (N.D.T.); antonia.silvestri@polito.it (A.S.); ywang2@houstonmethodist.org (Y.W.); xliu@houstonmethodist.org (X.L.)
2 University of Chinese Academy of Science (UCAS), Shijingshan, 19 Yuquan Road, Beijing 100049, China
3 Department of Electronics and Telecommunications, Polytechnic of Turin, 10129 Turin, Italy; danilo.demarchi@polito.it
4 Department of Surgery, Houston Methodist Hospital, Houston, TX 77030, USA
5 Department of Radiation Oncology, Houston Methodist Hospital, Houston, TX 77030, USA
* Correspondence: agrattoni@houstonmethodist.org

Abstract: Individualized long-term management of chronic pathologies remains an elusive goal despite recent progress in drug formulation and implantable devices. The lack of advanced systems for therapeutic administration that can be controlled and tailored based on patient needs precludes optimal management of pathologies, such as diabetes, hypertension, rheumatoid arthritis. Several triggered systems for drug delivery have been demonstrated. However, they mostly rely on continuous external stimuli, which hinder their application for long-term treatments. In this work, we investigated a silicon nanofluidic technology that incorporates a gate electrode and examined its ability to achieve reproducible control of drug release. Silicon carbide (SiC) was used to coat the membrane surface, including nanochannels, ensuring biocompatibility and chemical inertness for long-term stability for in vivo deployment. With the application of a small voltage ($\leq$ 3 V DC) to the buried polysilicon electrode, we showed in vitro repeatable modulation of membrane permeability of two model analytes—methotrexate and quantum dots. Methotrexate is a first-line therapeutic approach for rheumatoid arthritis; quantum dots represent multi-functional nanoparticles with broad applicability from bio-labeling to targeted drug delivery. Importantly, SiC coating demonstrated optimal properties as a gate dielectric, which rendered our membrane relevant for multiple applications beyond drug delivery, such as lab on a chip and micro total analysis systems (μTAS).

Keywords: electrostatic gating; nanofluidic diffusion; controlled drug release; silicon membrane; smart drug delivery

1. Introduction

Chronic pathologies affect nearly half of the population worldwide [1,2] and represent one of the leading causes of death and disability [3]. Management of chronic conditions is challenged by co-morbidities [4], poor adherence to treatment [5], and a lack of therapeutic technologies suitable to address the complexity of the disease [6]. Long-acting controlled therapeutic administration represents a promising strategy for medical conditions requiring repeated daily dosing [7,8]. In view of this, long-acting platforms for sustained drug release have been developed, leading to significant improvements in the management of conditions, such as hormone deficiency and infectious diseases [9–11]. However, the pathophysiology of most chronic diseases is determined by circadian biological cycles [12], which have a significant impact on the efficacy of treatment and associated adverse effects [13]. This is the case for pathologies, such as diabetes and metabolic disorders [14], hypertension, psychiatric and neurodegenerative conditions [15], rheumatoid arthritis [16], and chronic pain [17], to name a few, where the timing of drug administration is key to elicit the intended therapeutic effect.

Advanced technologies enabling personalized adjustments of therapeutic administration, both in time and dose, represent a desirable but unmet clinical need [18,19]. Ideally, these technologies should incorporate a drug delivery mechanism that can be rapidly and easily tuned to release the required dosage, at the right time, without requiring continuous external stimuli. Further, they should allow for pre-programmed dosing schedules as well as remote control capabilities, to enable healthcare providers to adjust medication through telemedicine approaches [20]. Devices with such capabilities could eradicate treatment compliance issues and dramatically improve the therapeutic index and the quality of life of patients, while substantially reducing healthcare expenditure.

Current approaches developed for controlled drug administration are based on modulation of permeability of membranes via sustained external stimuli. These systems mostly rely on polymeric membrane architectures and achieve changes in pore size and conformation via temperature variation triggered by a magnetic field [21], near-infrared irradiation [22–24], or ultrasound [25]. Other devices use a magnetic field to reversibly or irreversibly obstruct the pores of a membrane using microparticles [26] or low melting temperature polymers [27]. Albeit promising, these strategies are limited by the need for continuous external activation and associated cumbersome external equipment. Electrical actuation offers a solution to these limitations, enabling control via miniaturized circuitry and low energy radio-frequency (RF) communications. In this context, various technologies have been created, either integrating gate electrodes [28] or polypyrrole (PPy) [29,30] on anodic aluminum oxide (AAO) membranes. However, polydispersity in pore size common to AAO membranes represents a limitation to achieve fine control of drug release [28,31].

In this study, we investigated the performance of a silicon nanofluidic membrane that uses electrostatic gating [32] to modulate the transport of charged molecules by modifying nanochannel permeability. Microfabricated using standard semiconductor manufacturing techniques, this membrane features hundreds of thousands of identical slit-nanochannels geometrically distributed across the membrane surface to maximize porosity while maintaining mechanical integrity. A buried polysilicon layer extends over the entire nanochannel surface and acts as a single distributed gate electrode. An outermost layer of biocompatible silicon carbide (SiC) is adopted to bury and insulate the gate electrode and minimize leakage while providing chemical inertness for applications in vivo or in contact with biological fluids. SiC insulation properties were studied in comparison with silicon dioxide (SiO_2), the most common gate dielectric material in metal–oxide–semiconductor field-effect transistor (MOSFET). Further, energy consumption leakage current and gating performance were assessed at different gate potentials. Finally, we adopted two relevant model analytes—methotrexate and quantum dots—to assess the in vitro transport modulation performances. Methotrexate represents an important therapeutic agent commonly used for rheumatoid arthritis [33], whereas quantum dots are adopted for a variety of biomedical imaging applications as well as drug delivery and theranostics [34,35]. In light of the promising results and the ease of integration within implantable devices, our gated membrane might constitute a promising step forward in the development of flexible technologies for the treatment of chronic diseases. Further, our nanofluidic technology could be adopted in other applications for lab on a chip [36] and micro total analysis systems (μTAS) devices for electrokinetic separation processes [37], bio-sample sorting and analysis [38], among others.

2. Materials and Methods

2.1. *Nanofluidic Membrane Fabrication*

Silicon membranes fabrication was performed using standard semiconductor techniques. The fabrication process is described step-by-step elsewhere [39]. Briefly, a dense array of nanochannels (500 nm width, 6 μm length) was obtained by vertically etching via deep reactive ion etching (DRIE) the device layer (10 μm) of a silicon on insulator (SOI) wafer (total thickness 411 μm). The etching was stopped at the middle oxide layer (1 μm). The handle wafer (400 μm) on the opposite side of the SOI was etched using DRIE up to the oxide layer to create a hexagonal pattern of densely packed circular microchannels. To connect the nanochannels to the microchannels, the buried oxide layer was etched by a buffered oxide etchant solution (BOE). The resulting nanochannels size (770 nm) was reduced by three subsequent processes. First, wet thermal oxidation generated a 175 nm layer of SiO_2, and then a 121 nm layer of polycrystalline silicon (poly-Si) was obtained via low-pressure chemical vapor deposition (LPCVD). Plasma-enhanced chemical vapor deposition (PECVD) was then used for the silicon carbide coating (SiC, 64 nm). Electrode pads were exposed via selective etching of SiC via fluorine-based RIE. Wafers were then diced into individual membranes (ADT 7100 Dicing Saw, Advanced Dicing Technologies, Zhengzhou, China), obtaining individual silicon membranes of 6 mm × 6 mm × 411 μm. Each membrane featured a total of 278,600 identical slit nanochannels 10 μm long and 6 μm wide. Nanochannels were arranged in groups of 1400, where each group led to one circular microchannel on the opposite side of the chip. Finally, microchannels were geometrically organized in a hexagonal pattern to maximize porosity and structural integrity. In this study, membranes with a final layer of SiO_2 were also used and obtained by wet thermal oxidation of poly-Si.

2.2. Assessment of Membrane Structure

Morphological assessment and characterization of the nanochannel multi-layer structure were performed via scanning electron microscopy (SEM). A focused ion beam (FIB) system FEI 235 (Nanofabrication facility of the University of Houston, Houston, TX, USA) was used to simultaneously create nanochannels' cross-sections and acquire images. Gallium ion milling was performed on the micromachine parts of the membrane and to expose the nanochannel cross-section. Imaging was then performed at a 52° angle.

2.3. Electrode Connection

Electrical wires (36 AWG, McMaster Carr, Elmhurst, IL, USA) were epoxied to the membrane pads using a silver-based conductive adhesive (H20E, Epoxy Technology, Inc., Billerica, MA, USA) and cured at 150 °C for 1 h. Electrode insulation was achieved by applying a thin layer of UV epoxy (OG116, Epoxy Technologies, Inc. Billerica, MA, USA) over the conductive pad and UV-curing (UVP UVL-18 EL Series, Analytik Jena US LLC, Upland, CA, USA) for 120 min. The correct electrode connection was tested by measuring the resistance between the two connection pads with a Fluke 177 True RMS Multimeter (Fluke Corporation, Everett, WA, USA).

2.4. Electrochemical Characterization

A custom dual-reservoir polymethyl methacrylate (PMMA) apparatus [39] was employed to perform electrochemical measurements. Membranes were clamped between the two 2 mL reservoirs of the testing apparatus, each containing two Ag/AgCl electrodes (64-1313, Harvard Apparatus, Holliston, MA, USA). All measurements were performed in PBS, except for conductance studies, where KCl solutions at different concentrations (from 10^{-6} to 10^{-1} M) were used. A benchtop electrochemical tester (CH Instruments, Inc. 660E, Austin, TX, USA) was used in either 3 or 4 electrode configurations.

Impedance was measured with a 4-electrodes configuration. A 50 mV perturbation signal was applied through the electrochemical analyzer within a frequency window from 10 mH to 10 kH. The measurements were performed with a superimposed DC voltage in the range −3 V to 3 V in steps of 1 V. Fittings to a Randles cell model were performed with the CHI 660E software (CH Instruments, Inc. 660E, Austin, TX, USA).

Leakage current was measured with a 3-electrodes configuration. Voltages were applied using the CHI 660E between the electrode pad and Ag/AgCl electrodes in solution at a distance of ~1 cm from the membrane. Measurements were performed in the −3 V to +3 V range in 1 V steps, and each step lasted for 120 s, allowing for transient phenomena to resolve and obtain a stable measurement.

For conductance experiments, we employed a 4-electrodes configuration. Measurements were performed for KCl concentrations from 1 μM to 100 mM from the lower to the highest ionic strength. Reservoirs were rinsed with deionized water for 1 min, and the solution was replaced after each measurement. Steps of 400 mV were applied using the CHI 660E from −2 V to 2 V, with 30 s pauses to exhaust possible transient effects. Conductance measurements were performed with a floating gate, and the values calculated for each step and averaged.

Cyclic voltammetry measurements were conducted with a 3-electrodes configuration and a scanning rate of 50 mV/s within the interval −2 V to 2 V. Electrochemical measurements were carried out on membranes with a final dielectric layer of both SiC and SiO_2.

2.5. *In Vitro Release Modulation*

In vitro release modulation experiments were performed employing a custom dual-reservoir device described in detail elsewhere [40]. Nanochannel membranes were individually clamped between a 250 μL drug reservoir and a UV-Vis transparent macro-cuvette serving as the sink reservoir. Two O-rings were used to prevent fluid leakage between membranes and the reservoir. Fluid evaporation was prevented by sealing a drug reservoir with biocompatible silicone plugs (McMaster Carr, Elmhurst, IL, USA).

Experiments were performed using SiC-coated membranes with ~300 nm nanochannels. To ensure proper channel wetting, membranes were immersed in isopropyl alcohol for 1 h and then rinsed three times in deionized H_2O. Membranes were then placed overnight in 0.01 × PBS or 1 × PBS in preparation for quantum dots and methotrexate release, respectively. Sink reservoirs (4.45 mL) were filled with matching PBS solutions. After fixture assembly, the source reservoir was loaded with either 1 mg/mL 0.01 × PBS solution of quantum dots (CdTe core-type, COOH functionalized, 777978-10MG, Sigma Aldrich, St. Louis, MO, USA) or 2.5 mg/mL PBS solution of methotrexate (13960, Cayman Chemical, Ann Arbor, MI, USA). Both molecules possess a negative charge at pH 7.4, with methotrexate presenting a stable −2q charge (-3.2×10^{-19} C) and quantum dots having a charge that ranges from −5q to −15q depending on pH and ionic strength [41]. Methotrexate has a molar mass of 454 Da and an estimated diameter of 1.6 nm [42], while quantum dots have an estimated molar mass of 200 kDa and an estimated diameter of 4.7 nm [43]. An Ag/AgCl reference electrode (Harvard Apparatus, Holliston, MA, USA) was used and placed in the source drug reservoir.

Absorbance measurements of every sample were performed at 5 min intervals using a custom UV-vis spectrophotometer apparatus consisting of a robotic carousel [44] connected to an Agilent Cary 50 spectrophotometer (Agilent, Technologies, Santa Clara, CA, USA). Sink solution homogeneity was maintained by constant magnetic stirring (600 rpm). Methotrexate absorbance was measured at 373 nm, while quantum dots at 240 nm. An electrical potential (0, −1.5, or −3 V DC) was applied between the Ag/AgCl and the membrane electrodes through a waveform generator (33522A, Keysight Technologies, Santa Clara, CA, USA). Passive (0 V) and active (−1.5 or −3 V) phases were alternated at regular intervals. For methotrexate, phases were alternated every 6 h between passive and active (0 and −3 V DC, respectively). For quantum dots, 12 h passive phases were alternated with 8 h of active applied potential (−1.5 V).

2.6. *Statistical Analysis*

Statistical analysis was performed using GraphPad Prism 8 (version 8.1.1; GraphPad Software, Inc., San Diego, CA, USA). Mean ± SD values were calculated for all results. Further statistical significance was assessed, adopting the two-tailed paired t-tests (** $p \leq 0.01$; **** $p \leq 0.0001$). Cumulative releases were split into phases, and each fitted by a first-order polynomial (MATLAB® polyfit, MathWorks, Natick, MA, USA). Slopes of cumulative release curves were normalized and displayed as a percentage of the passive release profiles.

3. Results and Discussion

3.1. Nanofluidic Membrane

Prior to investigating the electrical performance of the membranes, we sought to analyze the quality of the membrane fabrication process (Figure 1). Individual silicon membranes were first visually inspected to assess integrity. Figure 1A shows a stereomicroscope picture of a single membrane, highlighting the conductive electrode pads at the top right and bottom left edges. The hexagonal arrangement of microchannels allowed us to maximize packing density without compromising mechanical robustness. By measuring transmembrane nitrogen gas flow and adopting our predictive model for nanofluidic gas transport [45], we obtained an indirect measurement for the size of nanochannels (~300 nm). Sample membranes were further analyzed with SEM imaging. Figure 1B shows the tightly packed nanochannel arranged in arrays of 19 rows and 96 columns with a horizontal pitch of 2 μm and a vertical pitch of 10 μm. No macroscopic defects or pinholes were observed across wafers, which indicated that the fabrication protocol was repeatable.

The analysis of the membrane cross-sections obtained via FIB milling was performed to evaluate the uniformity of layer deposition at different nanofabrication steps. SiO_2 growth via thermal oxidation resulted in a highly uniform layer along the whole length of the vertical nanochannels (Figure 1C). Thermal oxidation is a slow process that enables precise control over layer thickness. Thus, it allowed us to accurately and homogeneously reduce the size of nanochannels. The subsequent deposition of poly-Si (Figure 1D) was used to create a gate electrode that coats the whole nanofluidic structure with the objective of maximizing the electrostatic gating performances. Uniform poly-Si deposition through the chemical vapor deposition-based (CVD) process in high-aspect-ratio hollow structures can be challenging. However, our imaging analysis showed that the deposited layer was uniform (Figure 1D), except for a slight increase in thickness at the nanochannel outlet (bottom right). Finally, a thin layer of SiC (Figure 1E) was used to coat the conductive poly-Si and act as an insulating and chemical inert layer. Despite the high-aspect-ratio of the slit nanochannels, the deposition of SiC was also achieved with good uniformity (Figure 1E). Slight material accumulations at the inlet and outlet of nanochannels were expected. While we did not generate these intentionally, we noted that a local restriction at the nanochannel extremities could improve gating performance.

All materials used for the fabrication of the nanofluidic membrane have previously been demonstrated to be biocompatible using ISO 10993 standards by Kotzar et al. [46]. A subset of these materials has also been investigated in vivo in rodents and has shown biocompatibility and low biofouling [47]. Moreover, in our fabrication protocol, silicon carbide completely encapsulates the membrane and, therefore, is the only material exposed to the environment. Silicon carbide was specifically chosen for this encapsulation purpose as it's considered a versatile material for biomedical applications where extended exposure to physiological fluids is needed [48,49]. Additionally, in vivo biocompatibility of SiC was demonstrated by Cogan et al. [50], who subcutaneously implanted SiC discs in New Zealand White rabbit, the histological evaluation showed no chronic inflammatory response, and a capsule thickness comparable to controls was found.

Furthermore, silicon carbide has previously been shown to offer reduced biofouling when compared to other biocompatible materials, such as silicon or silicon dioxide [51]. Although complete protection against protein adsorption could not be achieved [52], we previously showed that biofouling did not negatively affect the function of our devices. Specifically, nanofluidic membranes, similar to the one presented in this study, have been used in-vivo in rats for up to 6 months [53] and in non-human primates for up to 4 months [54] with no alteration of drug release from biofouling or fibrotic tissue encapsulation.

When compared to membrane architectures previously developed in our lab [55–57], this membrane presented a less cumbersome fabrication process, thanks to the direct alignment of nanochannels and microchannels [58,59]. Further, a substantially higher nanochannels density [55,60] was achieved. In contrast with other gated membrane based on porous alumina (AAO) [29], presenting an irregular pore size distribution [28], our structure achieved a monodispersed nanochannel size that could aid in better control of molecular transport. In its current configuration, featuring 278,600 nanochannels, our membrane configuration was designed to achieve high mass transport rates per unit surface area. This is typically preferable in the context of implantable drug delivery application, where miniaturization is a requirement [39]. However, in light of its modular structure, the same fabrication process could be employed to create alternative configurations with a different number of channels for adoption in electrokinetic-enabled molecular manipulation or sorting applications. For these purposes, the large gate electrode surface area might provide increased electrostatic control of fluid molecules as compared to common Polydimethylsiloxane-glass (PDMS-glass) systems [61,62] which feature localized gate electrodes.

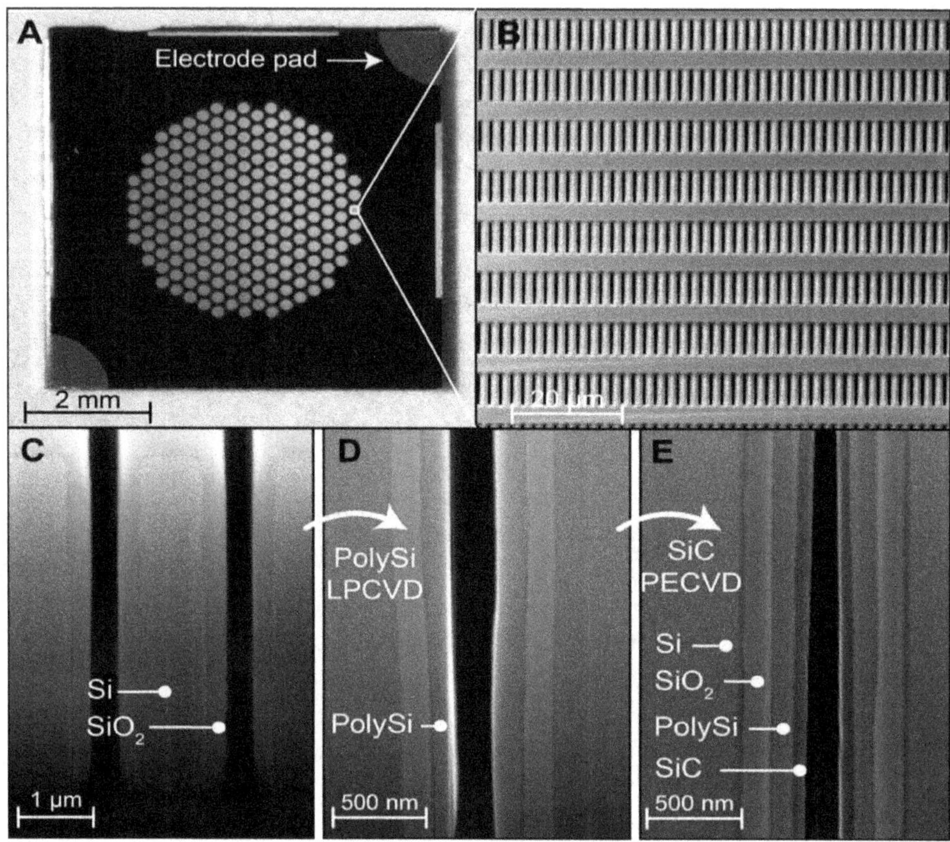

Figure 1. Nanochannel membrane structure. (**A**) Optical image of a silicon nanofluidic membrane, presenting electrode pads with exposed conductive polysilicon. (**B**) SEM micrograph, showing the array of nanochannel inlets. (**C**,**D**,**E**) Vertical cross-section image (SEM) obtained along the length of nanochannel, showing the membrane fabrication at different stages. Micrographs were color-enhanced for clarity of visualization. (**C**) Thermally grown SiO_2 layer (~175 nm, blue); (**D**) Low-pressure chemical vapor deposition (LPCVD)-deposited poly-Si layer (~121 nm, red); (**E**) Plasma-enhanced-CVD deposited SiC coating (~64 nm, gray). Images **C**, **D**, and **E** do not picture the same membrane location.

3.2. Solid–Liquid Interface, SiO_2 vs SiC

To evaluate SiC properties as a gate dielectric in contact with ionic solutions, we compared its insulation performance to SiO_2, which is a broadly used gate dielectric in solid electronics [63]. SiO_2 and other metal oxides, such as alumina and hafnium dioxide, owe their success to their high dielectric constants that allow for low leakage currents. Even though these materials excel in solid electronic manufacturing, they either lack biocompatibility or chemical inertness and durability in aqueous environments [50].

Leakage current measurements (Figure 2A) performed with our membranes did not show substantial differences between SiO_2 and SiC, except for 3 V. However, the steep increase in leakage observed for SiC between 2 and 3 V, emphasized by the electrolytic solution environment, suggests that the molecular arrangement in the dielectric layer is not ideal [64]. The literature on gate dielectric leakage in ionic solutions is scarce, and the available models for a solid-state field-effect transistor (FET) are unable to account for the effect of the electrolyte solution environment. In aqueous solutions, currents in the order of μA were measured for electric fields as low as 0.5 MV cm^{-1} (Figure 2A). In contrast, for solid-state FET, currents in the order of magnitude of μA are only expected for electric fields greater than 15 and 2 MV cm^{-1} for SiO_2 and SiC, respectively. High leakage currents are usually attributed to the formation of conductive filaments within the oxide, whereby electrons are trapped and form clusters within defects in the material. When clusters are at tunneling distance, a conductive path can form, leading to high leakage currents [65,66]. The proportional increase in leakage currents at increasing ionic strength of the solution, previously reported by this group [39], provides further support for this phenomenon.

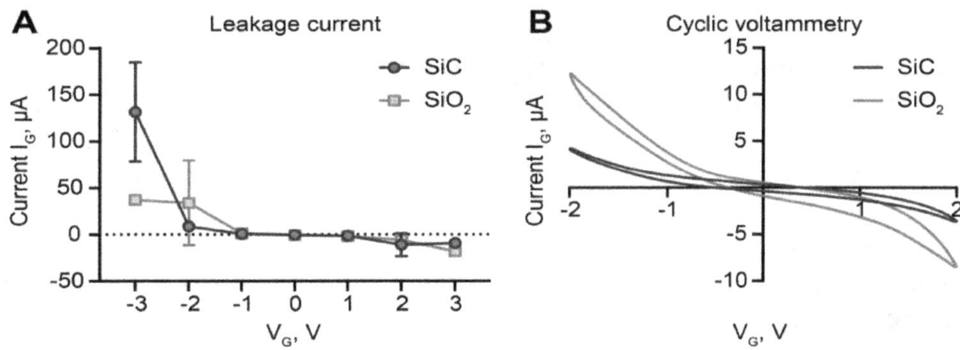

Figure 2. Leakage current and cyclic voltammetry. (**A**) Comparison of gate leakage current for SiO_2 and silicon carbide (SiC) dielectric. (**B**) Cyclic voltammetry comparison between SiO_2 and SiC.

In the voltage range between −2 and 2 V, SiC and SiO_2 exhibited similar values of leakage currents. Thus, to closer investigate differences in performances, we used cyclic voltammetry (CV). As compared to SiO_2-coated membranes, lower currents were measured for SiC at each applied voltage (Figure 2B). Interestingly, we observed a non-linear proportional relationship between voltage and current for both materials. SiC exhibited a steep increase in current for voltages higher than 1 V in absolute value. This suggested that for small applied voltages, no faradaic currents occurred, and the material behaved almost as an ideal capacitor. For voltages above ± 1 V, electrochemical reactions between the surface groups (C, SiO^-) and reactive species in the electrolyte solution (Cl^-, HO^-) led to increased currents.

In contrast, the significant current increase observed for the leakage currents (Figure 2A) for voltages over 2 V was likely related to material deterioration and conductive filament formation. The asymmetry between results obtained with positive and negative voltages provided further support for this theory. Higher currents for negative applied voltages were observed in both measurements. For negative voltages, positive species were attracted to the surface. The percolation model suggests that in the presence of strong electrostatic attraction, protons can diffuse in the insulator, starting a percolating path that can lead to the formation of a conductive filament [65]. Instead, for positive potentials, proton repulsion may cause a reversible interruption of the conductive filament, effectively decreasing leakage [67]. Additionally, the difference in hysteresis between the two CV profiles (Figure 2B) was suggestive of differences in surface charge accumulation between the two materials. A thinner CV profile usually correlates with low charge accumulation. Collectively, the results showed that SiC suffered lower leakage currents in the −2 V to 2 V range, exhibiting better insulation performance than SiO_2.

3.3. Electrochemical Characterization: Conductance

To further investigate the surface properties of SiC, we performed conductance measurements of SiC-coated membranes in the ionic concentration range between 1 μM and 100 mM. We employed a custom fixture [39] that allowed us to limit wetting to the nanochannel part of the membrane. The results are shown in Figure 3A. At high ionic strengths (>10^{-4} M), conductance measurements displayed a linear dependence on the ionic strength. In these conditions, the Debye length was significantly smaller than the size of nanochannels. Accordingly, the results were consistent with the bulk electrolyte conductance (red dashed line in Figure 3A). In contrast, at low ionic strengths (≤10^{-4} M), we observed a plateau in conductance (in the log-log scale). This occurred when the Debye length approached the nanochannel dimension, and the excess of counter-ions balanced the surface charge, reaching channel electroneutrality [68]. Here, as it directly related to the conductance, the surface charge could be calculated by fitting the results to the equation [69]:

$$\frac{I}{V} = 2F\mu\sqrt{\left(\frac{\Sigma}{2}\right)^2 + c_0^2}\,\frac{wh}{l} \quad (1)$$

In Equation (1), F, μ, and Σ are the Faraday's constant, ionic mobility, and the volume charge density, respectively. Further, c_0 is the solution molarity, and w, h, and l are the nanochannels' width, height, and length, respectively. Using the relation $zF\Sigma = -2\sigma_s/h$, we obtained a surface charge value of $\sigma_s = 1.81$ μC/m^2, which was consistent with the previously reported data for SiC surfaces [70]. Our SiC coating exhibited a surface charge orders of magnitude smaller than SiO_2 (1–100 mC/m^2) [71], which correlated with better performance in electrostatic gating control. In fact, chemically reactive surfaces act as charge buffers. An externally applied electric field is quickly compensated by protonation or deprotonation of reactive groups on the surface, limiting charge rearrangement in the electrical double layer (EDL) [72]. Thus, to minimize surface charge, materials are often artificially treated [28].

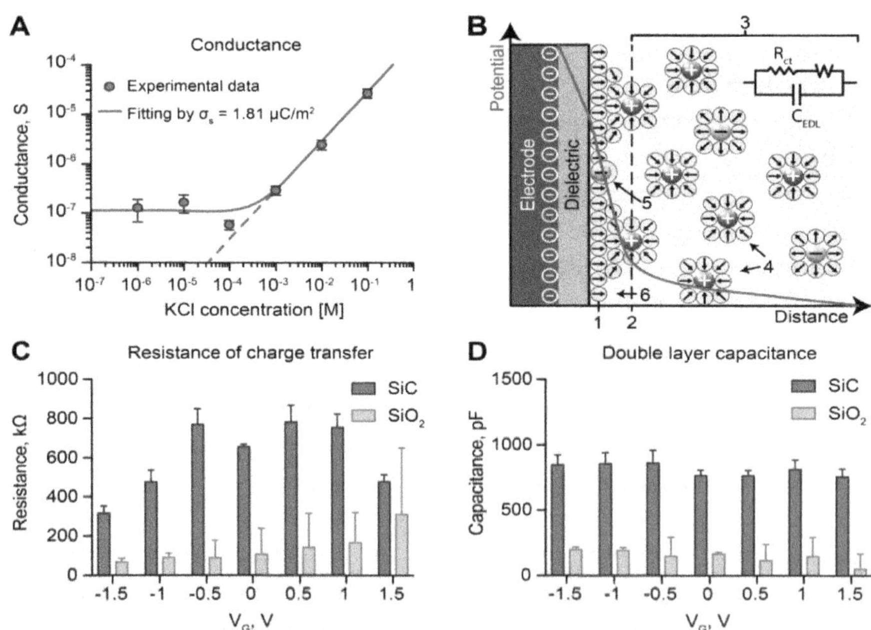

Figure 3. Electrochemical measurements. (**A**) Measured transmembrane ionic conductance. (**B**) Schematic of the electric double layer and relative model. (1) Inner Helmholtz plane; (2) Outer Helmholtz plane; (3) Diffuse layer; (4) Solvated ion; (5) Specifically adsorbed ion; (6) Molecules of the electrolyte solvent. (**C**) Fitted resistance of charge transfer (R_{ct}) of SiO_2-coated membranes versus SiC-coated membranes. (**D**) Fitted double-layer capacitance (C_{dl}) of SiO_2-coated membranes versus SiC-coated membranes.

3.4. Electrochemical Characterization: Electrochemical Impedance Spectroscopy

To investigate dielectric/liquid interface properties with the application of an external voltage, we performed electrochemical impedance spectroscopy (EIS) measurements. Specifically, we compared the resistance to charge transfer and the double layer capacitance at different gate voltages. A comparative assessment was conducted using SiC- and SiO_2-coated chips. Figure 3B shows a schematics of the electrical double layer (EDL), which described the ionic distribution that occurres at the solid–liquid interface of a charged surface to maintain local electroneutrality. The EDL is usually described by that Grahame model, which identifies three main layers consisting of 1) non-hydrated ions adsorbed to the surface, ii) hydrated immobile ions, iii) free moving hydrated ions [73]. The first and second layers of immobile ions are often referred to as the Stern layer. The EDL region is modeled by a series of capacitors, referred to as double-layer capacitance (C_{EDL}), where the Stern layer (~0.2 nm) [74] corresponds to the most significant contribution. As current can flow across the interface upon application of a DC potential, a resistive path is considered in parallel to the capacitance. This is usually referred to as a charge-transfer resistance (R_{ct}). R_{ct} can vary substantially depending on the material ability to exchange electrons with the electrolyte solution. Upon application of an external DC potential, if electrons cannot be easily exchanged, an overpotential builds up at the interface. In non-polarizable materials, such as Ag/AgCl, small R_{ct} permits high currents. In contrast, polarizable materials present high R_{ct}, and the current exchange is limited.

By fitting our EIS measurements to the model described above (Figure 3B), we calculated R_{ct} and C_{EDL} for both a SiO_2- and a SiC-coated membrane at different gate voltages (V_G) applied (Figure 3C,D). Depending on the applied potential, SiC showed an R_{ct} 1.5 to 8 times bigger than SiO_2 (Figure 3C). Interestingly, both materials showed a clear dependence of R_{ct} with the applied voltage. SiO_2 exhibited a monotonic increase of R_{ct} with the applied voltage, where more positive voltages resulted in higher R_{ct}. In contrast, SiC showed a decrease in R_{ct} proportional to the absolute value of the applied voltage. We attributed these phenomena to the difference in surface charge between SiO_2 and SiC. In fact, a higher number of available SiO^- sites on the SiO_2 surface allowed for increased electron exchange.

C_{EDL} did not exhibit a correlation with the applied gate voltage for either material (Figure 3D). Moreover, we unexpectedly found six times higher C_{EDL} for SiC with respect to SiO_2. As C_{EDL} mainly depends on the surface area and EDL thickness, our results could be explained in the context of the material porosity [75]. By presenting a larger surface area, pores displayed increased capacity. Overall, the low surface charge exposed by SiC and the high resistance to charge transfer qualified SiC as a polarizable interface suitable for electrostatic gating.

3.5. Mechanism of Analyte Flow Control through Electrostatic Gating

Nanofluidic systems present high surface to volume ratios. In light of this, charged species diffusing in nanoconfinement exhibit unique behaviors [76,77]. Electrostatic, steric, and hydrodynamic interactions with the nanochannel walls influence local molecular concentration and effective diffusivity. Depending on solution properties, such as ionic strength, pH, and surface charge density, the EDL can extend from a fraction to hundreds of nm in the fluid. Both SiC and SiO_2 surface expose native silanol groups, resulting in a net negative surface charge at pH 7.4 [78]. In proximity to the surface, charged species redistribute to reach electroneutrality [73]. While counter-ions concentration increases, co-ions are depleted following distribution with a characteristic dimension equal to the Debye length.

Once solution properties are defined, the surface charge is the only parameter that has a significant effect on the distribution of charges in the fluid. Thus, nanochannel charge-selectivity can be altered by controlling the channel surface charge. An applied difference in potential between a buried gate electrode and an electrode in solution creates an overpotential at the surface. We employed this strategy to modulate the diffusive transport of analytes through our nanofluidic membrane. With no applied voltage, molecules diffused through the channel unperturbed. By applying a negative gate potential, the transmembrane transport of co-ions was substantially reduced.

3.6. *In Vitro Release Modulation of Methotrexate*

To investigate the effectiveness of electrostatic gating on controlling trans-membrane transport of a small charged analyte, we performed an in vitro diffusion study using methotrexate. Methotrexate has a molecular weight of 454 Da and is a good representative of small molecules (<900 Da) therapeutics, which accounts for the majority of pharmaceuticals [79]. Clinically, methotrexate is used as a chemotherapeutic agent for the treatment of various cancers, as well as in the management of rheumatoid arthritis [33].

Figure 4A shows the normalized release rates for four consecutive cycles alternating between passive and active phases. During the passive phases, negatively charged molecules (−2q for methotrexate) diffused trough the nanochannels freely, largely unaffected by the low native charge of the SiC surfaces. When a negative voltage was applied (−3 V), an increase in negative surface charge repelled methotrexate molecules, reducing their release. The four alternation cycles between passive and active phases demonstrated that electrostatic gating allowed for repeatability of release modulation.

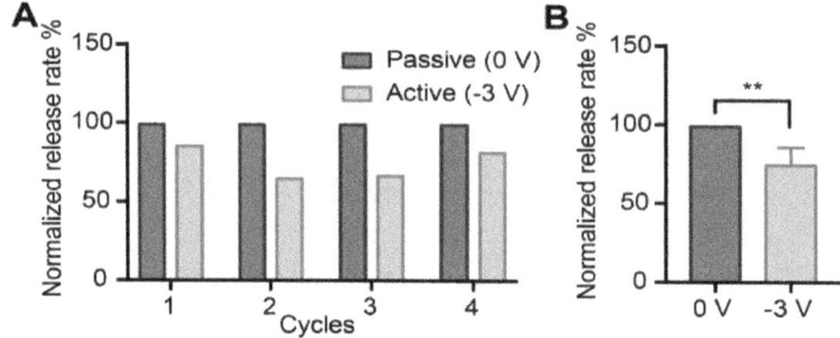

Figure 4. Electrostatically controlled release of methotrexate. (**A**) The normalized release rate of methotrexate for four cycles between free diffusion (Passive) and gated diffusion (Active). (**B**) Release rates grouped by phase typology (** $p \leq 0.01$).

We observed a statistically significant (** $p \leq 0.01$) difference in release rate between active and passive phases, whereby the applied potential −3 V yielded a decrease in the release rate of ~35%. During the passive phase, an average release rate of 10 μg/day was obtained, which was consistent with daily doses used to treat rheumatoid arthritis in pre-clinical testing [80]. Other small molecule therapeutics, including glucocorticoids [81], hormone therapeutics [82], and antivirals [83], present effective daily doses in the order of micrograms. This indicates that the current membrane architecture could, in principle, be adopted for various therapeutic applications. However, further testing with different pharmaceutical agents is warranted.

3.7. *In Vitro Controlled Release of Quantum Dots*

To assess the ability of our membrane to modulate the release rate of larger molecules, we performed an in vitro release study with quantum dots. Quantum dots possess broad applicability in bioengineering, including imaging [84], theranostics [85], cell labeling for in vivo tracking [86], tissue staining [87]. They have also been investigated as biomarkers for cancer detection and for targeted drug delivery [35]. Figure 5A shows the normalized release rate of each phase, where passive (0 V) and active phases (−1.5 V) were alternated over three cycles.

The application of the negative gate potential drastically reduced the release of quantum dots from the membrane. Subsequent cycles demonstrated consistent and reproducible release rate reduction, suggesting that the membrane and the gating performance were consistent over time. A statistically significant difference (**** $p \leq 0.0001$) in the release between active and passive phases (84%) was observed (Figure 5B). When compared to methotrexate, quantum dots clearly showed a more effective electrostatic modulation, which could be attributed to higher particle charge and lower ionic strength of the solution. Specifically, the high exposed charge is due to the carboxylic functionalization, where several groups result in a negative net charge that ranges from −5 to −15 depending on pH and ionic strength [41]. Moreover, the low ionic strength solution (0.01 × PBS) has a Debye length 10 times greater than the 1 × PBS. These two properties contribute to enhance the electrostatic interactions between the wall and the solute. Thus, the application of the gate potential resulted in increased efficacy of release modulation.

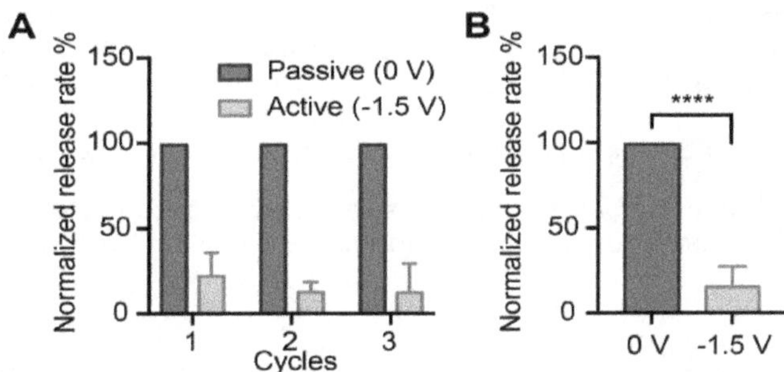

Figure 5. Electrostatically controlled release of quantum dots. (**A**) The normalized release rate of quantum dots for three cycles between free diffusion (Passive) and gated diffusion (Active). (**B**) Release rates grouped by phase typology (**** $p \leq 0.0001$).

3.8. Considerations on Electrostatic Gating Performance

To achieve efficient devices for tunable molecular diffusion via electrostatic gating, various parameters need to be optimized. Of utmost importance is the choice of dielectric material to insulate the buried gate electrode. In this study, we investigated SiC as it conciliates the need for low leakage currents, with a dielectric constant similar to SiO_2 (4.4–4.9) [88], and offers chemical inertness in aqueous solutions [48]. Moreover, SiC offers a low native charge; therefore, it minimizes unwanted non-linearities connected to the buffer capacity of strongly charged surfaces [72].

Further, efficient electrostatic flow modulation is strictly connected to the nanochannel size to the Debye length ratio (h/λ). Our membrane was designed for medical applications, where the ionic strength and pH were bound to physiological values. Our future investigations focus on manufacturing membranes with smaller nanochannels to be able, in principle, to completely stop analyte diffusion. Finally, as flow control trough electrostatic gating is mainly based on coulombic interactions, analytes that expose high surface charges are more suitable for gate modulation. Therefore, drug encapsulation with highly charged polymers can significantly improve administration control of small analytes.

4. Conclusions

In this work, we investigated a SiC-coated nanofluidic membrane capable of the reproducible control of analyte transport via electrostatic gating. The application of a low-intensity electrical potential to the gate electrode allowed us to alter nanochannel surface charge, leading to tunable membrane charge-selectivity, and control over the release of methotrexate and quantum dots. Electrochemical characterization showed that SiC dielectric coating exhibited low leakage current and reduced intrinsic charge as compared to SiO_2. Moreover, SiC offered chemical bioinertness, which rendered it an ideal candidate for use in biomedical devices for therapeutic delivery based on electrostatic-gating. In this context, our membranes could be employed as actuators for remotely controlled drug delivery systems. The low voltage needed to modulate the release rate could be provided via small scale and low-power circuitry. This investigation might pave the way for the development of the next generation of drug delivery systems, enabling pre-programmed or remotely managed pharmaceutic administration. Further, our gated nanofluidic membrane might find applicability in molecular sieving and lab on a chip diagnostic.

5. Patents

Grattoni, A.; Liu, X.; Ferrari, M. Gated Nanofluidic Valve For Active And Passive Electrosteric Control Of Molecular Transport, And Methods Of Fabrication, U.S. Provisional Pat. Ser. No. 62/961,437, filed Jan 15. (2020).

Author Contributions: Conceptualization, N.D.T., A.S., X.L., and A.G.; Data curation, N.D.T; Formal analysis, N.D.T and A.S.; Funding acquisition, X.L. and A.G.; Investigation, N.D.T., A.S., and Y.W.; Methodology, N.D.T., A.S., Y.W., and X.L.; Project administration, A.G.; Resources, X.L., and A.G.; Software, N.D.T.; Supervision, D.D. and A.G.; Validation, D.D., X.L., and A.G.; Visualization, N.D.T.; Writing—original draft, N.D.T.; Writing—review and editing, A.G. All authors have read and agreed to the published version of the manuscript.

Acknowledgments: We thank Valentina Serafini for her support in experimental studies and Jianhua (James) Gu from the electron microscopy core of the Houston Methodist Research Institute.

References

1. Hajat, C.; Stein, E. The global burden of multiple chronic conditions: A narrative review. *Prev. Med. Rep.* **2018**, *12*, 284–293. [CrossRef] [PubMed]
2. Yach, D.; Leeder, S.R.; Bell, J.; Kistnasamy, B. Global chronic diseases. *AAAS.* **2005**, *307*, 317. [CrossRef] [PubMed]
3. World Health Organization. *Global Status Report on Noncommunicable Diseases 2014*; WHO Press: Geneva, Switzerland, 2014.
4. Divo, M.; Cote, C.; de Torres, J.P.; Casanova, C.; Marin, J.M.; Pinto-Plata, V.; Zulueta, J.; Cabrera, C.; Zagaceta, J.; Hunninghake, G. Comorbidities and risk of mortality in patients with chronic obstructive pulmonary disease. *Am. J. Respi. Crit. Care Med.* **2012**, *186*, 155–161. [CrossRef] [PubMed]
5. Lemstra, M.; Nwankwo, C.; Bird, Y.; Moraros, J. Primary nonadherence to chronic disease medications: A meta-analysis. *Patient Prefer. Adherence* **2018**, *12*, 721. [CrossRef]
6. García-Lizana, F.; Sarría-Santamera, A. New technologies for chronic disease management and control: A systematic review. *J. Telemed. Telecare.* **2007**, *13*, 62–68. [CrossRef]
7. Desai, T.A.; Hansford, D.J.; Ferrari, M. Micromachined interfaces: New approaches in cell immunoisolation and biomolecular separation. *Biomol. Eng.* **2000**, *17*, 23–36. [CrossRef]
8. Peng, L.; Mendelsohn, A.D.; LaTempa, T.J.; Yoriya, S.; Grimes, C.A.; Desai, T.A. Long-term small molecule and protein elution from TiO2 nanotubes. *Nano Lett* **2009**, *9*, 1932–1936. [CrossRef]
9. Pons-Faudoa, F.P.; Ballerini, A.; Sakamoto, J.; Grattoni, A. Advanced implantable drug delivery technologies: Transforming the clinical landscape of therapeutics for chronic diseases. *Biomed. Microdevices* **2019**, *21*, 47. [CrossRef]
10. Chua, C.Y.X.; Jain, P.; Ballerini, A.; Bruno, G.; Hood, R.L.; Gupte, M.; Gao, S.; Di Trani, N.; Susnjar, A.; Shelton, K.; et al. Transcutaneously refillable nanofluidic implant achieves sustained level of tenofovir diphosphate for HIV pre-exposure prophylaxis. *J. Controlled Release* **2018**, *286*, 315–325. [CrossRef]
11. Ballerini, A.; Chua, C.Y.X.; Rhudy, J.; Susnjar, A.; Di Trani, N.; Jain, P.R.; Laue, G.; Lubicka, D.; Shirazi-Fard, Y.; Ferrari, M. Counteracting Muscle Atrophy on Earth and in Space via Nanofluidics Delivery of Formoterol. *Adv. Ther.* **2020**, *3*, 2000014. [CrossRef]
12. Hermida, R.C.; Ayala, D.E.; Smolensky, M.H.; Mojón, A.; Fernández, J.R.; Crespo, J.J.; Moyá, A.; Rios, M.T.; Portaluppi, F. Chronotherapy improves blood pressure control and reduces vascular risk in CKD. *Nat. Rev. Nephrol.* **2013**, *9*, 358. [CrossRef] [PubMed]
13. Lin, S.-Y.; Kawashima, Y. Current status and approaches to developing press-coated chronodelivery drug systems. *J. Controlled Release* **2012**, *157*, 331–353. [CrossRef] [PubMed]
14. Iwasaki, Y.; Sendo, M.; Dezaki, K.; Hira, T.; Sato, T.; Nakata, M.; Goswami, C.; Aoki, R.; Arai, T.; Kumari, P. GLP-1 release and vagal afferent activation mediate the beneficial metabolic and chronotherapeutic effects of D-allulose. *Nat. Commun.* **2018**, *9*, 1–17. [CrossRef] [PubMed]
15. Fifel, K.; Videnovic, A. Chronotherapies for Parkinson's disease. *Prog. Neurobiol.* **2019**, *174*, 16–27. [CrossRef]
16. Kaur, G.; Phillips, C.; Wong, K.; Saini, B. Timing is important in medication administration: A timely review of chronotherapy research. *Int J. Clin. Pharm.* **2013**, *35*, 344–358. [CrossRef]
17. Sprintz, M.; Tasciotti, E.; Allegri, M.; Grattoni, A.; Driver Larry, C.; Ferrari, M. Nanomedicine: Ushering in a new era of pain management. *Eur. J. Pain Suppl.* **2012**, *5*, 317–322. [CrossRef]

18. Celler, B.G.; Lovell, N.H.; Basilakis, J. Using information technology to improve the management of chronic disease. *Med. J. Aust.* **2003**, *179*, 242–246. [CrossRef]
19. Milani, R.V.; Bober, R.M.; Lavie, C.J. The role of technology in chronic disease care. *Prog. Cardiovasc. Dis.* **2016**, *58*, 579–583. [CrossRef]
20. Coye, M.J.; Haselkorn, A.; DeMello, S. Remote patient management: Technology-enabled innovation and evolving business models for chronic disease care. *Health Aff.* **2009**, *28*, 126–135. [CrossRef]
21. Hoare, T.; Timko, B.P.; Santamaria, J.; Goya, G.F.; Irusta, S.; Lau, S.; Stefanescu, C.F.; Lin, D.; Langer, R.; Kohane, D.S. Magnetically triggered nanocomposite membranes: A versatile platform for triggered drug release. *Nano Lett.* **2011**, *11*, 1395–1400. [CrossRef]
22. Timko, B.P.; Arruebo, M.; Shankarappa, S.A.; McAlvin, J.B.; Okonkwo, O.S.; Mizrahi, B.; Stefanescu, C.F.; Gomez, L.; Zhu, J.; Zhu, A.; et al. Near-infrared-actuated devices for remotely controlled drug delivery. *Proc. Natl. Acad. Sci. USA* **2014**, *111*, 1349–1354. [CrossRef] [PubMed]
23. Kim, K.; Jo, M.-C.; Jeong, S.; Palanikumar, L.; Rotello, V.M.; Ryu, J.-H.; Park, M.-H. Externally controlled drug release using a gold nanorod contained composite membrane. *Nanoscale* **2016**, *8*, 11949–11955. [CrossRef] [PubMed]
24. Kumeria, T.; Yu, J.; Alsawat, M.; Kurkuri, M.D.; Santos, A.; Abell, A.D.; Losic, D. Photoswitchable Membranes Based on Peptide-Modified Nanoporous Anodic Alumina: Toward Smart Membranes for On-Demand Molecular Transport. *Adv. Mater.* **2015**, *27*, 3019–3024. [CrossRef]
25. Ferrara, K.W. Driving delivery vehicles with ultrasound. *Adv. Drug Deliver Rev.* **2008**, *60*, 1097–1102. [CrossRef]
26. Lee, S.H.; Piao, H.; Cho, Y.C.; Kim, S.N.; Choi, G.; Kim, C.R.; Ji, H.B.; Park, C.G.; Lee, C.; Shin, C.I.; et al. Implantable multireservoir device with stimulus-responsive membrane for on-demand and pulsatile delivery of growth hormone. *Proc. Natl. Acad. Sci. USA* **2019**, *116*, 11664–11672. [CrossRef] [PubMed]
27. Farina, M. Remote magnetic switch off microgate for nanofluidic drug delivery implants. *Biomed. Microdevices* **2017**, *19*, 42. [CrossRef]
28. Kim, S.; Ozalp, E.I.; Darwish, M.; Weldon, J.A. Electrically gated nanoporous membranes for smart molecular flow control. *Nanoscale* **2018**, *10*, 20740–20747. [CrossRef]
29. Jeon, G.; Yang, S.Y.; Byun, J.; Kim, J.K. Electrically actuatable smart nanoporous membrane for pulsatile drug release. *Nano Lett.* **2011**, *11*, 1284–1288. [CrossRef]
30. Zhang, Q.; Kang, J.; Xie, Z.; Diao, X.; Liu, Z.; Zhai, J. Highly Efficient Gating of Electrically Actuated Nanochannels for Pulsatile Drug Delivery Stemming from a Reversible Wettability Switch. *Adv. Mater.* **2018**, *30*, 1703323. [CrossRef]
31. Kostaras, C.; Dellis, S.; Christoulaki, A.; Anastassopoulos, D.L.; Spiliopoulos, N.; Vradis, A.; Toprakcioglu, C.; Priftis, G.D. Flow through polydisperse pores in an anodic alumina membrane: A new method to measure the mean pore diameter. *J. Appl. Phys.* **2018**, *124*, 204307. [CrossRef]
32. Grattoni, A.; Liu, X.; Ferrari, M. Gated Nanofluidic Valve For Active And Passive Electrosteric Control Of Molecular Transport, And Methods Of Fabrication. U.S. Patent 62/961,437, 15 January 2020.
33. Lopez-Olivo, M.A.; Siddhanamatha, H.R.; Shea, B.; Tugwell, P.; Wells, G.A.; Suarez-Almazor, M.E. Methotrexate for treating rheumatoid arthritis. *Cochrane Database Syst. Rev.* **2014**. [CrossRef] [PubMed]
34. Matea, C.T.; Mocan, T.; Tabaran, F.; Pop, T.; Mosteanu, O.; Puia, C.; Iancu, C.; Mocan, L. Quantum dots in imaging, drug delivery and sensor applications. *Int J. Nanomed.* **2017**, *12*, 5421–5431. [CrossRef]
35. Cheki, M.; Moslehi, M.; Assadi, M. Marvelous applications of quantum dots. *Eur Rev. Med. Pharmacol. Sci.* **2013**, *17*, 1141–1148. [PubMed]
36. Napoli, M.; Eijkel, J.C.; Pennathur, S. Nanofluidic technology for biomolecule applications: A critical review. *Lab Chip* **2010**, *10*, 957–985. [CrossRef] [PubMed]
37. Lu, Y.; Liu, T.; Lamanda, A.C.; Sin, M.L.; Gau, V.; Liao, J.C.; Wong, P.K. AC electrokinetics of physiological fluids for biomedical applications. *J. Lab. Autom.* **2015**, *20*, 611–620. [CrossRef] [PubMed]
38. Gao, J.; Riahi, R.; Sin, M.L.; Zhang, S.; Wong, P.K. Electrokinetic focusing and separation of mammalian cells in conductive biological fluids. *Analyst* **2012**, *137*, 5215–5221. [CrossRef]
39. Di Trani, N.; Silvestri, A.; Sizovs, A.; Wang, Y.; Erm, D.R.; Demarchi, D.; Liu, X.; Grattoni, A. Electrostatically gated nanofluidic membrane for ultra-low power controlled drug delivery. *Lab Chip* **2020**, *20*, 1562–1576. [CrossRef]

40. Grattoni, A.; Gill, J.; Zabre, E.; Fine, D.; Hussain, F.; Ferrari, M. Device for rapid and agile measurement of diffusivity in micro- and nanochannels. *Anal. Chem.* **2011**, *83*, 3096–3103. [CrossRef]
41. Voráčová, I.; Klepárník, K.; Lišková, M.; Foret, F. Determination of ζ-potential, charge, and number of organic ligands on the surface of water soluble quantum dots by capillary electrophoresis. *Electrophoresis* **2015**, *36*, 867–874. [CrossRef]
42. Swain, M. Chemicalize.org. *J. Chem. Inf. Model.* **2012**, *52*, 613–615. [CrossRef]
43. Haro-González, P.; Martínez-Maestro, L.; Martín, I.; García-Solé, J.; Jaque, D. High-Sensitivity Fluorescence Lifetime Thermal Sensing Based on CdTe Quantum Dots. *Small* **2012**, *8*, 2652–2658. [CrossRef] [PubMed]
44. Geninatti, T.; Small, E.; Grattoni, A. Robotic UV-Vis apparatus for long-term characterization of drug release from nanochannels. *Meas. Sci. Technol.* **2014**, *25*. [CrossRef]
45. Scorrano, G.; Bruno, G.; Di Trani, N.; Ferrari, M.; Pimpinelli, A.; Grattoni, A. Gas Flow at the Ultra-nanoscale: Universal Predictive Model and Validation in Nanochannels of Ångstrom-Level Resolution. *ACS Appl. Mater. Interfaces* **2018**, *10*, 32233–32238. [CrossRef] [PubMed]
46. Kotzar, G.; Freas, M.; Abel, P.; Fleischman, A.; Roy, S.; Zorman, C.; Moran, J.M.; Melzak, J. Evaluation of MEMS materials of construction for implantable medical devices. *Biomaterials* **2002**, *23*, 2737–2750. [CrossRef]
47. Voskerician, G.; Shive, M.S.; Shawgo, R.S.; Von Recum, H.; Anderson, J.M.; Cima, M.J.; Langer, R. Biocompatibility and biofouling of MEMS drug delivery devices. *Biomaterials* **2003**, *24*, 1959–1967. [CrossRef]
48. Oliveros, A.; Guiseppi-Elie, A.; Saddow, S.E. Silicon carbide: A versatile material for biosensor applications. *Biomed. Microdevices* **2013**, *15*, 353–368. [CrossRef] [PubMed]
49. Mahmoodi, M.; Ghazanfari, L. *Physics and Technology of Silicon Carbide Devices*; Hijikata, Y, Ed.; InTech: Vienna, Austria, 2012.
50. Cogan, S.F.; Edell, D.J.; Guzelian, A.A.; Ping Liu, Y.; Edell, R. Plasma-enhanced chemical vapor deposited silicon carbide as an implantable dielectric coating. *J. Biomed. Mater. Res.* **2003**, *67*, 856–867. [CrossRef]
51. Zorman, C.A.; Eldridge, A.; Du, J.G.; Johnston, M.; Dubnisheva, A.; Manley, S.; Fissell, W.; Fleischman, A.; Roy, S. *Amorphous Silicon Carbide as a Non-Biofouling Structural Material for Biomedical Microdevices*; Materials Science Forum, Trans Tech Publications Ltd.: Stafa-Zurich, Switzerland, 2012; pp. 537–540. [CrossRef]
52. Takami, Y.; Yamane, S.; Makinouchi, K.; Otsuka, G.; Glueck, J.; Benkowski, R.; Nosé, Y. Protein adsorption onto ceramic surfaces. *J. Biomed. Mater. Res.* **1998**, *40*, 24–30. [CrossRef]
53. Ferrati, S.; Nicolov, E.; Zabre, E.; Geninatti, T.; Shirkey, B.A.; Hudson, L.; Hosali, S.; Crawley, M.; Khera, M.; Palapattu, G.; et al. The Nanochannel Delivery System for Constant Testosterone Replacement Therapy. *J. Sex. Med.* **2015**, *12*, 1375–1380. [CrossRef]
54. Pons-Faudoa, F.P.; Sizovs, A.; Shelton, K.A.; Momin, Z.; Bushman, L.R.; Chua, C.Y.X.; Nichols, J.E.; Hawkins, T.; Rooney, J.F.; Marzinke, M.A. Preventive efficacy of a tenofovir alafenamide fumarate nanofluidic implant in SHIV-challenged nonhuman primates. *BioRxiv.* **2020**. [CrossRef]
55. Bruno, G.; Canavese, G.; Liu, X.; Filgueira, C.S.; Sacco, A.; Demarchi, D.; Ferrari, M.; Grattoni, A. The active modulation of drug release by an ionic field effect transistor for an ultra-low power implantable nanofluidic system. *Nanoscale* **2016**, *8*, 18718–18725. [CrossRef] [PubMed]
56. Ferrati, S.; Fine, D.; You, J.; De Rosa, E.; Hudson, L.; Zabre, E.; Hosali, S.; Zhang, L.; Hickman, C.; Sunder Bansal, S.; et al. Leveraging nanochannels for universal, zero-order drug delivery in vivo. *J. Controlled Release* **2013**, *172*, 1011–1019. [CrossRef] [PubMed]
57. Di Trani, N.; Jain, P.; Chua, C.Y.X.; Ho, J.S.; Bruno, G.; Susnjar, A.; Pons-Faudoa, F.P.; Sizovs, A.; Hood, R.L.; Smith, Z.W.; et al. Nanofluidic microsystem for sustained intraocular delivery of therapeutics. *Nanomed. Nanotechnol. Biol. Med.* **2019**, *16*, 1–9. [CrossRef] [PubMed]
58. Fine, D.; Grattoni, A.; Hosali, S.; Ziemys, A.; De Rosa, E.; Gill, J.; Medema, R.; Hudson, L.; Kojic, M.; Milosevic, M.; et al. A robust nanofluidic membrane with tunable zero-order release for implantable dose specific drug delivery. *Lab Chip* **2010**, *10*, 3074–3083. [CrossRef] [PubMed]
59. Di Trani, N.; Silvestri, A.; Bruno, G.; Geninatti, T.; Chua, C.Y.X.; Gilbert, A.; Rizzo, G.; Filgueira, C.S.; Demarchi, D.; Grattoni, A. Remotely controlled nanofluidic implantable platform for tunable drug delivery. *Lab.Chip* **2019**, *19*, 2192–2204. [CrossRef] [PubMed]
60. Fine, D.; Grattoni, A.; Zabre, E.; Hussein, F.; Ferrari, M.; Liu, X. A low-voltage electrokinetic nanochannel drug delivery system. *Lab Chip* **2011**, *11*, 2526–2534. [CrossRef]
61. Prakash, S.; Conlisk, A.T. Field effect nanofluidics. *Lab Chip* **2016**, *16*, 3855–3865. [CrossRef]

62. Plecis, A.; Tazid, J.; Pallandre, A.; Martinhon, P.; Deslouis, C.; Chen, Y.; Haghiri-Gosnet, A. Flow field effect transistors with polarisable interface for EOF tunable microfluidic separation devices. *Lab Chip* **2010**, *10*, 1245–1253. [CrossRef]
63. Robertson, J. High dielectric constant gate oxides for metal oxide Si transistors. *Rep. Prog. Phys.* **2005**, *69*, 327–396. [CrossRef]
64. Padovani, A.; Gao, D.Z.; Shluger, A.L.; Larcher, L. A microscopic mechanism of dielectric breakdown in SiO2 films: An insight from multi-scale modeling. *J. Appl. Phys.* **2017**, *121*, 155101. [CrossRef]
65. Yao, J.; Zhong, L.; Natelson, D.; Tour, J.M. In situ imaging of the conducting filament in a silicon oxide resistive switch. *Sci. Rep.* **2012**, *2*, 1–5. [CrossRef] [PubMed]
66. Tung, C.H.; Pey, K.L.; Tang, L.J.; Radhakrishnan, M.K.; Lin, W.H.; Palumbo, F.; Lombardo, S. Percolation path and dielectric-breakdown-induced-epitaxy evolution during ultrathin gate dielectric breakdown transient. *Appl. Phys. Lett.* **2003**, *83*, 2223–2225. [CrossRef]
67. Chen, X.; Wang, H.; Sun, G.; Ma, X.; Gao, J.; Wu, W. Resistive switching characteristic of electrolyte-oxide-semiconductor structures. *J. Semicond.* **2017**, *38*, 8. [CrossRef]
68. Daiguji, H.; Yang, P.; Majumdar, A. Ion transport in nanofluidic channels. *Nano Lett.* **2004**, *4*, 137–142. [CrossRef]
69. Yossifon, G.; Mushenheim, P.; Chang, Y.-C.; Chang, H.-C. Nonlinear current-voltage characteristics of nanochannels. *Phys. Rev. E* **2009**. [CrossRef]
70. Grosjean, A.; Rezrazi, M.; Tachez, M. Study of the surface charge of silicon carbide (SIC) particles for electroless composite deposits: Nickel-SiC. *Surf. Coat. Technol.* **1997**, *96*, 300–304. [CrossRef]
71. Karnik, R.; Fan, R.; Yue, M.; Li, D.; Yang, P.; Majumdar, A. Electrostatic control of ions and molecules in nanofluidic transistors. *Nano lett.* **2005**, *5*, 943–948. [CrossRef]
72. Jiang, Z.; Stein, D. Electrofluidic Gating of a Chemically Reactive Surface. *Langmuir* **2010**, *26*, 8161–8173. [CrossRef]
73. Schoch, R.B.; Han, J.; Renaud, P. Transport phenomena in nanofluidics. *Rev. Mod. Phys.* **2008**, *80*, 839–883. [CrossRef]
74. Herbowski, L.; Gurgul, H.; Staron, W. Experimental determination of the Stern layer thickness at the interface of the human arachnoid membrane and the cerebrospinal fluid. *Z. Med. Phys.* **2009**, *19*, 189–192. [CrossRef]
75. Lu, P.; Dai, Q.; Wu, L.; Liu, X. Structure and Capacitance of Electrical Double Layers at the Graphene–Ionic Liquid Interface. *Appl. Sci.* **2017**, *7*, 939. [CrossRef]
76. Bruno, G.; Di Trani, N.; Hood, R.L.; Zabre, E.; Filgueira, C.S.; Canavese, G.; Jain, P.; Smith, Z.; Demarchi, D.; Hosali, S. Unexpected behaviors in molecular transport through size-controlled nanochannels down to the ultra-nanoscale. *Nat. Commun.* **2018**, *9*, 1682. [CrossRef] [PubMed]
77. Di Trani, N.; Pimpinelli, A.; Grattoni, A. Finite-Size Charged Species Diffusion and pH Change in Nanochannels. *ACS Appl. Mater. Interfaces* **2020**, *12*, 12246–12255. [CrossRef] [PubMed]
78. Behrens, S.H.; Grier, D.G. The charge of glass and silica surfaces. *J Chem. Phys.* **2001**, *115*, 6716–6721. [CrossRef]
79. Veber, D.F.; Johnson, S.R.; Cheng, H.-Y.; Smith, B.R.; Ward, K.W.; Kopple, K.D. Molecular Properties That Influence the Oral Bioavailability of Drug Candidates. *J. Med. Chem.* **2002**, *45*, 2615–2623. [CrossRef]
80. Liu, D.Y.; Lon, H.K.; Wang, Y.L.; DuBois, D.C.; Almon, R.R.; Jusko, W.J. Pharmacokinetics, pharmacodynamics and toxicities of methotrexate in healthy and collagen-induced arthritic rats. *Biopharm. Drug Dispos.* **2013**, *34*, 203–214. [CrossRef]
81. Yasin, M.N.; Svirskis, D.; Seyfoddin, A.; Rupenthal, I.D. Implants for drug delivery to the posterior segment of the eye: A focus on stimuli-responsive and tunable release systems. *J. Controlled Release* **2014**, *196*, 208–221. [CrossRef]
82. Langer, R.D. Efficacy, Safety, and Tolerability of Low-Dose Hormone Therapy in Managing Menopausal Symptoms. *J Am. Board Fam. Med.* **2009**, *22*, 563. [CrossRef]
83. Charles, N.C.; Steiner, G.C. Ganciclovir intraocular implant. A clinicopathologic study. *Ophthalmology* **1996**, *103*, 416–421. [CrossRef]
84. Li, J.; Zhu, J.-J. Quantum dots for fluorescent biosensing and bio-imaging applications. *Analyst* **2013**, *138*, 2506–2515. [CrossRef] [PubMed]
85. Ho, Y.-P.; Leong, K.W. Quantum dot-based theranostics. *Nanoscale* **2010**, *2*, 60–68. [CrossRef]

86. Kim, J.; Song, S.H.; Jin, Y.; Park, H.-J.; Yoon, H.; Jeon, S.; Cho, S.-W. Multiphoton luminescent graphene quantum dots for in vivo tracking of human adipose-derived stem cells. *Nanoscale* **2016**, *8*, 8512–8519. [CrossRef] [PubMed]
87. Bajwa, N.; Mehra, N.K.; Jain, K.; Jain, N.K. Pharmaceutical and biomedical applications of quantum dots. *Artif. Cells Nanomed. Biotechnol.* **2016**, *44*, 758–768. [CrossRef]
88. Hsu, J.-M.; Tathireddy, P.; Rieth, L.; Normann, A.R.; Solzbacher, F. Characterization of a-SiCx: H thin films as an encapsulation material for integrated silicon based neural interface devices. *Thin Solid Films* **2007**, *516*, 34–41. [CrossRef] [PubMed]

6

Versatile Layer-By-Layer Highly Stable Multilayer Films: Study of the Loading and Release of FITC-Labeled Short Peptide in the Drug Delivery Field

Kun Nie [1], Xiang Yu [1,*], Navnita Kumar [2] and Yihe Zhang [1,*]

[1] Beijing Key Laboratory of Materials Utilization of Nonmetallic Minerals and Solid Wastes, National Laboratory of Mineral Materials, School of Materials Science and Technology, China University of Geosciences (Beijing), Beijing 100083, China; nk@cugb.edu.cn

[2] Department of Chemistry and Biochemistry, University of California, Los Angeles, CA 90095, USA; navnitakumar77@gmail.com

* Correspondence: yuxiang@cugb.edu.cn (X.Y.); zyh@cugb.edu.cn (Y.Z.)

Abstract: A viable short FITC-peptide immobilization is the most essential step in the fabrication of multilayer films based on FITC-peptide. These functional multilayer films have potential applications in drug delivery, medical therapy, and so forth. These FITC-peptides films needed to be handled with a lot of care and precision due to their sensitive nature. In this study, a general immobilization method is reported for the purpose of stabilizing various kinds of peptides at the interfacial regions. Utilizing Mesoporous silica nanoparticles can help in the preservation of these FITC-peptides by embedding themselves into these covalently cross-linked multilayers. This basic outlook of the multilayer films is potent enough and could be reused as a positive substrate. The spatio-temporal retention property of peptides can be modulated by varying the number of capping layers. The release speed of guest molecules such as tyrosine within FITC-peptide or/and adamantane (Ad)-in short peptides could also be fine-tuned by the specific arrangements of the multilayers of mesoporous silica nanoparticles (MSNs) and hyaluronic acid- cyclodextrin (HA-CD) multilayer films.

Keywords: mesoporous silica; layer-by-layer; FITC-peptide; hyaluronic acid; multilayer film; host-guest interaction

---

1. Introduction

Layer-by-layer self-assembly technology is a useful method to prepare multilayer films with a thickness which can be controlled even down to the nanoscale [1–5], and is among one of the most widely used techniques to weave the organic-inorganic multilayer films together [6–10]. Mesoporous silica nanoparticles (MSNs) have been widely used in adsorption and drug delivery due to their unique pore structure, large specific surface area and good biocompatibility [11]. Some of these can directly act as catalysts as well because the ordered mesoporous material can accelerate the diffusion rate of the product. The selectivity is 100% and the conversion rate is up to 90%. Due to the flexibility of the structure and the narrow pore distribution, the doping of metal oxide and other complexes to these ordered mesoporous material matrix makes them better catalysts. Biological macromolecules, such as enzymes, proteins, nucleic acids, etc., have molecular sizes less than 10 nm, while viruses have sizes around 30 nm. However, the ordered mesoporous materials have quite a range of pore sizes between 2 and 50 nm. Due to the non-toxicity of these MSNs, they play an important role in the decomposition and fixation of enzymes, proteins and other substances. The mesoporous silica used for a particular function needs to be of a particle size, otherwise it will have an adverse effect [11–13]. A lot of research has been done in the area of multilayer films conjoining polymer and inorganic nanoparticles [14–16], and this can be attributed to the variable functionalities from the organic and inorganic parts of multilayer films [17–20]. The multilayer films which incorporate different inorganic parts can generally be prepared either by forming a covalent cross-link or by utilizing the non-covalent interactions between the polymer and the inorganic parts [21–25]. According to the literature, under ultraviolet irradiation, poly (allylamine hydrochloride) (PAH) and 4,4′-diazostilbene-2,2′-disulfonic acid disodium salt (DAS) can form covalent cross-linked layers in situ [26]. Non-covalent multilayer films have been obtained by using different kinds of supramolecular interactions [27–29], electrostatic interactions [30], hydrophobic interactions [29], host–guest interactions [30–32] and so on and so forth.

The knowledge of diffusion mechanism of fluorescent agent in these multilayers is very important and can provide a deeper perspective into the molecular interaction in organisms, soft material systems, and various advanced functional films [33–35]. Due to their good absorptivity, water solubility, and fluorescence quantum yield, Fluorescein derivatives, especially Fluorescein Isothiocyanate (FITC) have become the most popular fluorescent reagents in this field. Owing to their wide fluorescence emission range, their good performance on photo-bleaching and fluorescence quenching on conjugation to biopolymers, the scope of the application can be widened for FITC-based dyes and their conjugates [36].

Hyaluronic acid (HA) consists of repeatable disaccharides of the β-glucuronic acid and N-acetyl-d-glucosamine [37]. Hyaluronic gel is found in synovial fluid and is the main component of a glycosaminoglycan superstructure complex which is associated with different polysaccharides such as the chondroitin sulfate [38]. Hyaluronic acid can anchor to the surface of the cell by attaching itself to the cell surface receptors. HA is an upcoming drug delivery molecule for soft tissue repair and regeneration [39]. Studies to control the host-guest interaction within supramolecular structures are gradually rising because of their potential application as stimuli-responsive hydrogels, nanoparticles, smart biosensor devices and so on [40,41].

Amino-betacyclodextrin (CD) is a member of cyclic oligosaccharides and consists of the lipophilic central cavity and a hydrophilic outer surface [42,43]. Amino-betacyclodextrin has a large structure with a many hydrogen donors and acceptor groups. However, these groups are impermeable to the lipophilic films, making them difficult to use as a drug delivery vehicle. To enhance aqueous solubility of those poorly soluble drugs and to also raise their bioavailability, cyclodextrin has been utilized as a complexing agent [44]. CD can be grafted onto HA by chemical synthesis, and then the properties of both the moieties in the complex can be utilized. The grafting rate can be measured by ^{1}H NMR [45]. In addition, there is supramolecular hydrophobic host-guest interaction between adamantine (Ad) and cyclodextrin (CD) [46]. Peptides with Ad can be used as targets to study the effect of host-guest interactions in molecular diffusion. At present, there are many reported articles on the host-guest inclusion phenomena that delays the release of peptides [47].

In this paper, we have explored a new method to construct multilayer film materials that effectively preserves different kinds of short peptides. Mesoporous silica serves as a short peptide-container and functional multilayers were embedded in these via electrostatic interactions. Because of the exquisite film structure, the magnitude of the supramolecular interactions within the multilayer films can be modulated. The release curves of the short peptides vary with the number of laminated multilayers. The supramolecular force-delayed molecular release was taken as an example to further demonstrate the functions of the reported peptides immobilization strategy. This technique can be utilized to prepare multilayers which can further be used to control the fabrication of these versatile multilayer films.

2. Materials and Methods

2.1. Materials and Instruments

The following chemicals were used without any further treatment: Sodium hyaluronate (HA, 95%), amino-betacyclodextrin, fluorescein isothiocyanate (FITC, purity > 90), phosphate buffer solution (PBS) and peptides (FITC-RGD & FITC-RGD-Ad) modified with fluorescein isothiocyanate were provided by Sinopharm Chemical Reagent Beijing Co., Ltd (Beijing, China). Mono-(6-Amino-6-deoxy)-Beta-cyclodextrin was bought from Shandong Binzhou Zhiyuan Biotechnology Co., Ltd (Shandong, China). Peptides (FITC-$(SGGYGGS)_4$ & FITC-$(SGGSGGS)_4$) were bought from LifeTein LLC (Beijing, China). Cetyltrimethylammonium bromide surfactant ($CH_3(CH_2)_{15}N(CH_3)_3Br$, CTAB), tetraethoxysilane (TEOS) and Poly(allylamine hydrochloride) (PAH, Mw = 15,000) were purchased from Sigma-Aldrich (St. Louis, MO, USA). 4,4′-diazostilbene-2,2′-disulfonic acid disodium salt (DAS), N-Hydroxy succinimide (NHS) and 1-(3-Dimethylaminopropyl)-3-ethylcarbodiimide hydrochloride (EDC) were purchased from TCI (Tokyo Chemical Industry, Tokyo, Japan). Only deionized water was used for all the syntheses.

UV-vis spectra were obtained using a Hitachi U-3900 spectrophotometer (Hitachi, Tokyo, Japan). The Surface morphologies of multilayer films were characterized using transmission electron microscope (TEM) (TEM, Tecnai T12, Field Electron and Ion Company, FEI, Hillsboro, OR, USA). TEM experiments were carried out on a Titan S/TEM (Field Electron and Ion Company, FEI, Hillsboro, OR, USA) microscope. ^1H NMR spectra were obtained on Bruker Avance III 400MHz WB (Bruker, Baden, Switzerland). The Brunauer-Emmett-Teller(BET)-Barret-Joyner-Halenda(BJH) BET-BJH data were obtained from the Autosorb-iQ2 (Quantachrome, Boynton Beach, FL, USA).

2.2. The Preparation of HA-β-CD Gels

HA-CD gel was prepared according to literature [48]. In a 100 mL Erlenmeyer flask, 0.3 g of sodium hyaluronate and 50 mL of morpholinoethanesulfonic buffer (MES) were added and rapid stirred for 6 h. Subsequently, 0.285 g of NHS and 0.342 g of EDC were added into the Erlenmeyer flask. Then the mixture was stirred for another hour. To the mixture, 0.1686 g of amino cyclodextrin was added, followed by stirring for 24 h. The detailed experimental procedure and the sample codes are listed in Table S1. ^1H NMR spectroscopy was used to determine the degree of grafting of HA-CD. The graft ratio was calculated by using the integral area of the ^1H NMR spectrum. As shown in Figure S1, the peak at 5.10 ppm represents the proton of amino (NH) (5.10 ppm) group and its integral area was 0.11. Therefore, the integral area of each hydrogen atom of the aminocyclodextrin was 0.11/7. Similarly, the peak at 2.05 ppm represents the proton of CH_3 (2.05 ppm) group and its integral area was 1.00. Therefore, the integral area of each hydrogen atom of hyaluronic acid was 1/3. Grafting ratio was obtained by dividing the integral area of each hydrogen atom of amino cyclodextrin by the integral area of each hydrogen atom of hyaluronic acid. So, according to the ^1H NMR (400 MHz, D_2O) data, the grafting rate of HA-CD was 4.71%.

2.3. The Synthesis of Mesoporous Silica Nanoparticles (MSNs)

MSNs were synthetized according to the literature [49]. In brief, an aqueous solution containing of 2.0 g CTAB, 7.0 mL NaOH (2 mol L^{-1}) and H_2O (480 g) was heated for 30 min at 80 degrees with rapid stirring. To this solution, 8.31 g ethyl orthosilicate was added. The white solid appeared within two minutes. The product was further stirred at 80 degrees for two more hours, followed by centrifugation, washing with a lot of ultra-pure water, and drying in vacuum oven for 12 h. The CTAB extraction was carried at 60-degrees Celsius. This white powder was added to a mixture of ethanol (120 mL) and concentrated hydrochloric acid (1.0 mL) and stirred for 8 h at 60 degrees Celsius. The product was then centrifuged and washed with a lot of water and ethanol, followed by drying under vacuum. The diameter of meso-SiO_2 is about 100 nm as seen in TEM images shown in Figure 1c. The surface area of the MSN is 646.715 m^2 g^{-1} and the pore diameter of the MSN was about 3.4 nm, which was characterized via the BET instrument.

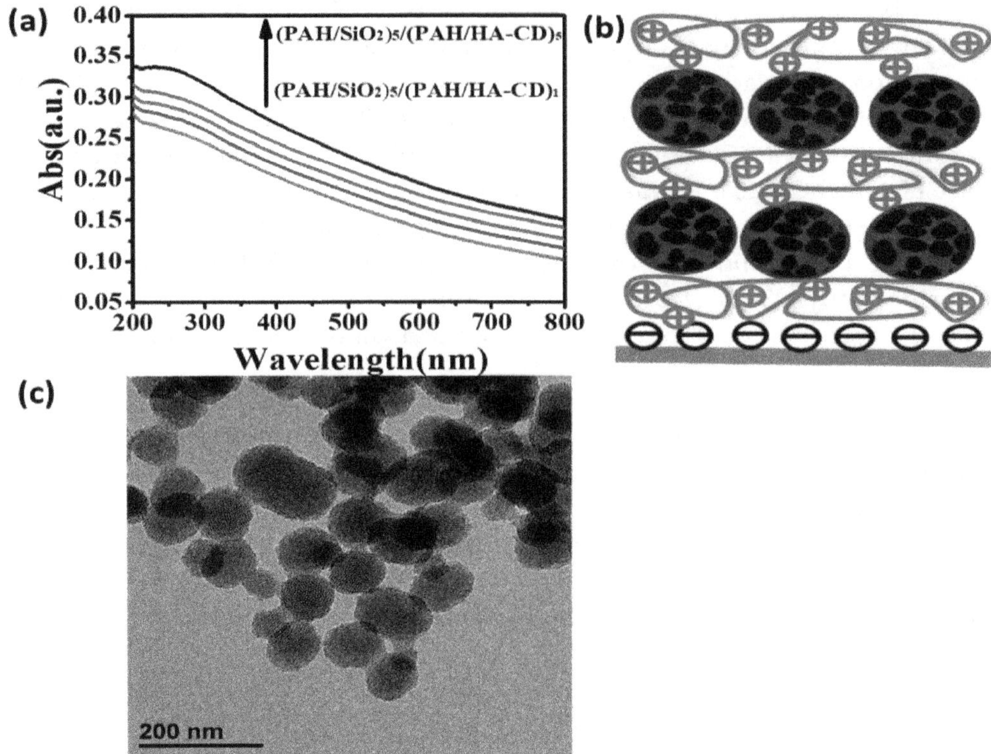

Figure 1. (**a**) Assembly process followed by UV-vis spectrum of $(SiO_2/PAH)_5/(PAH/HA\text{-}CD)_5/(PAH/DAS)_5$ multilayers; (**b**) Cartoon showing the process of layer-by-layer self-assembly; (**c**) TEM image of MSNs.

2.4. Layer-By-Layer Assembly Multilayer

Quartz slides cleaned by piranha solution (concentrated H_2SO_4/H_2O_2 (v:v = 7:3)) for 10 h were immersed in PAH (aq., MW = 15,000, 1 mg ml^{-1}, pH = 9) for 25 min in a typical layer-by-layer cycle. They were rinsed in ultrapure water and then dried with nitrogen. After that, the slides were dipped into the SiO_2 solution for 25 min and rinsed and dried as before. The cycle was continued until desirable thickness was obtained and the related coating film will be designated as $(PAH/SiO_2)_n$. Generally, the LBL film was assembled in pH = 9 solution. The substrate was immersed in PAH (aq., MW = 15,000, 1 mg mL^{-1}, pH = 9) for 25 min, rinsed in ultrapure water, and then dried with nitrogen. Subsequently, these slides were soaked into the HA-CD (1 mg mL^{-1}) solution for 25 min, rinsed and dried as before so that (PAH/HA-CD) LBL films could be deposited onto the surface of the $(PAH/SiO_2)_n$ films. The film should be fixed on the quartz substrate to avoid bending during handling so that the good quality of multilayers on the quartz substrate can be guaranteed.

2.5. Peptide Loading and Release

1 mg of FITC-labeled peptide solution was dissolved in 10 mL of PBS buffer solution (pH = 7.4) in a 20 mL glass beaker at room temperature. The quartz sheets with the multilayers on the surface were then immersed in the peptide solution for 24 h. The quartz sheets were then removed and the surface was immediately rinsed with deionized water and blown dry with nitrogen. Finally, these quartz sheets were used for release experiments in PBS buffer solution.

3. Results and Discussions

The surfaces of PAH and DAS are positively charged. PAH and DAS can form covalent cross-linked layers in situ under ultraviolet irradiation. The versatile multilayer films reported here were built by integrating MSN, which act as the storage space of polypeptide of FITC-peptide-Ad and the covalently cross-linking multilayers to increase the stability of the whole system of the multilayer films

(Scheme 1). A multilayer film of $(PAH/SiO_2)_5/(PAH/HA\text{-}CD)_5$ was prepared as illustrated in Figure 1a. The formation of this multilayer was monitored by UV-vis spectroscopy. The cartoon as shown in Figure 1b, displays the process of layer by layer self-assembly between MSN and PAH. The MSN used in the experiment were synthesized in our laboratory. The diameters for these MSNs vary from small to 100 nm as shown in Figure 1c. The thickness of the cross-section of multilayer films prepared on the silica substrate was about 140 nm with surface roughness of around 35 nm (Figure S2). As compared to uncross-linked $(PAH/DAS)_5$ films, the stability of the $(PAH/SiO_2)_5$ multilayer films is not great and could not be enhanced, and the absorbance of the basic solution remains 32.26% of the original absorbance after the immersion as shown by the UV-vis spectra (Figure 2a,b).

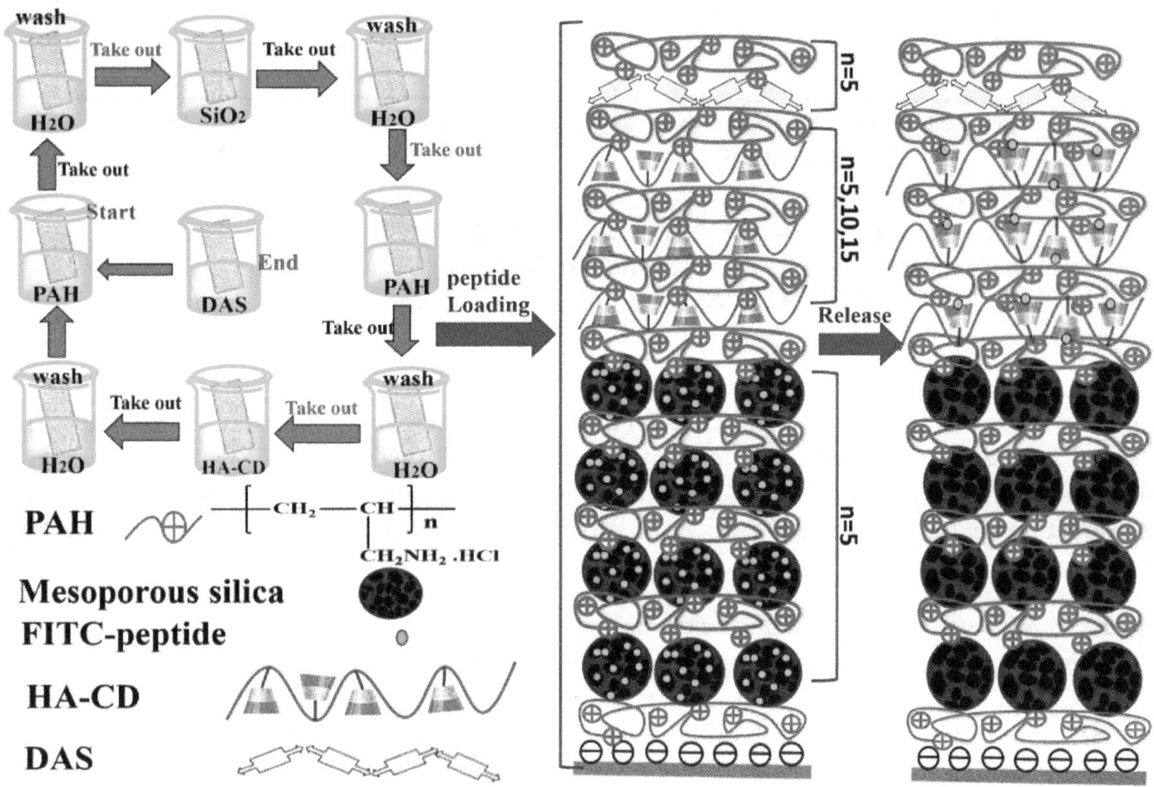

Scheme 1. Description of the loading and release using multilayer film: polymer layers and the mesoporous silica reservoir both play an important role in fabricating functional and stable multilayer films.

UV irradiation was used to enhance the stability of the multilayer films. $(PAH/DAS)_5$ multilayer films were subsequently prepared by a self-assembly method on the top of the $(PAH/SiO_2)_5/(PAH/HA\text{-}CD)_5$ multilayers, and cross-link of $(PAH/DAS)_5$ multilayer films was analyzed using UV spectra. The decrease of the absorbance peak at 340 nm indicates that the DAS decomposes and forms covalent cross-linkages within the $(PAH/DAS)_5$ films. The stability of these films can be verified by soaking the cross-linked multilayer films into the basic solution. After the treatment with basic solution for 2 h, the peak absorbance of the multilayer films increased by 94.12% (Figure 2a).

The result shows that the covalently cross-linked $(PAH/DAS)_5$ acts as an outermost film which contributes in the enhancement of the stability of the multilayer films within the MSNs. Based on these results, the presence of $(PAH/DAS)_5$ multilayer films can enhance the stability of the uncross-linked multilayer films. It was supposed that the nano-net effect resulted in the ability of $(PAH/DAS)_5$ multilayer films to improve the stability of the films by incorporating silica underneath. In addition, DAS could enter the multilayer films and also enhance the stability of the multilayer films through covalent cross-linking bonding. This effective and facile strategy can play an important role in practical purposes because of its ability in stabilizing different kinds of multilayer films.

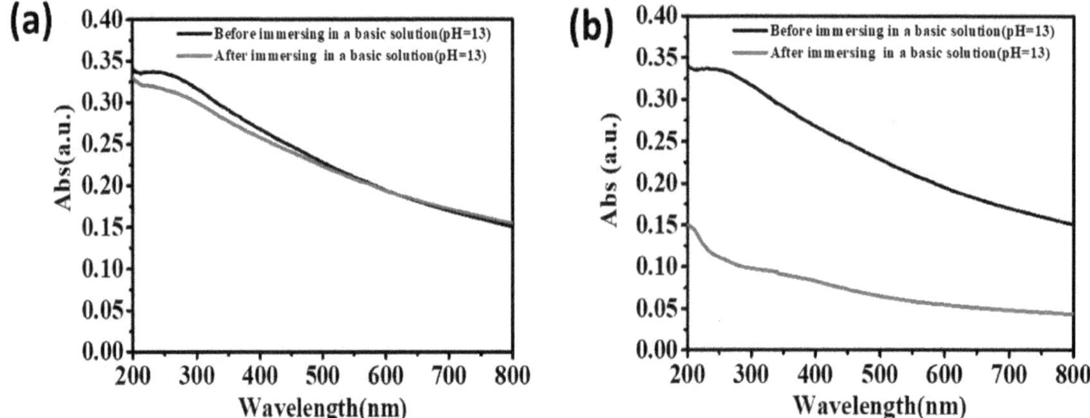

Figure 2. (**a**) UV-vis spectrum of the cross-linked $(SiO_2/PAH)_5(PAH/HA\text{-}CD)_5(PAH/DAS)_5$ film before (black) and after (red) immersion in a basic solution (pH = 13); (**b**) UV-vis spectrum of the uncross-linked $(SiO_2/PAH)_5/(PAH/HA\text{-}CD)_5/(PAH/DAS)_5$ film before (black) and after (red) immersion in a basic solution (pH = 13).

In consideration of the above facts, a model multilayer film for the release of FITC-labeled peptides can be employed as a model drug. The host-guest interaction between CD and Ad existed on the three-dimensional scale. The cyclodextrin molecule is hydrophilic from outside and hydrophobic from inside. It indicates that the CD possesses the external hydrophilic surface and the hydrophobic central cavity.

Figure 3 shows the short peptides release profiles from cross-linked multilayer films. Figure 3a clearly shows that the drug release rate of FITC-RGD is faster than the drug release rate of FITC-RGD-Ad. The release curve clearly shows the release time of FITC-RGD from $(SiO_2/PAH)_5/(PAH/HA\text{-}CD)_5/(PAH/DAS)_5$ is about 180 min (in the red line) (Figure 3a); however, the release time of FITC-RGD-Ad from $(SiO_2/PAH)_5/(PAH/HA\text{-}CD)_5/(PAH/DAS)_5$ is about 360 min (in the black line) (Figure 3a). As shown in Figure 3b, the release time of FITC-RGD and FITC-RGD-Ad is about 360 min and 480 min, respectively. As shown in Figure S3, ten layers of multilayers were used for experiments to prove that the molecular size had little effect on the release rate. As shown in Figure S3, the release time of both FITC-RGD and FITC-RGD-Ad is about 480 min. As illustrated in Figure 3c, it takes about 480 min for the release of FITC-RGD, and 720 min for FITC-RGD-Ad from $(SiO_2/PAH)_5/(PAH/HA\text{-}CD)_5/(PAH/DAS)_5$ multilayer film. Moreover, it shows that the release profiles are very smooth in Figure 3. Despite the number of multilayers in the film being same, the release speed and release time is different. The delayed effect of the films was caused by the host-guest supramolecular interactions between cyclodextrin and adamantane and also the release process increased with number of the multilayers. In addition, the release time of different kinds of multilayer is summarized in Figure 3d. In the experiment, the controlled variable method was used to study the release of peptide. Figure 4a is the same as Figure 3a. Compared with the release profiles in Figures 3 and 4a, Figure 4b clearly shows that the peptide release speed of FITC-RGD is faster than the release speed of FITC-RGD-Ad. The release time of FITC-RGD and FITC-RGD-Ad is about 210 min and 400 min, respectively. As seen in Figure 4c, the release time of FITC-RGD and FITC-RGD-Ad is 350 min and 470 min, respectively. Delayed effect of the multilayer films resulted from the host-guest supramolecular interactions, which show an increase in the release process with an increasing number of multilayers.

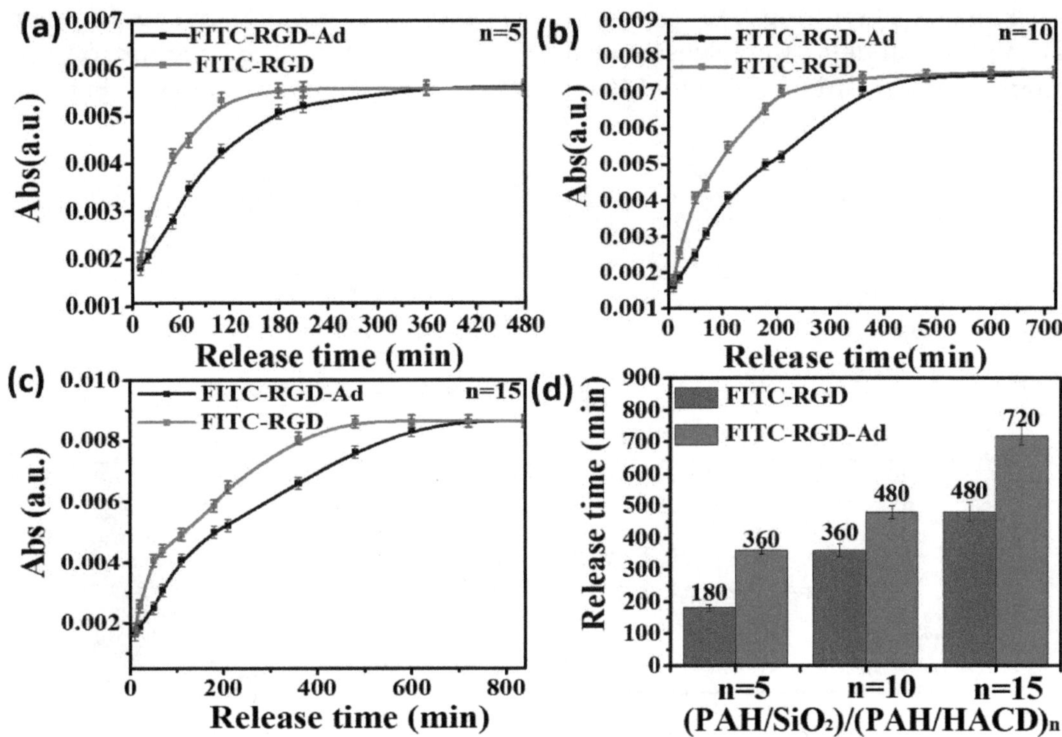

Figure 3. Release profiles of FITC-RGD-Ad and FITC-RGD from the cross-linked (**a**) $(SiO_2/PAH)_5/(PAH/HA\text{-}CD)_5/(PAH/DAS)_5$; (**b**) $(SiO_2/PAH)_5/(PAH/HA\text{-}CD)_{10}/(PAH/DAS)_5$ and (**c**) $(SiO_2/PAH)_5/(PAH/HA\text{-}CD)_{15}/(PAH/DAS)_5$ multilayer films. (**d**) the release time of FITC-RGD-Ad and FITC-RGD from different kinds of multilayer films.

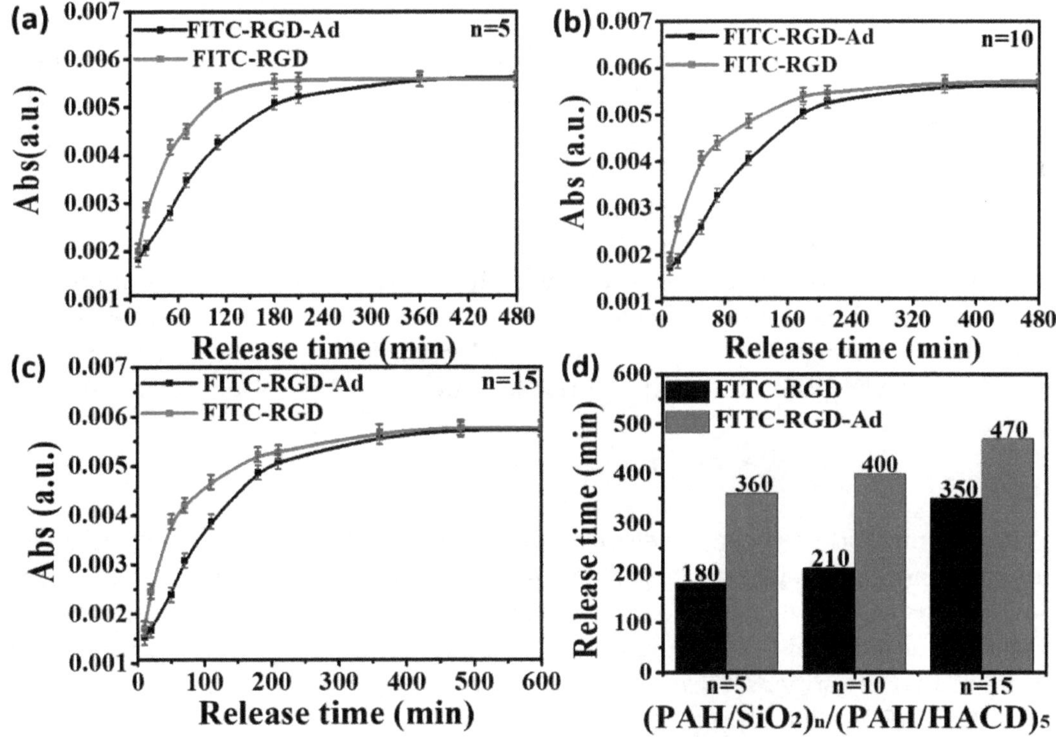

Figure 4. Release profiles of FITC-RGD-Ad and FITC-RGD from the cross-linked (**a**) $(SiO_2/PAH)_5/(PAH/HA\text{-}CD)_5/(PAH/DAS)_5$. (**b**) $(SiO_2/PAH)_{10}/(PAH/HA\text{-}CD)_5/(PAH/DAS)_5$ and (**c**) $(SiO_2/PAH)_{15}/(PAH/HA\text{-}CD)_5/(PAH/DAS)_5$ multilayer films. (**d**) The release time of FITC-RGD-Ad and FITC-RGD from different kinds of multilayer films.

It is well known that tyrosine (Y) is a hydrophobic amino acid. We infer that host-guest interactions between CD and Y will delay the release speed of Y-based peptide. For proof of concept, different kinds of multilayers were immersed into different solution of peptide, as shown in Figure 5.

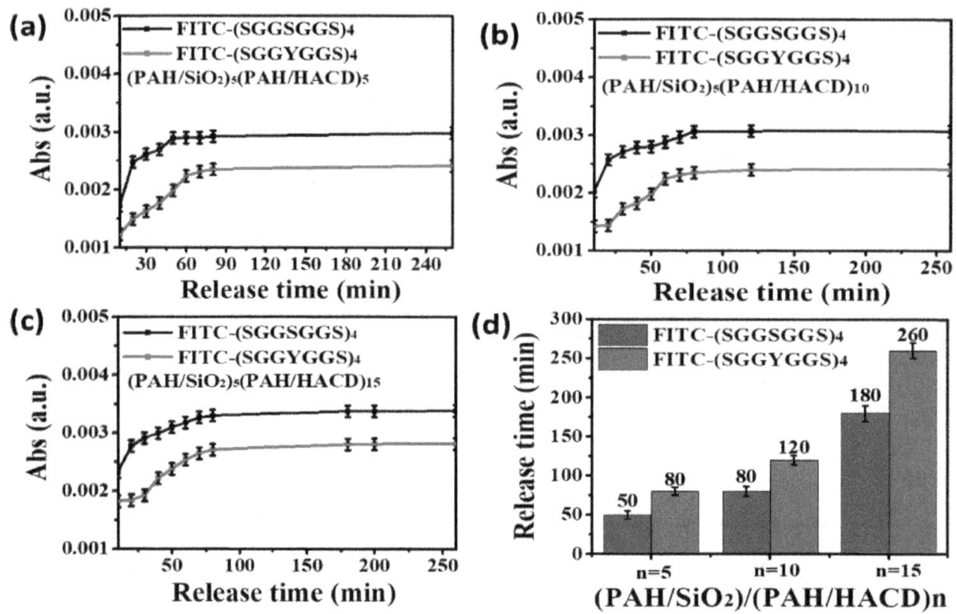

Figure 5. Release profiles of FITC-$(SGGSGGS)_4$ or FITC-$(SGGYGGS)_4$ from the cross-linked (**a**) $(SiO_2/PAH)_5/(PAH/HA\text{-}CD)_5/(PAH/DAS)_5$ (**b**) $(SiO_2/PAH)_5/(PAH/HA\text{-}CD)_{10}/(PAH/DAS)_5$ and (**c**) $(SiO_2/PAH)_5/(PAH/HA\text{-}CD)_{15}/(PAH/DAS)_5$ multilayer films. (**d**) The release time of FITC-RGD-Ad and FITC-RGD from different kinds of multilayer films.

As illustrated in Figure 5a, the release time of FITC-$(SGGYGGS)_4$ from $(SiO_2/PAH)_5(PAH/HA\text{-}CD)_5(PAH/DAS)_5$ is about 50 min. This is the time taken to obtain saturated release of fluorescent probe. For FITC-$(SGGSGGS)_4$ from $(SiO_2/PAH)_5(PAH/HA\text{-}CD)_5(PAH/DAS)_5$ this release time is 80 mins. As shown in Figure 5b, the release time of FITC-$(SGGYGGS)_4$ from $(SiO_2/PAH)_5(PAH/HA\text{-}CD)_{10}(PAH/DAS)_5$ is about 80 min and around 120 min for FITC-$(SGGYGGS)_4$ from $(SiO_2/PAH)_5(PAH/HA\text{-}CD)_{10}(PAH/DAS)_5$. Figure 5c shows that it takes around 180 min for the release of FITC-$(SGGSGGS)_4$ and 260 min for FITC-$(SGGYGGS)_4$ from $(SiO_2/PAH)_5(PAH/HA\text{-}CD)_{15}(PAH/DAS)_5$ multilayer films. The more the number of the multilayers in the film, the greater the host-guest interactions. By changing variables and adjusting parameters, it is proved that upon coming in contact with supramolecular forces, host-guest interactions between HA-CD and FITC-$(SGGYGGS)_4$ delayed the release speed of fluorescent molecules as shown in Figure 5.

4. Conclusions

In this study, a method has been developed which can raise the stability of multilayer films made up of polymer and inorganic nanoparticles. The covalently cross-linked super stratum was formed on outermost layer of the multilayer films so that the structure of multilayers can be stabilized. The super stratum acts as a nano-net which prevents the diffusion of the nanoparticles from the substrate. It is worth mentioning that the super stratum possesses permeability for small molecules like FITC-RGD, FITC-RGD-Ad, FITC-$(SGGYGGS)_4$ or FITC-$(SGGSGGS)_4$. The difference in permeability of the super stratum towards nanoparticles and small molecules is utilized to synthesize a functional system for drug delivery incorporating mesoporous silica as the molecule reservoir. The construction of functional multilayer films that incorporate inorganic nanoparticles has potential promotional value benefitting from the mild synthesis conditions of the super stratum.

Author Contributions: K.N., X.Y., N.K. and Y.Z. conceived and designed the experiments; K.N. conducted the experiments and analyzed the data; K.N. wrote the draft, and K.N., N.K. and X.Y. improved it.

Acknowledgments: This work was supported by the NSFC (21303169, 21673209) and the National Scholarship Fund of China Scholarship Council (CSC). I am very grateful to Jeffrey I. Zink and Navnita Kumar for helping me to polish and revise the paper. Navnita Kumar is a postdoctoral faculty in the Department of Chemistry and Biochemistry at University of California, Los Angeles (UCLA).

References

1. Manna, U.; Bharani, S.; Patil, S. Layer-by-Layer Self-Assembly of Modified Hyaluronic Acid/Chitosan Based on Hydrogen Bonding. *Biomacromolecules* **2009**, *10*, 2632–2639. [CrossRef]
2. Campbell, M.G.; Liu, Q.; Sanders, A.; Evans, J.S.; Smalyukh, I.I. Preparation of nanocomposite plasmonic films made from cellulose nanocrystals or mesoporous silica decorated with unidirectionally aligned gold nanorods. *Materials* **2014**, *7*, 3021–3033. [CrossRef]
3. Nie, K.; An, Q.; Tao, S.Y.; Zhang, Z.P.; Luan, X.L.; Zhang, Q.; Zhang, Y.H. Layer-by-layer reduced graphene oxide (rGO)/gold nanosheets (AuNSs) hybrid films: significantly enhanced photothermal transition effect compared with rGO or AuNSs films. *RSC Adv.* **2015**, *5*, 57389–57394. [CrossRef]
4. Anirudhan, T.S.; Vasantha, C.S.; Sasidharan, A.V. Layer-by-layer assembly of hyaluronic acid/carboxymethylchitosan polyelectrolytes on the surface of aminated mesoporous silica for the oral delivery of 5-fluorouracil. *Eur. Polym. J.* **2017**, *93*, 572–589. [CrossRef]
5. Wang, D.G.; Sheridan, M.V.; Shan, B.; Famum, B.H.; Marquard, S.L.; Sherman, B.D.; Eberhart, M.S.; Nayak, A.; Dares, C.J.; Das, A.K.; Bullock, R.M.; Meyer, T.J. Layer-by-Layer Molecular Assemblies for Dye-Sensitized Photoelectrosynthesis Cells Prepared by Atomic Layer Deposition. *J. Am. Chem. Soc.* **2017**, *139*, 14518–14525. [CrossRef]
6. Kang, E.H.; Bu, T.J.; Jin, P.C.; Sun, J.Q.; Yang, Y.Q.; Shen, J.C. Layer-by-layer deposited organic/inorganic hybrid multilayer films containing noncentrosymmetrically orientated azobenzene chromophores. *Langmuir* **2007**, *23*, 7594–7601. [CrossRef]
7. Wang, H.J.; Ishihara, S.; Ariga, K.; Yamauchi, Y. All-Metal Layer-by-Layer Films: Bimetallic Alternate Layers with Accessible Mesopores for Enhanced Electrocatalysis. *J. Am. Chem. Soc.* **2012**, *134*, 10819–10821. [CrossRef]
8. Nie, K.; An, Q.; Zhang, Y.H. A functional protein retention and release multilayer with high stability. *Nanoscale* **2016**, *8*, 8791–8797. [CrossRef]
9. Xu, Q.W.; Li, X.; Jin, Y.Y.; Sun, L.; Ding, X.X.; Liang, L.; Wang, L.; Nan, K.H.; Ji, J.; Chen, H.; Wang, B.L. Bacterial self-defense antibiotics release from organic-inorganic hybrid multilayer films for long-term anti-adhesion and biofilm inhibition properties. *Nanoscale* **2017**, *9*, 19245–19254. [CrossRef]
10. Slowing, I.I.; Vivero-Escoto, J.L.; Wu, C.W.; Lin, V.S.Y. Mesoporous silica nanoparticles as controlled release drug delivery and gene transfection carriers. *Adv. Drug Deliv. Rev.* **2008**, *60*, 1278–1288. [CrossRef]
11. Lau, H.H.; Murney, R.; Yakovlev, N.L.; Novoselova, M.V.; Lim, S.H.; Roy, N.; Singh, H.; Sukhorukov, G.B.; Haigh, B.; Kiryukhin, M.V. Protein-tannic acid multilayer films: A multifunctional material for microencapsulation of food-derived bioactives. *J. Colloid Interface Sci.* **2017**, *505*, 332–340. [CrossRef]
12. Nguyen, T.T.T.; Belbekhouche, S.; Dubot, P.; Carbonnier, B.; Grande, D. From the functionalization of polyelectrolytes to the development of a versatile approach to the synthesis of polyelectrolyte multilayer films with enhanced stability. *J. Mater. Chem. A* **2017**, *5*, 24472–24483. [CrossRef]
13. Jin, W.; Shi, X.Y.; Caruso, F. High activity enzyme microcrystal multilayer films. *J. Am. Chem. Soc.* **2001**, *123*, 8121–8122. [CrossRef]
14. Kanazawa, A.; Ikeda, T.; Abe, J. Supramolecular polar thin films built by surfactant liquid crystals: Polarization-tunable multilayer self-assemblies with in-plane ferroelectric ordering of ion-based dipoles. *J. Am. Chem. Soc.* **2001**, *123*, 1748–1754. [CrossRef]
15. Ma, R.Z.; Sasaki, T.; Bando, Y. Layer-by-layer assembled multilayer films of titanate nanotubes, Ag- or Au-loaded nanotubes, and nanotubes/nanosheets with polycations. *J. Am. Chem. Soc.* **2004**, *126*, 10382–10388. [CrossRef]
16. Ribeiro, T.; Baleizao, C.; Farinha, J.P.S. Functional films from silica/polymer nanoparticles. *Materials* **2014**, *7*, 3881–3900. [CrossRef]

17. Rest, C.; Kandanelli, R.; Fernandez, G. Strategies to create hierarchical self-assembled structures via cooperative non-covalent interactions. *Chem. Soc. Rev.* **2015**, *44*, 2543–2572. [CrossRef]
18. Sakata, S.; Inoue, Y.; Ishihara, K. Molecular Interaction Forces Generated during Protein Adsorption to Well-Defined Polymer Brush Surfaces. *Langmuir* **2015**, *31*, 3108–3114. [CrossRef]
19. Zhang, D.W.; Tian, J.; Chen, L.; Zhang, L.; Li, Z.T. Dimerization of Conjugated Radical Cations: An Emerging Non-Covalent Interaction for Self-Assembly. *Chem. Asian J.* **2015**, *10*, 56–68. [CrossRef]
20. Ma, X.X.; Mei, L.F.; Liu, H.K.; Liao, L.B.; Liu, Y.Q.; Nie, K.; Li, Z.H. Structure and fluorescent properties of Ba3Sc(PO4)(3):Sm3+ red-orange phosphor for n-UV w-LEDs. *Chem. Phys. Lett.* **2016**, *653*, 212–215. [CrossRef]
21. Steiner, C.; Gebhardt, J.; Ammon, M.; Yang, Z.C.; Heidenreich, A.; Hammer, N.; Gorling, A.; Kivala, M.; Maier, S. Hierarchical on-surface synthesis and electronic structure of carbonyl-functionalized one- and two-dimensional covalent nanoarchitectures. *Nat. Commun.* **2017**, *8*, 14765. [CrossRef]
22. Zhang, X.S.; Jiang, C.; Cheng, M.J.; Zhou, Y.; Zhu, X.Q.; Nie, J.; Zhang, Y.J.; An, Q.; Shi, F. Facile Method for the Fabrication of Robust Polyelectrolyte Multilayers by Post-Photo-Cross-Linking of Azido Groups. *Langmuir* **2012**, *28*, 7096–7100. [CrossRef]
23. Nguyen, H.D.; Dang, D.T.; van Dongen, J.L.J.; Brunsveld, L. Protein Dimerization Induced by Supramolecular Interactions with Cucurbit[8]uril. *Angew. Chem. Int. Edit.* **2010**, *49*, 895–898. [CrossRef]
24. Boraste, D.R.; Chakraborty, G.; Ray, A.K.; Shankarling, G.S.; Pal, H. Supramolecular host-guest interaction of antibiotic drug ciprofloxacin with cucurbit[7]uril macrocycle: Modulations in photophysical properties and enhanced photostability. *J. Photoch. Photobio. Chem.* **2018**, *358*, 26–37. [CrossRef]
25. Conesa-Egea, J.; Redondo, C.D.; Martinez, J.I.; Gomez-Garcia, C.J.; Castillo, O.; Zamora, F.; Amo-Ochoa, P. Supramolecular Interactions Modulating Electrical Conductivity and Nanoprocessing of Copper-Iodine Double-Chain Coordination Polymers. *Inorg. Chem.* **2018**, *57*, 7568–7577. [CrossRef]
26. Lee, H.Y.; Park, S.H.; Kim, J.H.; Kim, M.S. Temperature-responsive hydrogels via the electrostatic interaction of amphiphilic diblock copolymers with pendant-ion groups. *Polymer Chem.* **2017**, *8*, 6606–6616. [CrossRef]
27. Derbenev, I.N.; Filippov, A.V.; Stace, A.J.; Besley, E. Electrostatic interactions between charged dielectric particles in an electrolyte solution: constant potential boundary conditions. *Soft Matter* **2018**, *14*, 5480–5487. [CrossRef]
28. Mishra, A.K.; Weissman, H.; Krieg, E.; Votaw, K.A.; McCullagh, M.; Rybtchinski, B.; Lewis, F.D. Self-Assembly of Perylenediimide-Single-Strand-DNA Conjugates: Employing Hydrophobic Interactions and DNA Base-Pairing To Create a Diverse Structural Space. *Chem. Eur. J.* **2017**, *23*, 10328–10337. [CrossRef]
29. Moon, S.; Park, S.O.; Ahn, Y.H.; Kim, H.; Shin, E.; Hong, S.; Lee, Y.; Kwak, S.K.; Park, Y. Distinct hydrophobic-hydrophilic dual interactions occurring in the clathrate hydrates of 3,3-dimethyl-1-butanol with help gases. *Chem. Eng. J.* **2018**, *348*, 583–591. [CrossRef]
30. Shumilova, T.A.; Ruffer, T.; Lang, H.; Kataev, E.A. Straightforward Design of Fluorescent Receptors for Sulfate: Study of Non-Covalent Interactions Contributing to Host-Guest Formation. *Chem. Eur. J.* **2018**, *24*, 1500–1504. [CrossRef]
31. Xue, F.C.; Wang, Y.Q.; Zhang, Q.X.; Han, S.L.; Zhang, F.Z.; Jin, T.T.; Li, C.W.; Hu, H.Y.; Zhang, J.X. Self-assembly of affinity-controlled nanoparticles via host-guest interactions for drug delivery. *Nanoscale* **2018**, *10*, 12364–12377. [CrossRef]
32. Furchner, A.; Kroning, A.; Rauch, S.; Uhlmann, P.; Eichhorn, K.J.; Hinrichs, K. Molecular Interactions and Hydration States of Ultrathin Functional Films at the Solid-Liquid Interface. *Anal. Chem.* **2017**, *89*, 3240–3244. [CrossRef]
33. Palao, E.; Sola-Llano, R.; Tabero, A.; Manzano, H.; Agarrabeitia, A.R.; Villanueva, A.; Lopez-Arbeloa, I.; Martinez-Martinez, V.; Ortiz, M.J. Acetylacetonate BODIPY-Biscyclometalated Iridium(III) Complexes: Effective Strategy towards Smarter Fluorescent Photosensitizer Agents. *Chem. Eur. J.* **2017**, *23*, 10139–10147. [CrossRef]
34. Schwenck, J.; Maier, F.C.; Kneilling, M.; Wiehr, S.; Fuchs, K. Non-invasive In Vivo Fluorescence Optical Imaging of Inflammatory MMP Activity Using an Activatable Fluorescent Imaging Agent. *Jove-J. Vis. Exp.* **2017**, *123*, e55180. [CrossRef]
35. Luan, L.; Lin, Z.J.; Wu, G.H.; Huang, X.L.; Cai, Z.M.; Chen, X. Encoding electrochemiluminescence using $Ru(bpy)(_3)(^{2+})$ and fluorescein isothiocyanate co-doped silica nanoparticles. *Chem. Commun.* **2011**, *47*, 3963–3965. [CrossRef]

36. Tang, A.M.; Mei, B.; Wang, W.J.; Hu, W.L.; Li, F.; Zhou, J.; Yang, Q.; Cui, H.; Wu, M.; Liang, G.L. FITC-quencher based caspase 3-activatable nanoprobes for effectively sensing caspase 3 in vitro and in cells. *Nanoscale* **2013**, *5*, 8963–8967. [CrossRef]
37. Tay, A.; Sohrabi, A.; Poole, K.; Seidlits, S.; Di Carlo, D. A 3D Magnetic Hyaluronic Acid Hydrogel for Magnetomechanical Neuromodulation of Primary Dorsal Root Ganglion Neurons. *Adv. Mater.* **2018**, *30*, 1800927. [CrossRef]
38. Souchek, J.J.; Wojtynek, N.E.; Payne, W.M.; Holmes, M.B.; Dutta, S.; Qi, B.W.; Datta, K.; LaGrange, C.A.; Mohs, A.M. Hyaluronic acid formulation of near infrared fluorophores optimizes surgical imaging in a prostate tumor xenograft. *Acta Biomater.* **2018**, *75*, 323–333. [CrossRef]
39. Hunt, J.A.; Joshi, H.N.; Stella, V.J.; Topp, E.M. Diffusion and Drug Release in Polymer-Films Prepared from Ester Derivatives of Hyaluronic-Acid. *J. Control. Release* **1990**, *12*, 159–169. [CrossRef]
40. Pitarresi, G.; Palumbo, F.S.; Albanese, A.; Fiorica, C.; Picone, P.; Giammona, G. Self-assembled amphiphilic hyaluronic acid graft copolymers for targeted release of antitumoral drug. *J. Drug Target* **2010**, *18*, 264–276. [CrossRef]
41. Ramamurthy, V.; Jockusch, S.; Pore, M. Supramolecular Photochemistry in Solution and on Surfaces: Encapsulation and Dynamics of Guest Molecules and Communication between Encapsulated and Free Molecules. *Langmuir* **2015**, *31*, 5554–5570. [CrossRef]
42. Mondal, P.; Rath, S.P. Efficient Host-Guest Complexation of a Bisporphyrin Host with Electron Deficient Guests: Synthesis, Structure, and Photoinduced Electron Transfer. *Isr. J. Chem.* **2016**, *56*, 144–155. [CrossRef]
43. Kanagaraj, K.; Pitchumani, K. The Aminocyclodextrin/Pd(OAc)(2) Complex as an Efficient Catalyst for the Mizoroki-Heck Cross-Coupling Reaction. *Chem. Eur. J.* **2013**, *19*, 14425–14431. [CrossRef]
44. Kaur, N.; Garg, T.; Goyal, A.K.; Rath, G. Formulation, optimization and evaluation of curcumin-β-cyclodextrin-loaded sponge for effective drug delivery in thermal burns chemotherapy. *Drug Deliv.* **2016**, *23*, 2245–2254. [CrossRef]
45. Nakahata, M.; Takashima, Y.; Yamaguchi, H.; Harada, A. Redox-responsive self-healing materials formed from host-guest polymers. *Nat. Commun.* **2011**, *2*, 511. [CrossRef]
46. Wei, S.J.; Chu, H.M.; Xu, L.S.; Wang, Z.Z.; Huang, Q. Macrocyclic drug conjugates of metronidazole-cyclodextrin for colon-targeted delivery. *J. Control. Release* **2017**, *259*, E120–E121. [CrossRef]
47. Parlati, S.; Gobetto, R.; Barolo, C.; Arrais, A.; Buscaino, R.; Medana, C.; Savarino, P. Preparation and application of a beta-cyclodextrin-disperse/reactive dye complex. *J. Incl. Phenom. Macrocycl. Chem.* **2007**, *57*, 463–470. [CrossRef]
48. Nie, K.; An, Q.; Zink, J.I.; Yu, X.; Zhang, Y.H. Layer by Layer Mesoporous Silica-Hyaluronic Acid-Cyclodextrin Bifunctional "Lamination": Study of the Application of Fluorescent Probe and Host-Guest Interactions in the Drug Delivery Field. *Materials* **2018**, *11*, 1745. [CrossRef]
49. Trebosc, J.; Wiench, J.W.; Huh, S.; Lin, V.S.Y.; Pruski, M. Solid-state NMR study of MCM-41-type mesoporous silica nanoparticles. *J. Am. Chem. Soc.* **2005**, *127*, 3057–3068. [CrossRef]

7

Controlled Delivery of Insulin-like Growth Factor-1 from Bioactive Glass-Incorporated Alginate-Poloxamer/Silk Fibroin Hydrogels

Qing Min [1,†], Xiaofeng Yu [2,†], Jiaoyan Liu [2], Yuchen Zhang [1], Ying Wan [2,*] and Jiliang Wu [1,*]

1 School of Pharmacy, Hubei University of Science and Technology, Xianning 437100, China; baimin0628@hbust.edu.cn (Q.M.); zhangych@hbust.edu.cn (Y.Z.)

2 College of Life Science and Technology, Huazhong University of Science and Technology, Wuhan 430074, China; m201771729@hust.edu.cn (X.Y.); liujiaoyan@hust.edu.cn (J.L.)

* Correspondence: ying_wan@hust.edu.cn (Y.W.); jlwu@hbust.edu.cn (J.W.)

† These authors contributed equally to this work.

Abstract: Thermosensitive alginate–poloxamer (ALG–POL) copolymer with an optimal POL content was synthesized, and it was used to combine with silk fibroin (SF) for building ALG–POL/SF hydrogels with dual network structure. Mesoporous bioactive glass (BG) nanoparticles (NPs) with a high level of mesoporosity and large pore size were prepared and they were employed as a vehicle for loading insulin-like growth factor-1 (IGF-1). IGF-1-loaded BG NPs were embedded into ALG–POL/SF hydrogels to achieve the controlled delivery of IGF-1. The resulting IGF-1-loaded BG/ALG–POL/SF gels were found to be injectable with their sol-gel transition near physiological temperature and pH. Rheological measurements showed that BG/ALG–POL/SF gels had their elastic modulus higher than 5kPa with large ratio of elastic modulus to viscous modulus, indicative of their mechanically strong features. The dry BG/ALG–POL/SF gels were seen to be highly porous with well-interconnected pore characteristics. The gels loaded with varied amounts of IGF-1 showed abilities to administer IGF-1 release in approximately linear manners for a few weeks while effectively preserving the bioactivity of encapsulated IGF-1. Results suggest that such constructed BG/ALG–POL/SF gels can function as a promising injectable biomaterial for bone tissue engineering applications.

Keywords: alginate–poloxamer copolymer; silk fibroin; dual network hydrogel; mesoporous bioactive glass; insulin-like growth factor-1

---

1. Introduction

The extracellular matrix (ECM) is the noncellular component presenting within all tissues and organs, and it usually has three-dimensional porous architecture. It provides not only essential physical scaffolding for the cellular constituents but also initiates crucial processes that are required for tissue morphogenesis, differentiation, and homeostasis [1]. Each tissue has its own ECM with a unique composition and topology, generated during tissue development [2]. Cells interact with biochemical and biophysical cues in their ECM in highly dynamic and reciprocal manners, and such cell–ECM interactions play a critical role in cell behavior mediation, cell function normality and even cell fate decisions, involving quite complicated processes from quiescence to activation and progenitor state to terminal differentiation [1,2]. Accordingly, it is pivotal to harness the interactions between ECM and the resident cells in developing strategies for effectively regenerating tissue or regulating disease [1,2]. To data, many kinds of hard biomaterials have been employed in tissue engineering for various purposes, but their applications in ECM biomimicry have been limited because these hard biomaterials are lack of ability to adequately mimic the structure and properties of ECM in body tissues [3]. Polymer hydrogels, which behave like soft and elastic objects, are usually constructed by physically or chemically crosslinked macromolecules. They contain large amounts of water while having highly porous architecture with tailorable physiochemical properties and easy diffusivity of small molecules. These features make them attractive candidates for mimicking the dynamic ECM [3,4].

Injectable polymer hydrogels having in situ gelling properties under physiological conditions have received a great deal of attention in tissue engineering owing to their two advantageous characteristics [5]. One is that they can be conveniently used to deliver cells, bioactive compounds, and therapeutic drugs alone or in combination by simply mixing these consignments with polymer solutions prior to gelation; and another is that they can be injected to the defect site via minimally invasive surgery followed by formation into solid-like fillers with discretional shapes [5,6]. Nowadays, varied kinds of natural polymers have been commonly used in the form of hydrogels. Among them, alginate has been extensively investigated for its hydrogel applications. Physically crosslinked alginate hydrogels can be easily built by using certain divalent cations, typically calcium ions (Ca^{2+}), as a crosslinker. Despite the convenience of preparation, so constructed alginate hydrogels often undergo progressive disintegration in vivo due to the ionic exchange between Ca^{2+} in the gels and monovalent cations (such as Na^+ and K^+) coming from the host tissue surrounding the applied gels, which often results in their unstable dimension and uncontrolled properties [7,8]. Another type of physically crosslinked alginate hydrogel was engineered by grafting a type of thermosensitive polymer, poloxamer (Pluronic F127), onto alginate backbone, and the sol-gel transition of alginate–poloxamer (ALG–POL) hydrogels can be trigged by thermosensitive action arisen from the poloxamer component [9]. Despite easy-handled and safe advantages, ALG–POL gels appear to be weak and brittle in nature, and are apt to disintegrate due to its high percentage of Pluronic F127 [10]. Thus, ALG–POL gels are incompetent for certain applications in cartilage or bone tissue engineering where sufficient strength and persistent dimension stability are concomitantly required.

Many studies have revealed that hydrogels with dual or multiple networks could be largely enhanced in their stability and mechanical performance when compared to the single network gel [11]. In spite of the mentioned advantages, multiple network gels are not all suitable for tissue engineering applications as they are usually fabricated via chemical crosslinking, and the involved crosslinking reactions could possibly impair the loaded cells or the host tissue surrounding the applied gel [5,12]. Silk fibroin (SF) is a kind of natural fibrous protein and it can be processed into hydrogels via enzyme-catalyzed crosslinking of amino acid phenolic groups by the aid of H_2O_2, and the obtained SF hydrogels show tunable strength and elasticity [13]. In the case of in vivo usage, the applied amount of H_2O_2 for crosslinking SF gels has to be controlled at a safe level since the resulting SF gels could be cytotoxic if the applied dose of H_2O_2 is higher than certain thresholds [14]. As a result, so prepared SF gels were usually weak [15]. Taking into account the gelable characteristics of ALG–POL and SF through their respectively independent gelling mechanisms, it is feasible to construct a new type of ALG–POL/SF gel with dual network structure while having enhanced performance.

Some growth factors have been proved to be highly effective for promoting bone repair, especially taking advantage of the controlled factor release by way of proper carriers [16]. Among various kinds of growth factors, insulin-like growth factor-1 (IGF-1) is considered to be crucial for longitudinal bone growth, skeletal maturation, and bone mass acquisition not only in the bone growth phase of young individuals but also in the maintenance of bone in adult life [17]. In the situation of bone repair, in addition to promoting cell proliferation and matrix synthesis, the applied IGF-1 at the defect site can also induce the chemotactic migration of osteoblasts to the repair site via local concentration gradients established by factor diffusion [18]. Like many other growth factors, IGF-1 has a short half-life when exposed to the circulatory system [19]. Therefore, when the need arises to maintain sustained release of IGF-1 at the local site in vivo, one of the practical strategies for its administration is to encapsulate IGF-1 into certain vehicles to preserve its activity while managing to modulate its dose and action duration. It is generally realized that directly encapsulating growth factors into hydrogels would result in their burst release because hydrogels commonly have rather porous structures with high water content [7,20]. It has been suggested that release kinetics of growth factors delivered by a hydrogel system could be mediated to varied degrees by encapsulating the growth factor into certain microcarriers such as microspheres (MPs) and nanoparticles (NPs) first, and then, embedding the factor-loaded microcarrier into the hydrogel system [20–22].

Bioactive glasses (BGs) have now been widely used as an attractive inorganic biomaterial for bone repair since they have the ability to strongly bond bone tissue via a hydroxycarbonate apatite interface layer with composition and function similar to naturally occurring bone hydroxyapatite [23]. Mesoporous BG microspheres or nanoparticles can also serve as a reservoir for delivering therapeutic drugs or bioactive molecules besides their functions for acting as bone repair material [24]. In addition to regular BG MPs or NPs, many of them have been doped with different kinds of compounds, and their ionic dissolution products are capable of inducing osteogenesis or angiogenesis at the bone defect site, depending on the variety of doped elements [25]. In this context, it would be rational to load IGF-1 into porous BG NPs, and then, to incorporate the IGF-1-loaded BG NPs into above mentioned dual network ALG–POL/SF gels. On the basis of such designed strategy, a multifunctional composite hydrogel system with mechanically strong features and capabilities for administering the release of IGF-1 could be obtained. In this study, an attempt was made to achieve this goal. Some formulated IGF-loaded BG/ALG–POL/SF gels were found to be injectable and mechanically strong, and to have affirmative abilities to control the release of IGF-1 while preserving its bioactivity.

2. Materials and Methods

2.1. Materials

Sodium alginate (ALG, M_n: 1.3×10^5 Da), Poloxamer 407 (POL, M_n: 12,600 Da), 1-ethyl-3-(3-dimethylaminopropyl)-carbodiimide (EDC), horseradish peroxidase (HRP), and *N*-hydroxyl succinimide (NHS) were procured from Aladdin Inc (Shanghai, China). Recombinant human IGF-1 and IGF-1 enzyme-linked immunosorbent assay (ELISA) Kit were purchased from PeproTech Inc (Cranbury, NJ, USA) and R&D systems (Minneapolis, MN, USA), respectively. Other reagents and chemicals were of analytical grade and purchased from Sinopharm Inc (Shanghai, China).

SF was produced using Bombyx Mori cocoons according to the reported method [15]. Cocoons were degummed in a Na_2CO_3 solution (0.02 M) at 100 °C for 30 min, and the retrieved silk fibers were rinsed with ultrapure water followed by drying in a ventilated hood. The obtained SF fibers were then dissolved in a LiBr solution (9.3 M) at 60 °C with stirring for 5 h, and the prepared solution was dialyzed against distilled water for 2 days using membrane tubes (MW cutoff: 3500) to remove impurities. The achieved dilute SF solution was further concentrated to varied concentrations by immersing the solution-loaded membrane tubes in a 50% PEG20000 solution, and the concentrated SF solutions were stored at 4 °C for further use.

2.2. Synthesis of Alginate-Poloxamer Copolymers

A two-step method was used to synthesize alginate–poloxamer (ALG–POL) copolymers. POL was first modified into monoamine-terminated POL (MATP) following reported methods [26,27], and the obtained MAPT was then grafted onto alginate at a fixed feed mass ratio of alginate to MATP at 1:30 to achieve alginate–poloxamer copolymers. Details for the synthesis of MATP and ALG–POL can be found in the Supplementary Materials.

2.3. Preparation of Bioactive Mesoporous Glasses

Two kinds of porous mesoporous BG NPs (named as MBG-1 and MBG-2, respectively) with different pore-sizes were prepared following reported methods. MBG-1 NPs were prepared as follows [28]. One gram of hexadecyl-trimethylammonium bromide was dissolved in an emulsion consisted of 150 mL of H_2O, 2 mL of aqueous ammonia, 40 mL of ethyl ether, 20 mL of ethanol, and 0.1125 g of calcium nitrate ($Ca(NO_3)_2 \cdot 4H_2O$). 600 μL of tetraethyl orthosilicate (TEOS) was then added to the mixture at a molar Ca/Si ratio of 15:85. After stirring at 30 °C for 4 h, the white sediment was collected by filtration, washed with distilled water, and dried in air at 60 °C, and finally, calcined at 550 °C for 5 h. The same method was used to prepare MBG-2 NPs with slight modification [29]. The above prepared emulsion was vigorously stirred at room temperature for 30 min, and then, 600 μL of TEOS was added with vigorous stirring at 30 °C for 4 h. The resulting precipitate was collected and processed in the same way as that applied to MBG-1 NPs. Parameters for these BG NPs are given in Table 1.

Table 1. Parameters for bioactive glass (BG) nanoparticles.

Sample Name	Surface Area (m^2/g)	Pore Volume (mL/g)	Pore Size (nm)	ζ-Potential (mV)	Particle Size (nm)	PDI
MBG-1	562.4 ± 10.2	0.49 ± 0.02	6.1 ± 0.13	−14.9 ± 0.5	227.2 ± 10.3	0.11
MBG-2	498.3 ± 9.4	0.61 ± 0.03	10.3 ± 0.18	−17.1 ± 0.7	264.7 ± 12.1	0.13

Several IGF-1 solutions in PBS (pH 7.4) with varied concentration of 50 ng/mL (low dose), 100 ng/mL (medium dose), and 150 ng/mL (high dose) were first prepared. In a typical preparation process, 1 mL of any IGF-1 solutions was introduced into a vial with inner protein-resistant coating, and 10 mg of blank MBG-1 or MBG-2 NPs was then added. The mixture was allowed to incubate overnight on an orbital shaker at 37 °C. The IGF-1-loaded BG NPs were collected by centrifugation and washed with PBS followed by freeze-drying. The amount of IGF-1 loaded in BG NPs was measured basing on the difference of IGF-1 concentrations in the loading medium before and after soaking BG NPs by using IGF-1 ELISA Kit. Loading efficiency (LE) of BG NPs was calculated by the following equation:

$$\mathrm{LE}(\%) = (M_0/M_1) \times 100\% \tag{1}$$

where M_0 is the mass of IGF-1 encapsulated inside NPs, and M_1 is the feed mass of IGF-1. Parameters for the IGF-1oaded BG NPs are provided in Table 2.

Table 2. Parameters for insulin-like growth factor-1 (IGF-1)-loaded BG nanoparticles.

Sample Name	Feed Amount of IGF-1 (ng/mL)	Particle Size (nm)	PDI	ζ-Potential (mV)	LE (%)
BS1 (a)	50	229.1 ± 11.4	0.14	−10.3 ± 0.5	38.6 ± 1.7
BS2	100	230.4 ± 12.6	0.18	−9.1 ± 0.6	46.1 ± 2.1
BS3	150	232.7 ± 10.8	0.19	−8.6 ± 0.3	48.5 ± 2.5
BL1 (b)	50	265.3 ± 11.35	0.17	−10.5 ± 0.5	45.9 ± 2.4
BL2	100	268.2 ± 12.46	0.16	−8.1 ± 0.4	57.2 ± 1.9
BL3	150	267.9 ± 13.14	0.18	−7.2 ± 0.6	61.4 ± 2.3

(a) BS*i* (i = 1, 2 and 3) sample set was prepared using blank MBG-1 NPs. (b) BL*j* (j = 1, 2 and 3) sample set was prepared using blank MBG-2 NPs.

2.4. Preparation of Hydrogels

IGF-1-free composite solutions were prepared using ALG–POL, SF solution and blank BG NPs and they were used to construct blank BG/ALG–POL/SF gels for their compositional and structural optimization in order to save costly IGF-1. Some composite solutions containing IGF-1 were also prepared by directly adding IGF-1 or incorporating IGF-1-loaded BG NPs into the aqueous ALG–POL/SF mixture. These solutions were further processed into gels by incubating them in a water bath at 37 °C. The major parameters for them are summarized in Tables 3 and 4, respectively.

Table 3. Parameters for BG/alginate–poloxamer (ALG–POL)/silk fibroin (SF) hydrogels without factor loading [(a)].

Sample Name	SF (wt%)	ALG–POL (wt%)	Blank MBG-2 NPs (wt%) [(b)]	H_2O_2 (μL) [(c)]	HRP (μL) [(d)]	pH	Gelation Time (min) [(d)]	T_i (°C)
G-A	7.0	5.0	–	10	10	7.06 ± 0.09	11.75 ± 0.96	36.1 ± 0.42
G-B	7.0	5.0	1.0	10	10	7.13 ± 0.06	10.5 ± 1.29	35.2 ± 0.57
G-C	7.0	5.0	2.0	10	10	7.11 ± 0.07	9.75 ± 0.96	34.6 ± 0.49

(a) The full volume of solutions: 2mL. (b) See Table 1 for their parameters. (c) Concentration of H_2O_2: 500 mmol/L. (d) Concentration of HRP: 1000 U/mL. (e) Gelation time was determined by inverting vial every 1 min.

Table 4. Parameters for IGF-loaded BG/ALG–POL/SF hydrogels.

Sample Name	SF (wt%)	ALG–POL (wt%)	IGF-1-Loaded MBG-2 NPs (wt%) [(b)]	H_2O_2 (μL) [(c)]	HRP (μL) [(d)]	IGF-1 Content in Gel (ng/mL)
GEL-1 [(a)]	7.0	5.0	–	10	10	154.2 ± 11.27
GEL-2	7.0	5.0	–	10	10	512.9 ± 16.35
GEL-3	7.0	5.0	1.0	10	10	160.3 ± 10.84
GEL-4	7.2	5.0	2.0	10	10	520.7 ± 19.52

(a) GEL-1 and GEL-2 were directly loaded with prescribed amounts of IGF-1 for making comparisons. (b) IGF-1 load inside MBG-2 NPs was regulated by changing the IGF-1feed amount. (c) and (d) See Table 3 for their concentrations.

Gelation time was assessed using the inverted tube testing method. Typically, one of the IGF-1-free composite solutions (2.0 mL) was introduced into a glass vial and it was stirred in an ice/water bath for 5 min before being gelled. Fluidity of the composite solution was checked by regularly inverting the vial, and gelation time was recorded starting from the beginning of vial incubation in the water bath and ending at the point when the solution stopped flowing.

2.5. Characterization

Fourier transform infrared (FTIR) spectra of samples were performed on a spectrometer (Vertex 70, Bruker, Ettlingen, Germany). ^{1}H NMR spectra were recorded on a NMR spectrometer (Ascend TM 600 MHz, Bruker, Rheinstetten, Germany). The weight percentage of POL in ALG–POL copolymers was determined using an elemental analyzer (Vario EL III, Elementar, Hanau, Germany). The morphology of BG NPs was viewed with a transmission electron microscope (TEM, Tecnai G2, FEI, Hillsboro, OR, USA). Hydrodynamic size and zeta (ζ) potential of BG NPs were measured using a dynamic light scattering (DLS) instrument (Nano-ZS90, Malvern Instruments, Worcestershire, UK). A mass of BG NPs (100–150 mg) were dried for 12 h at 120 °C and degassed for 24 h at 200 °C under vacuum. The volume of nitrogen adsorbed and desorbed at different relative gas pressures was measured using a surface area and pore size analyzer (ASAP 2020 Plus, Micromeritics, Norcross, GA, USA), and it was then utilized to construct adsorption–desorption isotherms. The specific surface area was determined with the Brunauer–Emmett–Teller (BET) method. The pore volume and the mean pore size were derived from the adsorption branches of the isotherms using the Barrett–Joyner–Halanda (BJH) method. The porous cross-section structure of dry gels was examined by scanning electron microscopy (SEM, Quanta 200, FEI, Eindhoven, Netherlands). Dry gel samples with known weight (Wd, g) were immersed in PBS at 37 °C till they attained equilibrium, and their wet weight (Ws, g) was measured after removal of excess surface water with filter paper. Swelling index (SI) of gels was calculated using the following formula:

$$\mathrm{SI\ (g/g)} = (W_s - W_d)/W_d \tag{2}$$

2.6. Rheological Analysis

Rheological measurements of fluids or hydrogels were carried out using a rheometer (Kinexus Pro KNX2100, Southborough, MA, USA) equipped with a parallel-plate sample holder. The temperature sweep curve was recorded in the range of 25 to 45 °C by heating liquid samples at a rate of 1 °C/min, and the incipient gelling temperature (T_i) of liquid samples was determined at the intersection point of storage modulus (G′) and loss modulus (G″). Isothermal frequency sweep experiments were conducted using hydrogel discs (10 mm in diameter and ca. 4 mm in height) prepared with a punch, and the obtained data were plotted as a function of modulus versus frequency at predefined strain amplitude of 1%. Shear viscosity of liquid samples was measured at 23 °C in a shear rate range between 0.1/s and 400/s.

2.7. Release of IGF-1

In vitro IGF-1 release profiles for IGF-1-loaded MBG-1 and MBG-2 NPs were first tested to find out their difference in release rates. Measurements were conducted using several sets of eppendorf tubes, each filled with 500 µL PBS containing 1% (*w/v*) bovine serum albumin. To each eppendorf tube, 5 mg of IGF-I-loaded MBG-1 or MBG-2 NPs was added, and all sets of tubes were incubated in a shaking water bath at 37 °C and 60 rpm for various periods up to 6 days. At predetermined time intervals, eppendorf tubes were withdrawn by group and they were centrifuged for 5 min at around 1000 g to collect supernatants. The release amount of IGF-I was determined using IGF-1 ELISA kit.

In the case of IGF-1 release from gel samples, some cylindrical gel samples were first produced. Each (0.5 mL) of IGF-1-loaded composite solutions (see Table 4) was filled into a cylindrical mold (diameter: 10 mm) and incubated at 37 °C for 20 min for gel formation. The gel samples were then introduced into different vials filled with 3 mL of PBS, and the vials were vortexed on a shaking table at 37 °C and 60 rpm. At prescribed time points, 1 mL of medium was withdrawn with replenishing the same volume of fresh buffer. The released amount of IGF-1 was measured using IGF-1 ELISA Kit.

2.8. Bioactivity of Released IGF-1

The IGF-1's ability to promote the proliferation of osteoblasts was tested to access the bioactivity of released IGF-1 [30–32]. MC3T3-E1 cells (Type Culture Collection of the Chinese Academy of Sciences, Shanghai, China) were used as testing cells. Cells were expanded in DMEM supplemented with 10% fetal bovine serum, 1% penicillin/streptomycin in a 5% CO_2 humidified atmosphere at 37 °C. The expanded cells were resuspended in PBS for further use.

Cells were cultured in 96-well plates at a density of 5×10^4 cells/well in complete culture medium at 37 °C for 24 h. The cells were serum-starved for 24 h, after which the media was replaced with either serum-free media (denoted as control, 0 ng/mL), serum-free media with free IGF-1 (5 or 50 ng/mL), or serum-free media with released IGF-1 (5 or 50 ng/mL). The cells were cultured for varied durations up to 72 h, and their proliferation was determined by 3-(4,5-dimethyl-2-thiazolyl)-2,5-diphenyl-2-H-tetrazolium bromide (MTT, Dojindo, Japan) essay. Briefly, the media was aspirated from the 96-well plates after the prescribed culture period, and a 20 µL aliquot of MTT stock solution and 200 µL of serum-free medium was added to each well. After being further cultured for 4 h, the media was removed from the wells, and 150 µL of DMSO was added to each well with shaking at 37 °C for 15 min. After that, the optical density (OD) was determined at 590 nm using a microplate reader (PerkinElmer Inc, USA).

Cells were also cultured on the surface of gels for making further comparison. Briefly, two kinds of IGF-1-contained composite solutions with their compositions respectively matching with GEL-2 and GEL-4 gels (see Table 4), 200 µL apiece, were pipetted into wells of 24-well plates, and cultured at 37 °C for gel formation. Subsequently, volume of MC3T3-E1 cell suspension (100 µL) was added to each well (5×10^4 cells/well), and cells were then cultured with serum-free media (500 µL) at 37 °C for varied periods up to 72 h. Cell proliferation was assessed by OD measurement using above described MTT assay. Cell cultured under monolayer condition in serum-free media (0 ng/mL) without exposing to gels were used as control.

2.9. Statistical Analysis

Data were presented as mean ± standard deviation. Analysis of the difference between groups was performed using one-way ANOVA. The statistical difference was considered to be significant when the p-value was less than 0.05.

3. Results and Discussions

3.1. Analysis of ALG–POL

ALG–POL copolymer was synthesized by grafting MAPT onto the ALG backbone through EDC/NHS chemistry. Figure 1 presents a schematic illustration to show the synthesis route for MAPT and ALG–POL copolymer. A representative NMR spectrum for MAPT is provided in Figure S1 in which the typical peaks respectively assigning to methyl and methylene confirm the successful synthesis of MAPT. The preliminary experimental results indicated that the composition of ALG–POL exerted significant effects on the thermoresponsivity, degradation tolerance, and strength of resulting ALG–POL/SF gels. Accordingly, the proportion of ALG and POL components in ALG–POL copolymer was optimized via orthogonal design method. By changing the ratio of MATP to ALG in a range between 20 and 35 at a step size of 5 during the synthesis of ALG–POL copolymers, one of ALG–POL copolymers was thus screened out by setting the MATP/ALG ratio at 30. The POL content in such optimized ALG–POL copolymer was thus measured to be around 66 wt% via elemental analysis. Figure S2 presents FTIR spectra for POL, ALG and ALG–POL. The spectrum of POL is characterized by three typical bands at 2891 (C–H stretch aliphatic), 1345 (in-plane O-H bend) and 1112 cm^{-1} (C–O stretching). The ALG spectrum shows specific absorbance bands of its COOH stretching at 1610 cm^{-1} and C–O–C stretching at 1305 cm^{-1} [33], respectively. In the spectrum for ALG–POL, the carbonyl absorption band for carboxylate sodium salt originally showing in the ALG spectrum disappeared while a new characteristic amide I band appeared at around 1637 cm^{-1}, suggesting that amide bonds have formed between ALG and POL [9,33]. FTIR spectra demonstrate that the ALG–POL copolymer has been successfully synthesized.

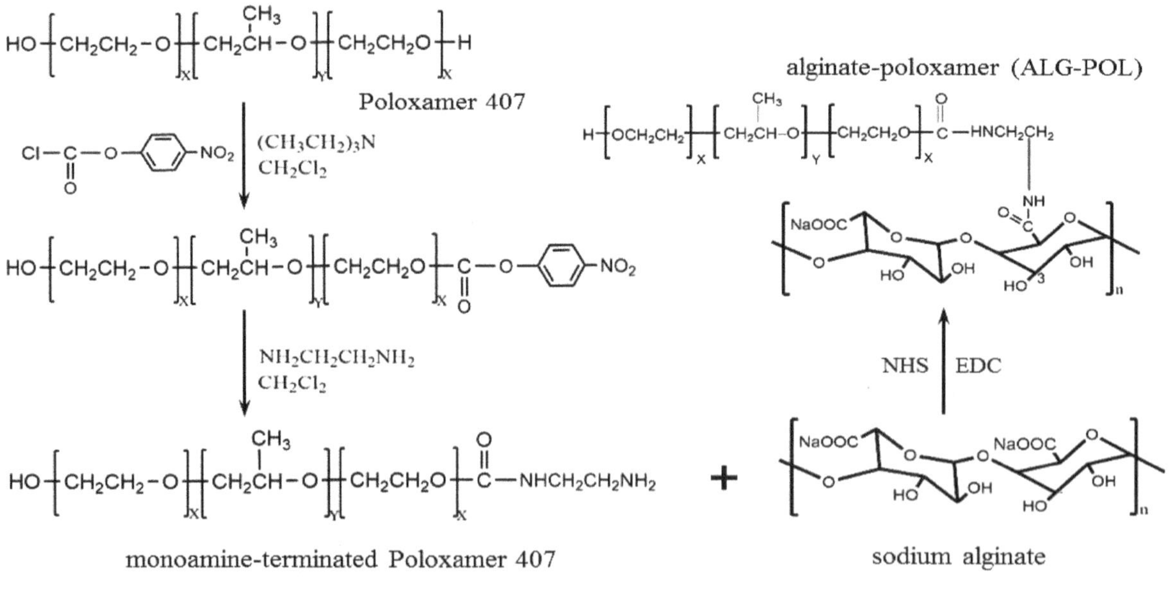

Figure 1. Schematic illustration for synthesis of alginate-poloxamer copolymer.

3.2. Parameters for Mesoporous BG Nanoparticles

Two kinds of mesoporous BG NPs were produced under slightly different processing conditions in order to attain certain BG NPs having proper pore-sizes and pore volumes for gaining high LE. Panels A and B in Figure 2 display two typical TEM micrographs for the prepared BG NPs, and these spherical BG NPs were seen to be porous with their size of about 200 nm. A mass of BG NPs were measured for their average particle size and ζ-potential, and relevant data are listed in Table 1. There were significant differences ($p < 0.05$) in the average size and ζ-potential of these BG NPs, signifying that the processing conditions significantly modulated their structure and property even though they were formulated with the same chemical composition [28,29]. Figure 2C displays the recorded N_2 adsorption–desorption isotherms for MBG-1 and MBG-2 NPs. Two isotherms exhibited their respective hysteresis loops of the desorption branch, indicative of the existence of large pores inside BG NPs [28,29]. In comparison to MBG-1 NPs, the hysteresis loop for MBG-2 NPs was shown to be steeper and its inception turning point was closer to the high pressure end of the N_2 isotherm, suggesting that MBG-2 NPs have more pores with larger size than MBG-1 NPs. Besides these differences, MBG-2 NPs also quite differed from MBG-1 NPs in pore volume and pore size distribution (Figure 2D). Two sets of BG NPs were measured for their major parameters and the obtained data are summarized in Table 1. It can be seen that the presently developed BG NPs had a high level of pore volume, large average pore size and negative ζ-potential, and thus, they could act as a practical vehicle for the IGF-1 delivery since IGF-1 is somewhat positively charged (isoelectric point, 8.6) at physiological pH and has its molecular weight of about 7.6 kD [34,35].

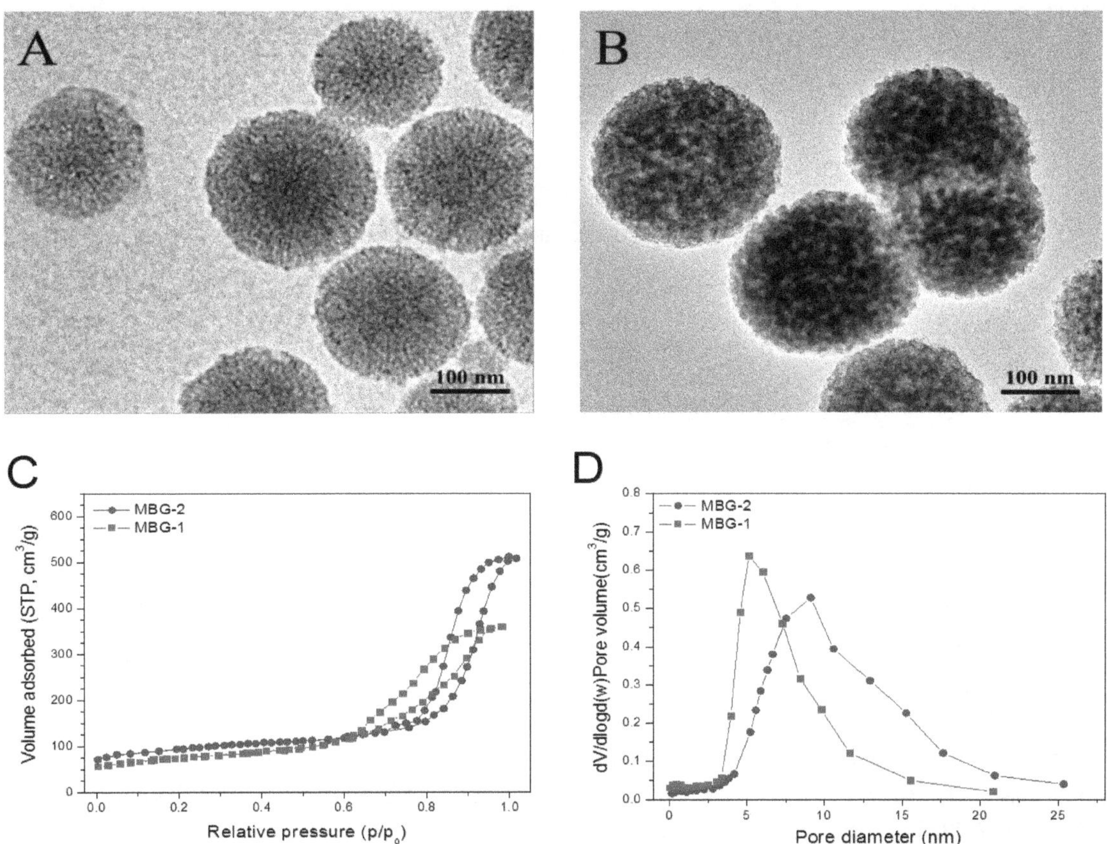

Figure 2. Images of MBG-1 (**A**) and MBG-2 (**B**) nanoparticles (NPs); N_2 adsorption isotherms (**C**) and pore size distribution (**D**) of NPs.

3.3. IGF-1 Release from BG Nanoparticles

Blank MBG-1 and MBG-2 NPs were loaded with IGF-1 under the condition of varying IGF-1 feed amounts, and two sets of IGF-1-loaded BG NPs were thus produced (Table 2). BS*i* (i = 1, 2 and 3) sample set was prepared by loading IGF-1 into MBG-1 NPs having smaller average pore size than that for MBG-2 NPs (see Table 1) whereas BL*j* (j = 1, 2 and 3) sample set was prepared by loading IGF-1 into MBG-2 NPs. Data in Table 2 reveal that these IGF-1-loaded NPs had similar average particle size ($p > 0.05$) but significantly higher ζ-potential ($p < 0.001$) as compared to their respective blank counterparts (see Table 1). The nearly unchanged average size for IGF-1-loaded NPs shown in Table 2 can be attributed to the very small IGF-1 mass when compared to NPs themselves, whereas the significantly increasing ζ-potential should be ascribed to the slightly positively charged nature of IGF-1 [34]. Table 2 indicates that the IGF-1-loaded NPs in BLj (j = 1, 2 and 3) set had significantly higher ($p < 0.05$) LE as compared to the counterpart in BSi (i = 1, 2 and 3) set. These differences are rational because the blank MBG-2 NPs used for preparing BLj (j = 1, 2 and 3) set have notably higher pore volume and larger pore size when compared to blank MBG-1 NPs used in BSi (i = 1, 2 and 3) set (see Table 1). Table 2 also shows that the IGF-1 feed amount exerted certain effects on LE, and this kind of effect would become insignificant once the IGF-1 feed amount reached 100 ng/mL or higher. It is worth mentioning that IGF-1 feed amounts were designated as such in order to test the LE for NPs. Actually, the IGF-1 load in these NPs can be effectively regulated by changing the feed amount of IGF-1.

The IGF-1 release patterns from IGF-1-loaded BG NPs are shown in Figure 3A,B. BS1, BS2, and BS3 NPs released around 50% of their initial IGF-1 load on the first day, and after 4-day release, the cumulative IGF-1 release amounted to about 70%. The IGF-1 load in these NPs did not impose any significant impacts on their release profiles. With respect to the cases associated with BL1, BL2, and BL3 NPs, their release profiles looked quite similar to that assigned for BS1, BS2, and BS3 NPs, respectively, with somewhat faster release rates (Figure 3B). Figure 3 verifies that these mesoporous BG NPs themselves are not able to effectively control the release kinetics of IGF-1 on account of their initial burst release features. LE is a key issue that is correlated to the rational use of IGF-1 because of high cost of IGF-1. In consideration of the similar release profiles illustrated in Figure 3 for both MBG-1 and MBG-2 NPs but significantly higher LE detected from MBG-2 NPs (see Table 2), MBG-2 NPs were thus chosen for the follow-up gel preparation.

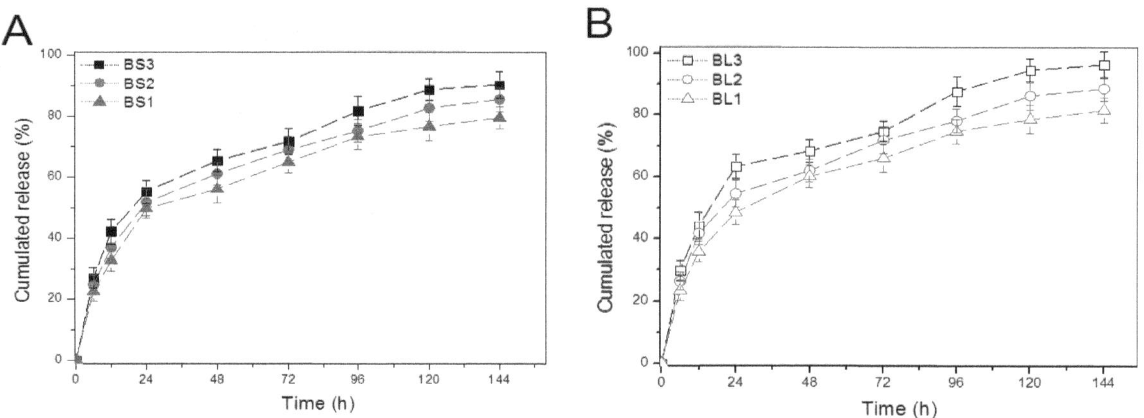

Figure 3. IGF-1 release profiles from 5 mg of BS1, BS2, and BS3 NPs ((**A**), initial IGF-1 load in BS1, BS2 and BS3 was 1.93, 4.61, and 7.27 ng/mg) and BL1, BL2, and BL3 NPs ((**B**), initial IGF-1 load in BL1, BL2, and BL3 was 2.29, 5.72, and 9.21 ng/mg) in 500 µL PBS (see Table 2 for their parameters).

3.4. Rheological Properties of BG/ALG–POL/SF Gels without IGF-1 Load

ALG–POL is a thermoresponsive copolymer and the thermal transition of ALG–POL solutions had strong concentration dependence. A previous study reported that ALG–POL was gelable when its solution concentration reached about 15 wt% or higher [9]. In the present study, the optimally synthesized ALG–POL copolymer was found to have clear sol-gel transition during a rational gelation period when its solution concentration reached 12 wt% or higher. Several optical images are presented in Figure S3 for showing changes of ALG–POL fluids after incubation. It can be noticed that the ALG–POL solution with its concentration of 9 wt% was remained as a fluid even though it was incubated at 37 °C for 60 min, and on the other hand, a 12 wt% ALG–POL solution was able to turn into gel via incubation at the same temperature during 14 min. Results in Figure S3 demonstrate that ALG–POL alone could be thermally gelable at 37 °C when its solution concentration is higher than a certain threshold.

In view of independent gelable mechanisms respectively belonging to ALG–POL and SF components, dual network gels with mechanically strong nature could be constructed by using ALG–POL and SF together. To achieve a ALG–POL/SF gel with required properties, a series of ALG–POL/SF composite solutions having their weight proportions of 4/8, 5/7, 6/6, and 7/5 was formulated for the preparation of blank ALG–POL/SF gels, and the optimal gel was sought out as 5 wt% for ALG–POL and 7 wt% for SF. Based on such designed composition for the ALG–POL/SF gel, blank MBG-2 NPs were embedded into the gel to fabricate three kinds of BG/ALG–POL/SF gels without IGF-1 load and the resulting gels were utilized to evaluate the rheological properties in order to save IGF-1. Major parameters for these blank BG/ALG–POL/SF gels are given in Table 3.

As seen from Table 3, G-A, G-B, and G-C gels had the same matrix and the difference in their composition was the percentage of blank MBG-2 NPs. Panels A, B, and C in Figure 4 elucidate the representative temperature sweep curves of G′ and G″ for different gels, and these gels were seen to respond to the thermal stimulus at different inception temperatures (T_i). G-A gel had its T_i at around 36 °C, whereas G-B and G-C gels showed their T_i near 35 °C, connoting that the introduction of BG NPs into the ALG–POL/SF gel has a very limited effect on their gelation temperature. It can be observed from Table 3 that the pH value and T_i of these gels were quite close to the physiological pH and temperature, and meanwhile, their gelation time was seen to be rational [5,6], suggesting their applicability under physiological conditions. Figure 4D presents the shear dependence of viscosity for different gels. Their viscosity was shown to be lower than 70 pa.s at 23 °C, and progressively decreased with rising shear rate, indicating their shear-thinning features. Given that the gel injection is usually performed at room temperature, curves graphed in Figure 4D validate that the presently formulated BG/ALG–POL/SF gels have well-defined injectability.

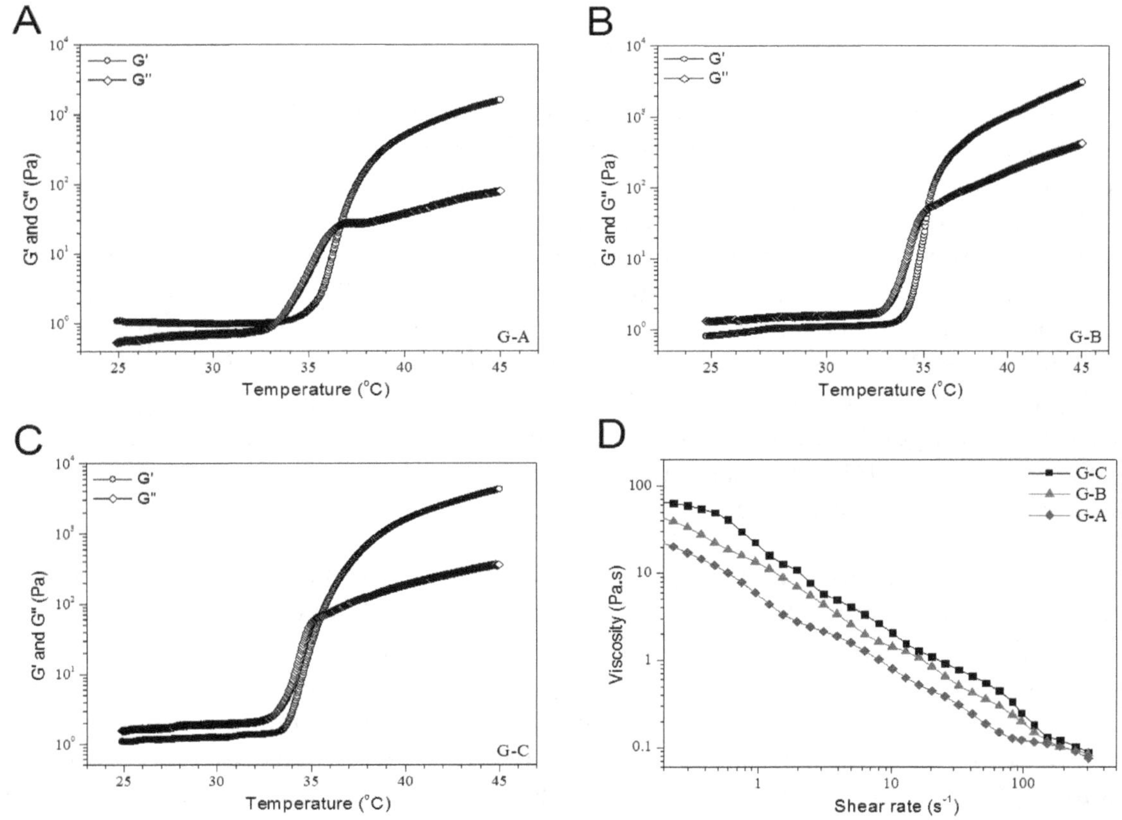

Figure 4. Temperature sweep curves (**A**–**C**) and shear viscosity ((**D**), 23 °C) for BG/ALG–POL/SF gels.

In principle, magnitude of G′ and G″ of hydrogels in the linear viscoelastic region (LVR) of their frequency sweep spectra together with G′/G″ ratio can be used to assess the gel strength [36]. In general, a strong hydrogel is characterized by high G′, and meanwhile, its G′ should be 1–2 orders of magnitude greater than its G″ [36]. Figure 5A,B show that at a fixed frequency in their respective LVR, for example, 1.0 HZ, three kinds of gels had their G′ of around 5 kPa or higher and their G″ greater than 300 Pa. The incorporation of BG NPs into the ALG–POL/SF gel seemed not to exert marked effects on G′ and G″ of the resulting gels. To make quantitative comparisons, G′ and G″ at 1.0 Hz for these gels were measured, and obtained average values are graphed in Figure 5C. The bar-graphs explicate that these gels had their G′ higher 5.5 kPa with the G′/G″ ratio greater than 15, verifying their mechanically strong features.

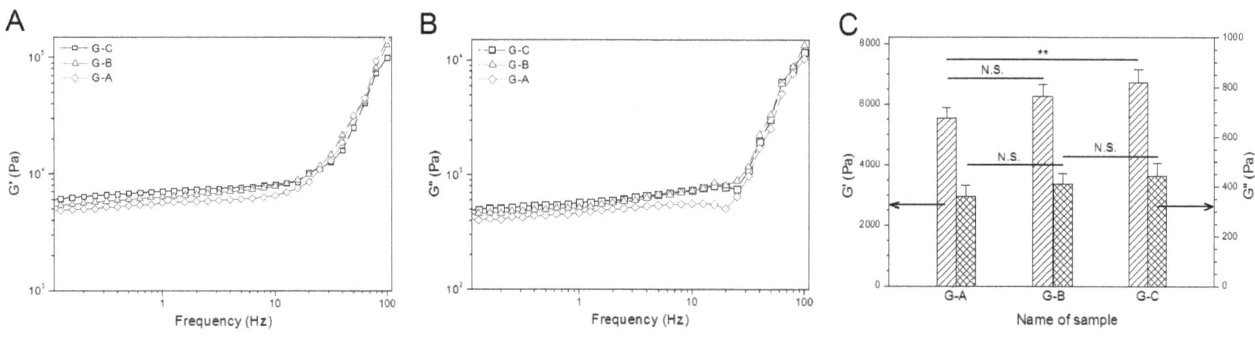

Figure 5. Frequency dependent functions (**A**,**B**) of modulus and average values (**C**) of modulus at 1.0 Hz and 37 °C for BG/ALG–POL/SF gels (**, $p < 0.001$; N.S., no significance).

3.5. Morphological Analysis of Dry Gels

The presently developed BG/ALG–POL/SF gels need to be porous because they are intended for use in bone repair where they will function as injectable materials for housing cells. G-A and G-C gels in Table 3 were selected and their lyophilized samples were examined to see their internal structures. A few SEM images for the dry gels are represented in Figure 6. These images show that dry gels were highly porous and their pore size changed from several tens of microns to more than two hundred microns with pore-interconnected characteristics. With respect to G-C gel, the incorporation of BG NPs did not significantly affect its pore structure when compared with G-A gel. The image with a larger magnification (Figure 6D) displays that the wall of pores in the gel was stuck or attached with many size-varied granules and these granules should be assigned to BG NPs or their aggregates. The average pore size for these dry gels is shown in Figure 6E. The dry gels had large average pore size without significant difference, which is advantageous for bone repair where large pore size and high porosity in the requisite gels are concurrently required.

SI of dry gels has been used as an approximate estimation for their porosity since the channels shaped inside the gels can regulate their swelling and deswelling behavior via water convection [37]. In general, dry gels with open-cell pores and high porosity have high SI and short swelling equilibrium time due to fast water convection [38]. The bar-graph in Figure 6F illustrates that these dry gels had their SI higher than 5, and meanwhile, the composition of the gels seemed not to exert significant impacts on their SI. In addition, it was found that these dry gels reached their respective swelling equilibrium in PBS less than 30 min. The similar SI together with their rapidly swollen features connotes that these gels have similar porosity.

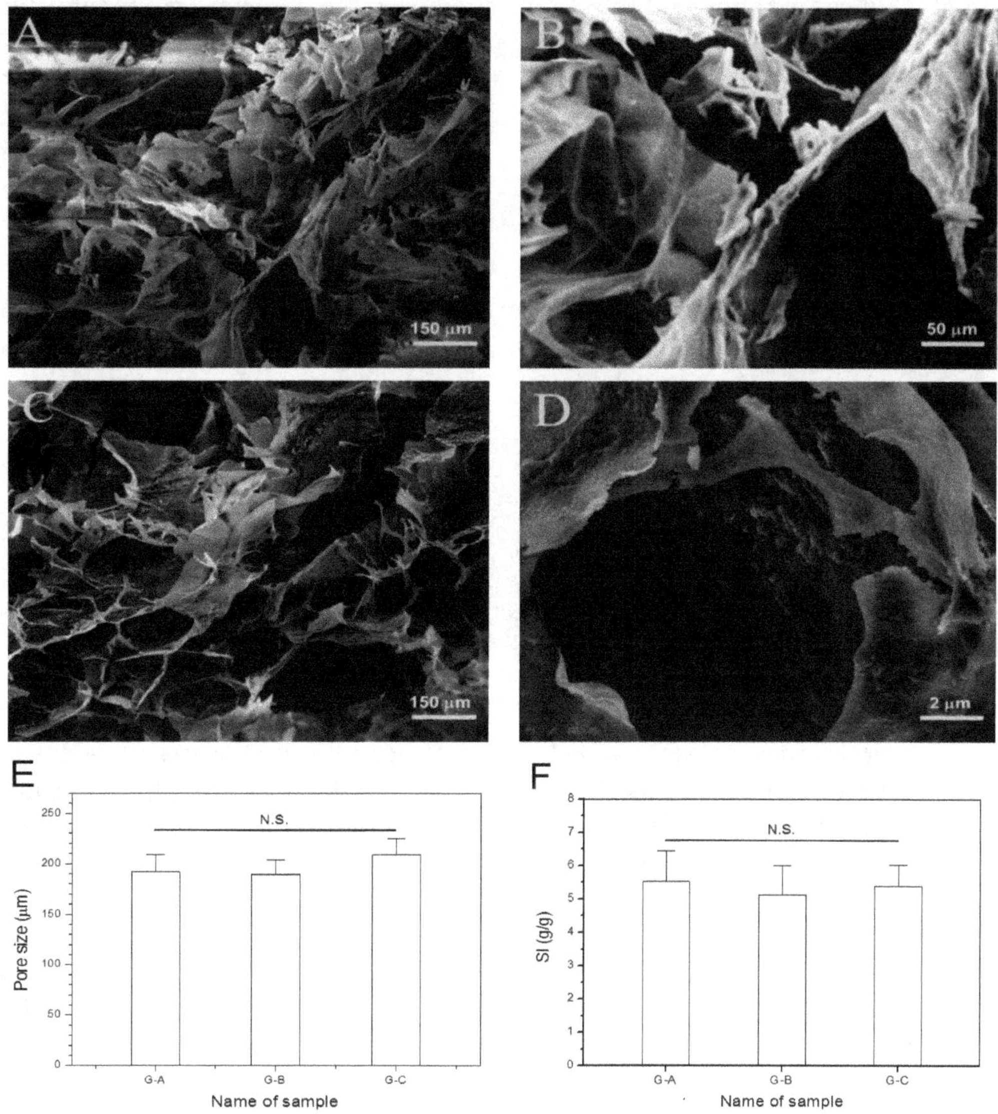

Figure 6. SEM micrographs ((**A**,**B**), G-A gel; (**C**,**D**), G-C gel), average pore-size (**E**) and swelling index (**F**) of BG/ALG–POL/SF dry gels (see Table 3 for parameters of gels; N.S., no significance).

3.6. IGF-1 Release of Gels

The gels were loaded with varied amounts IGF-1 in a designated way as illustrated in Table 4 and they were detected to access their capacity for administration of IGF-1 release. Release profiles for these gels are presented in Figure 7. Curves in Figure 7A exhibit that two kinds of gels directly loading with IGF-1 had fast IGF-1 release in the first few days at varied rates somewhat depending on their initial IGF-1 load, and their IGF-1 release became visibly slower after one-week release with similar release rate in the light of approximately constant distance between the two curves. In marked contrast to this observation, two gels embedded with IGF-1-loaded BG NPs behaved in quite different ways (Figure 7B). IGF-1 load of around 7% or less was released from the gels in the first day, and afterwards, the release patterns followed approximately linear behavior for a few weeks at various release rates. In comparison to the patterns shown in Figure 7A, the significantly reduced initial IGF-1 release and the subsequent release slowdown in Figure 7B can be attributed to the joint contribution of the gel matrix and BG NPs. As denoted in Table 4, GEL-3 and GEL-4 gels were prepared by embedding IGF-1-loaded BG NPs into ALG–POL/SF. In comparison to GEL-1 and GEL-2 gels, IGF-1 molecules in GEL-3 and GEL-4 gels will encounter increasing resistance derived from both BG NPs and gel matrix, which will certainly result in their release slowdown. When the release patterns in Figure 7B are compared each other, it can be observed that IGF-1 content in the gels remarkably affected the release rate. A possible reason could be ascribed to that the higher IGF-1 loading in a gel would form a larger IGF-1 concentration gradient inside the gel, which would force IGF-1 molecules to transport through the gel matrix faster and to reach the media earlier, leading to higher cumulative IGF-1 amount.

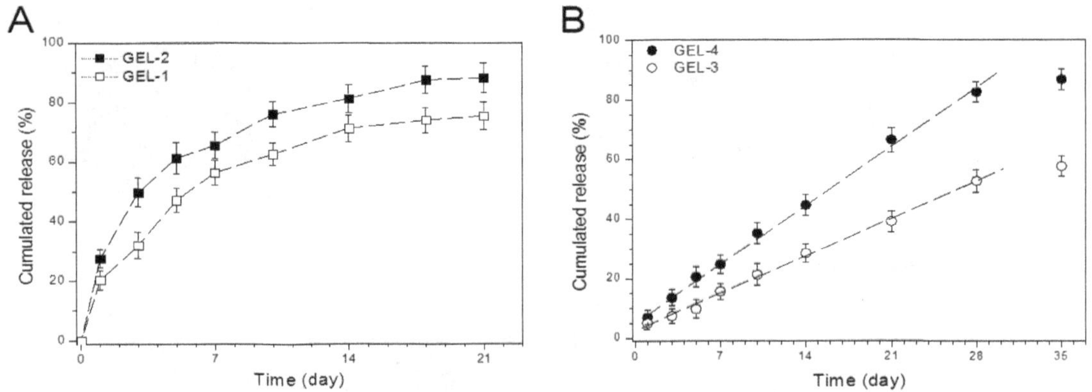

Figure 7. IGF-1 release patterns for gels directly loaded with IGF-1 (**A**) and for IGF-loaded BG/ALG–POL/SF gels (**B**).

3.7. *Bioactivity Assessment of IGF-1*

Bioactivity preservation of released IGF-1 is an important issue because it is closely correlated to the biological effects of IGF-1. In this study, MC3T3-E1 cells were used for assessment of IGF-1 bioactivity because IGF-1 is capable of promoting the proliferation of osteoid cells in dose-dependent manners [30–32]. To evaluate these gels on the same baseline, GEL-2 and GEL-4 gels were selected taking account of their similar and higher initial IGF-1 load. MC3T3-E1 cells were cultured with equivalent amount of released IGF-1 or free IGF-1 for varied durations up to 72 h and relevant results are elucidated in Figure 8. At a low level of IGF-1 (5 ng/mL), OD values matching with IGF-1-applied cell groups were remarkably higher than that of control group but no significant differences were detected among cell groups that were exposed to free IGF-1 or released IGF-1 as sampling time advanced (Figure 8A). By increasing the applied IGF-1 amount by 10 times (Figure 8B), the variation trend of OD values and their differences looked similar to that detected at the IGF-1 dosage of 5 ng/mL. In addition, by comparing each OD value in Figure 8B with the corresponding one in Figure 8A, IGF-1-dose dependent characteristics can be detected when the culture time reached 72h. These results support that the released IGF-1 was able to promote the proliferation of MC3T3-E1 cells in the way of dose-regulation, confirming that bioactivity of released IGF-1 can be well preserved.

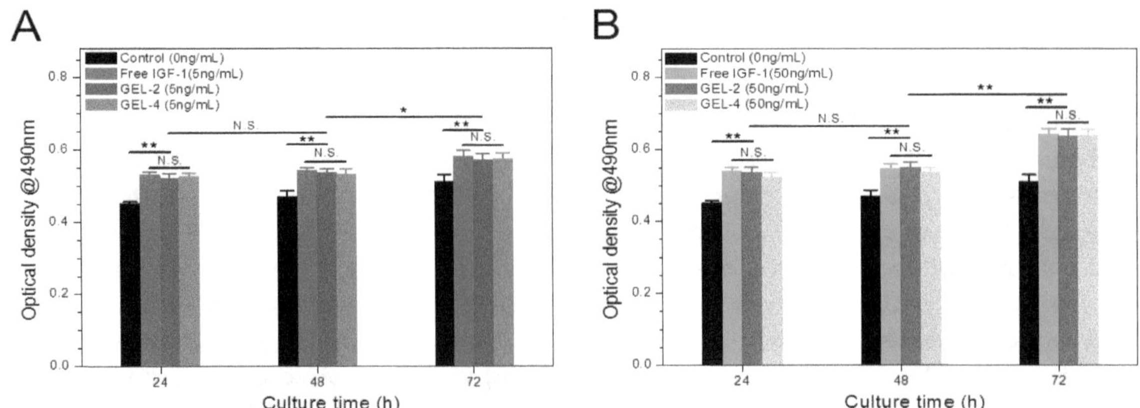

Figure 8. Response of MC3T3-E1 cells to 5 ng/mL (**A**) or 50 ng/mL (**B**) of free or released IGF-1 during various culture periods (*, $p < 0.05$; **, $p < 0.001$; N.S., no significance).

Besides these tests, MC3T3-E1 cells were also cultured on the surface of GEL-2 and GEL-4 gels for three days to further evaluate their growth, and the measured OD values are depicted in Figure 9. In these cases, the cumulated IGF-1 amount in the culture media would be dynamically altered because GEL-2 and GEL-4 gels would incessantly release IGF-1 at different rates despite their similar initial IGF-1 load. As shown in Figure 7, the cumulative amount of IGF-1 released from GEL-2 gel on the first, second and third days reached around 27, 39, and 50%, respectively; and the corresponding cumulative IGF-1 release from GEL-4 gel was about 7, 10, and 13%. Considering the patterns shown in Figure 7, it can be envisioned that in the current situation, the amount of available IGF-1 in GEL-2 group was significantly higher than that in GEL-4 group in the first three days. It can be seen that OD values measured from two gel groups were markedly higher than that detected from control group during the three sampling days, demonstrating that the released IGF-1 is bioactive and able to promote the growth of MC3T3-E1 cells (Figure 9). When GEL-2 and GEL-4 groups were compared each other, it shows that there was no significant difference in their OD value on the first day, but on the second and third days, OD value measured from GEL-2 group was notably larger than that detected from GEL-4 group. The possible reasons for these observations could be attributed to that (1) cells need a certain period of time to attach to the gels and to undergo recovery growth with low responsiveness to the released IGF-1 on the first day, resulting in insignificant difference in their OD value; and (2) after fully attaching and returning to their normal growth, cells seeded on GEL-2 gel would grow faster than those on GEL-4 gel because GEL-2 gel can release a notable higher IGF-1 amount than GEL-4 gel. These results further confirm that presently devised gels have ability to promote the proliferation of MC3T3-E1 cells.

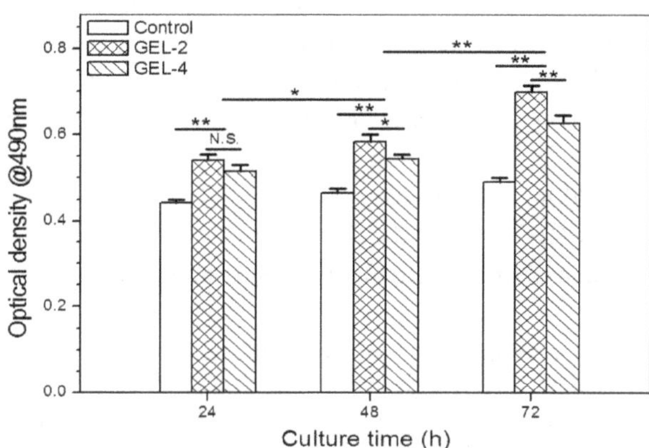

Figure 9. Optical density (OD) values of MC3T3-E1 cells cultured on the surface of gels during various periods (*, $p < 0.05$; **, $p < 0.001$; N.S., no significance).

4. Conclusions

Thermosensitive ALG–POL copolymer containing a necessitated percentage of POL was successfully synthesized. Such synthesized ALG–POL was found to be suitable for constructing hydrogels with dual network structure through combining with SF. The optimally obtained ALG–POL/SF gels were injectable at room temperature and mechanically strong with their sol-gel transition near physiological pH and temperature. Embedment of mesoporous BG nanoparticles into ALG–POL/SF gel did not significantly modify the gelation temperature, gelation time and pH of the resulting gels. The interior of the dry gels was seen to be highly porous with well-interconnected pore architecture. Direct incorporation of IGF-1 into ALG–POL/SF gels was inadvisable for administrating IGF-1 release. By embedding IGF-1-loaded BG nanoparticles into ALG–POL/SF gels, the resulting IGF-1-loaded BG/ALG–POL/SF gels showed a confirmative ability to administrate IGF-1 release in an approximately linear manner for a few weeks and their IGF-1 release rate could be effectively regulated by the IGF-1 load in BG nanoparticles. Cell tests confirmed that the released IGF-1 was bioactive as compared with the free IGF-1.

Supplementary Materials:
Figure S1. ^{1}H NMR spectra for monoamine-terminated poloxamer (MATP). Figure S2. FTIR spectra for poloxamer (A), alginate (B) and alginate-poloxamer (C). Figure S3. ALG-POL fluids and formed ALG-POL gel after incubation. (Concentration of ALG-POL: 9 wt% (A); and 12 wt% (B)).

Author Contributions: Q.M., Y.W., and J.W. conceived and designed the experiments; X.Y., J.L., and Y.Z. performed the experiments; Q.M., Y.W., and J.W. wrote the paper. All authors have read and agreed to the published version of the manuscript.

References

1. Jarvelainen, H.; Sainio, A.; Koulu, M.; Wight, T.N.; Penttinen, R. Extracellular matrix molecules: Potential targets in pharmacotherapy. *Pharmacol. Rev.* **2009**, *61*, 198–223. [CrossRef] [PubMed]
2. Frantz, C.; Stewart, K.M.; Weaver, V.M. The extracellular matrix at a glance. *J. Cell Sci.* **2010**, *123*, 4195–4200. [CrossRef] [PubMed]
3. Tibbitt, M.W.; Anseth, K.S. Hydrogels as extracellular matrix mimics for 3D cell. *Biotechnol. Bioeng.* **2009**, *103*, 655–663. [CrossRef] [PubMed]
4. Wang, C.; Varshney, R.R.; Wang, D.A. Therapeutic cell delivery and fate control in hydrogels and hydrogel hybrids. *Adv. Drug Delivery Rev.* **2010**, *62*, 699–710. [CrossRef]
5. Yang, J.A.; Yeom, J.; Hwang, B.W.; Hoffman, A.S.; Hahn, S.K. In situ-forming injectable hydrogels for regenerative medicine. *Prog. Polym. Sci.* **2014**, *39*, 1973–1986. [CrossRef]
6. Kretlow, J.D.; Klouda, L.; Mikos, A.G. Injectable matrices and scaffolds for drug delivery in tissue engineering. *Adv. Drug Deliv. Rev.* **2007**, *59*, 263–273. [CrossRef]
7. Tan, H.; Marra, K.G. Injectable, biodegradable hydrogels for tissue engineering applications. *Materials* **2010**, *3*, 1746–1767. [CrossRef]
8. Hermansson, E.; Schuster, E.; Lindgren, L.; Altskar, A.; Strom, A. Impact of solvent quality on the network strength and structure of alginate gels. *Carbohydr. Polym.* **2016**, *144*, 289–296. [CrossRef]
9. Chen, C.C.; Fang, C.L.; Al-Suwayeh, S.A.; Leu, Y.L.; Fang, J.Y. Transdermal delivery of selegiline from alginate-pluronic composite thermogels. *Int. J. Pharm.* **2011**, *415*, 119–128. [CrossRef]
10. Lin, H.R.; Sung, K.C.; Vong, W.J. In situ gelling of alginate/pluronic solutions for ophthalmic delivery of pilocarpine. *Biomacromolecules* **2004**, *5*, 2358–2365. [CrossRef]
11. Naseri, N.; Deepa, B.; Mathew, A.P.; Oksman, K.; Girandon, L. Nanocellulose-based interpenetrating polymer network (IPN) hydrogels for cartilage applications. *Biomacromolecules* **2016**, *17*, 3714–3723. [CrossRef] [PubMed]
12. Nie, J.; Pei, B.; Wang, Z.; Hu, Q. Construction of ordered structure in polysaccharide hydrogel: A review. *Carbohydr. Polym.* **2019**, *205*, 225–235. [CrossRef]
13. Partlow, B.P.; Hanna, C.W.; Rnjak-Kovacina, J.; Moreau, J.E.; Applegate, M.B.; Burke, K.A.; Marelli, B.; Mitropoulos, A.N.; Omenetto, F.G.; Kaplan, D.L.; et al. Highly tunable elastomeric silk biomaterials. *Adv. Funct. Mater.* **2014**, *24*, 4615–4624. [CrossRef] [PubMed]
14. Hopkins, A.M.; Laporte, L.D.; Tortelli, F.; Spedden, E.; Staii, C.; Atherton, T.J.; Hubbell, J.A.; Kaplan, D.L. Silk hydrogels as soft substrates for neural tissue engineering. *Adv. Funct. Mater.* **2013**, *23*, 5140–5149. [CrossRef]
15. Liu, J.; Yang, B.; Li, M.; Li, J.; Wan, Y. Enhanced dual network hydrogels consisting of thiolated chitosan and silk fibroin for cartilage tissue engineering. *Carbohydr. Polym.* **2020**, *227*, 115335. [CrossRef] [PubMed]
16. Santo, V.E.; Gomes, M.E.; Mano, J.F.; Reis, R.L. Controlled release strategies for bone, cartilage, and osteochondral engineering—Part II: Challenges on the evolution from single to multiple bioactive factor delivery. *Tissue Eng. Part B* **2013**, *19*, 327–352. [CrossRef] [PubMed]
17. Giustina, A.; Mazziotti, G.; Canalis, E. Growth hormone, insulin-like growth factors, and the skeleton. *Endocrine Rev.* **2008**, *29*, 535–559. [CrossRef]
18. Mantripragada, V.P.; Jayasuriya, A.C. IGF-1 release kinetics from chitosan microparticles fabricated using environmentally benign conditions. *Mater. Sci. Eng. C* **2014**, *42*, 506–516. [CrossRef]
19. Massicotte, F.; Fernandes, J.C.; Martel-Pelletier, J.; Pelletier, J.P.; Lajeunesse, D. Modulation of insulin-like growth factor 1 levels in human osteoarthritic subchondral bone osteoblasts. *Bone* **2006**, *38*, 333–341. [CrossRef]
20. Vo, T.N.; Kasper, F.K.; Mikos, A.G. Strategies for controlled delivery of growth factors and cells for bone regeneration. *Adv. Drug Deliv. Rev.* **2012**, *64*, 1292–1309. [CrossRef]

21. Wang, Z.; Wang, Z.; Lu, W.W.; Zhen, W.; Yang, D.; Peng, S. Novel biomaterial strategies for controlled growth factor delivery for biomedical applications. *NPG Asia Mater.* **2017**, *9*, e435. [CrossRef]
22. Min, Q.; Yu, X.; Liu, J.; Wu, J.; Wan, Y. Chitosan-based hydrogels embedded with hyaluronic acid complex nanoparticles for controlled delivery of bone morphogenetic protein-2. *Mar. Drugs* **2019**, *17*, 365. [CrossRef] [PubMed]
23. Hench, L.L. Bioceramics. *J. Am. Ceram. Soc.* **1998**, *81*, 1705–1728. [CrossRef]
24. Wu, C.; Chang, J. Multifunctional mesoporous bioactive glasses for effective delivery of therapeutic ions and drug/growth factors. *J. Control. Release* **2014**, *193*, 282–295. [CrossRef] [PubMed]
25. Boffito, M.; Pontremoli, C.; Fiorilli, S.; Laurano, R.; Ciardelli, G.; Vitale-Brovarone, C. Injectable thermosensitive formulation based on polyurethane hydrogel/mesoporous glasses for sustained co-delivery of functional ions and drugs. *Pharmaceutics* **2019**, *11*, 501. [CrossRef] [PubMed]
26. Cho, K.Y.; Chung, T.W.; Kim, B.C.; Kim, M.K.; Lee, J.H.; Wee, W.R.; Cho, C.S. Release of ciprofloxacin from poloxamer-graft-hyaluronic acid hydrogels in vitro. *Int. J. Pharm.* **2003**, *260*, 83–91. [CrossRef]
27. Hsu, S.H.; Leu, Y.L.; Hu, J.W.; Fang, J.Y. Physicochemical characterization and drug release of thermosensitive hydrogels composed of a hyaluronic acid/pluronic F127 graft. *Chem. Pharm. Bull.* **2009**, *57*, 453–458. [CrossRef]
28. Kim, T.H.; Singh, R.K.; Kang, M.S.; Kim, J.H.; Kim, H.W. Gene delivery nanocarriers of bioactive glass with unique potential to load BMP2 plasmid DNA and to internalize into mesenchymal stem cells for osteogenesis and bone regeneration. *Nanoscale* **2016**, *8*, 8300–8311. [CrossRef]
29. Mahapatra, C.; Singh, R.K.; Kim, J.J.; Patel, K.D.; Perez, R.A.; Jang, J.H.; Kim, H.W. Osteopromoting reservoir of stem cells: Bioactive mesoporous nanocarrier/collagen gel through slow-releasing FGF18 and the activated bmp signaling. *ACS Appl. Mater. Interfaces* **2016**, *8*, 27573–27584. [CrossRef]
30. Kim, S.K.; Kwon, J.Y.; Nam, T.J. Involvement of ligand occupancy in Insulin-like growth factor-I (IGF-I) induced cell growth in osteoblast like MC3T3-E1 cells. *BioFactors* **2007**, *29*, 187–202. [CrossRef]
31. Langdahl, B.L.; Kassem, M.; Moller, M.K.; Eriksen, E.F. The effects of IGF-I and IGF-II on proliferation and differentiation of human osteoblasts and interactions with growth hormone. *Eur. J. Clin. Invest.* **1998**, *28*, 176–183. [CrossRef] [PubMed]
32. Machwate, M.; Zerath, E.; Holy, X.; Pastoureau, P.; Marie, P.J. Insulin-like growth factor-I increases trabecular bone formation and osteoblastic cell proliferation in unloaded rats. *Endocrinology* **1994**, *134*, 1031–1038. [CrossRef] [PubMed]
33. Fang, J.Y.; Hsu, S.H.; Leu, Y.L.; Hu, J.W. Delivery of cisplatin from pluronic co-polymer systems: Liposome inclusion and alginate coupling. *J. Biomater. Sci. Polym. Ed.* **2009**, *20*, 1031–1047. [CrossRef] [PubMed]
34. Shavlakadze, T.; Winn, N.; Rosenthal, N.; Grounds, M.D. Reconciling data from transgenic mice that overexpress IGF-I specifically in skeletal muscle. *Growth Horm. IGF Res.* **2005**, *15*, 4–18. [CrossRef] [PubMed]
35. Rinderknecht, E.; Humbel, R.E. The amino acid sequence of human insulin like growth factor I and its structural homology, with proinsulin. *J. Biol. Chem.* **1978**, *253*, 2769–2776. [PubMed]
36. Clark, A.H.; Ross-Murphy, S.B. Structural and mechanical properties of biopolymer gel. *Adv. Polym. Sci.* **1987**, *83*, 60–192.
37. Yoshida, R.; Kaneko, Y.; Sakai, K.; Okano, T.; Sakurai, Y.; Bae, Y.H.; Kim, S.W. Positive thermo sensitive pulsatile drug release using negative thermosensitive hydrogels. *J. Control. Release* **1994**, *32*, 97–102. [CrossRef]
38. Dang, J.M.; Sun, D.D.N.; Shin-Ya, Y.; Sieber, A.N.; Kostuik, J.P.; Leong, K.W. Temperature-responsive hydroxybutyl chitosan for the culture of mesenchymal stem cells and intervertebral disk cells. *Biomaterials* **2006**, *27*, 406–418. [CrossRef]

Multivariate Design of 3D Printed Immediate-Release Tablets with Liquid Crystal-Forming Drug—Itraconazole

Witold Jamróz [1,*], Jolanta Pyteraf [1], Mateusz Kurek [1,*], Justyna Knapik-Kowalczuk [2,3], Joanna Szafraniec-Szczęsny [1], Karolina Jurkiewicz [2,3], Bartosz Leszczyński [4], Andrzej Wróbel [4], Marian Paluch [2,3] and Renata Jachowicz [1]

1 Department of Pharmaceutical Technology and Biopharmaceutics, Jagiellonian University Medical College, Medyczna 9, 30-688 Krakow, Poland; jolanta.pyteraf@uj.edu.pl (J.P.); joanna.szafraniec@uj.edu.pl (J.S.-S.); renata.jachowicz@uj.edu.pl (R.J.)

2 Division of Biophysics and Molecular Physics, Institute of Physics, University of Silesia, Uniwersytecka 4, 40-007 Katowice, Poland; justyna.knapik-kowalczuk@us.edu.pl (J.K.-K.); karolina.jurkiewicz@us.edu.pl (K.J.); marian.paluch@us.edu.pl (M.P.)

3 Silesian Center for Education and Interdisciplinary Research, University of Silesia, 75 Pulku Piechoty 1a, 41-500 Chorzow, Poland

4 Marian Smoluchowski Institute of Physics, Jagiellonian University, Łojasiewicza 11, 30-348 Krakow, Poland; bartosz.leszczynski@uj.edu.pl (B.L.); andrzej.wrobel@uj.edu.pl (A.W.)

* Correspondence: witold.jamroz@uj.edu.pl (W.J.); mateusz.kurek@uj.edu.pl (M.K.);

Abstract: The simplicity of object shape and composition modification make additive manufacturing a great option for customized dosage form production. To achieve this goal, the correlation between structural and functional attributes of the printed objects needs to be analyzed. So far, it has not been deeply investigated in 3D printing-related papers. The aim of our study was to modify the functionalities of printed tablets containing liquid crystal-forming drug itraconazole by introducing polyvinylpyrrolidone-based polymers into the filament-forming matrices composed predominantly of poly(vinyl alcohol). The effect of the molecular reorganization of the drug and improved tablets' disintegration was analyzed in terms of itraconazole dissolution. Micro-computed tomography was applied to analyze how the design of a printed object (in this case, a degree of an infill) affects its reproducibility during printing. It was also used to analyze the structure of the printed dosage forms. The results indicated that the improved disintegration obtained due to the use of Kollidon®CL-M was more beneficial for the dissolution of itraconazole than the molecular rearrangement and liquid crystal phase transitions. The lower infill density favored faster dissolution of the drug from printed tablets. However, it negatively affected the reproducibility of the 3D printed object.

Keywords: 3D printing; fused deposition modeling; hot-melt extrusion; solid dosage forms; itraconazole

1. Introduction

Additive manufacturing has huge potential to revolutionize the methods of drug delivery system formation. It was proven for mass-scale drug production by Aprecia Pharmaceuticals, which registered the first 3D printed drug, Spritam®, in 2015. However, the use of additive manufacturing also enables the preparation of small batches of customized, on-demand-prepared formulations—for example, in the treatment of patients with rare diseases or for clinical trials. The great applicability of 3D printing (3DP) in the pharmaceutical field results from the simplicity of object shape modification, which allows the production of dosage forms of complex shape and internal structure, containing one or more active pharmaceutical ingredients (APIs) [1,2]. Moreover, the differences in shape and infill density of tablets, which cannot be achieved in compressed tablets, lead to alternation in the surface-to-volume ratio and allow us to produce printlets with desired drug dosages and dissolution profiles [3–5]. Although the issue of the correlation between the internal structure of printed tablets and their properties, particularly the dissolution characteristics, has been explored by several research teams, there is still deficiency in studies on the actual microstructure and quality of printed objects and the mechanisms driving the release of the drug from printed dosage forms [6–9].

In the case of nearly all 3DP methods, the object is built layer by layer based on the computer aided design (CAD) model. However, various printing technologies vary between each other regarding used materials and process conditions such as temperature. The 3D printing methods can operate with a powder, which is bound with a liquid binder or sintered with a laser, a photosensitive resin, a thermoplastic material, or a semi-solid formulation extruded through the printer nozzle. Several techniques, such as stereolithography [10–14], selective laser sintering [8,15] digital light processing [16,17], binder jetting, [18,19], and extrusion-based methods including direct powder extrusion [20,21], semi-solid extrusion [22–26], and fused deposition modeling (FDM) [27,28], have been investigated for application in the pharmaceutical industry. The 3DP methods which can be introduced in the high-scale manufacturing process should be characterized by the high-speed production of uniform objects [29,30]. In the case of most of the abovementioned printing methods, process conditions may cause amorphization of the active ingredient, which increases its solubility [31,32].

Various dosage forms, such as orodispersible films [33], mucoadhesive films [34], immediate and modified-release tablets [35,36], capsules [37,38], implants [39], or even formulations imitating sweets [40], have been recently developed using fused deposition modeling. In the printed dosage forms, drug release modification is obtained mostly by selecting either the filament-forming polymers characterized by suitable pH-dependent solubility [41] or the printlet shape and geometry, i.e., the presence of channels [42], empty cavities (floating tablets) [43,44], variations in the infill degree or shape as well as the use of shape-memory polymers to prepare retentive drug delivery systems (4D printing) [45,46]. Despite the fabrication of dosage forms by means of 3DP, this technique can be used for capsular shell fabrication [47] to control the API's dissolution process as well as mold preparation to create custom-made, patient-oriented drugs [48]. The 3D printed molds can be also used in a range of science and technology sectors including electrochemical electrical applications—for example, flexible sensor prototypes [49,50].

The application of FDM printing technology in the manufacturing of dosage forms requires the use of previously prepared drug-loaded filament. Filaments are produced mostly in the hot-melt extrusion process (HME), which is also the method applied to increase drug solubility. During this process, a mixture of drug and thermoplastic polymer is heated and blended, and the molten mass is pushed through a nozzle to form a filament [51]. Instead of drugs, other substances can be used in the HME process, e.g., insoluble hydroxyapatite for filament fabrication, which can be used in bone tissue engineering [52]. One of the most important advantages is that this process does not require the use of organic solvents, such as the preparation of amorphous solid dispersion (ASD) by spray drying. However, HME operates at high temperatures, which are required to melt the formulation components [53]. In some cases, it is necessary to add plasticizers to the formulation to lower the process temperature in order to protect the thermolabile active ingredient and improve filament printability [36,54,55]. The combination of HME and FDM can induce phase transitions, including amorphization, which results in increased drug solubility. Further drug dissolution modification can be also achieved by changing the shape and surface of the printed dosage form [26].

Itraconazole (ITR) is an oral antifungal agent used in the treatment of systemic and superficial fungal infections, commercially available in the form of 65 mg and 100 mg capsules, 200 mg tablets, and 10 mg/mL solutions. It is a highly lipophilic, weakly alkaline drug with very low water solubility of 1 ng/mL at pH 7 and 4 μg/mL at pH 1. ITR is classified as a Biopharmaceutics Classification System (BCS) class II substance [56], which means it has solubility-limited bioavailability. The drug exhibits three polymorphs varying in stability and solubility [57]. Moreover, ITR can form liquid crystals, which are particularly interesting from the perspective of pharmaceutical sciences. Liquid crystals can adopt various molecular arrangements (nematic and smectic in the case of ITR), which affect the free energy of the system and thus the dissolution performance. Due to the relatively high glass transition temperature ($T_g = 59\ ^{\circ}C$), ITR can be also transformed into a stable amorphous state, usually in the form of amorphous solid dispersions with polymers or co-amorphous systems with small molecules [58].

Soluplus® [59–61], Eudragit® L [62], polyvinylpyrrolidone (PVP) [63], Kollidon® VA64 [64,65], polyvinyl alcohol (PVA) [65,66], as well as semi-synthetic cellulose derivatives such as hydroxypropyl cellulose [67] and hydroxypropyl methylcellulose acetate succinate [53,54,68–70], are examples of pharmaceutical polymers tested for preparing itraconazole amorphous solid dispersions (ASD) and also suitable as filament-forming polymers for FDM. Although many papers described the formation of amorphous solid dispersions with ITR, including the use of the hot-melt extrusion process [61], only two considered the formation of dosage forms using 3D printing. Kimura et al. reported that it is possible to use fused deposition modeling to prepare zero-order sustained-release floating tablets containing itraconazole [43]. They were able to control floating time by printing tablets with empty cavities inside and to modify the drug dissolution rate by changing the tablet surface and wall thickness. Goyanes et al. prepared tablets containing amorphous solid dispersions of itraconazole in different grades of hydroxypropylcellulose using direct powder extrusion 3D printing—a novel, single-step 3D printing process. In contrast to FDM, this 3D printer tool head is equipped with single screw extruder, which allows it to print directly using mixed powders or pellets, without preparing filaments [20].

In this paper, we describe for the first time the liquid crystal phase transitions of itraconazole in 3D printed tablets. The drug was combined with polymers, formed into filaments via hot-melt extrusion and then printed using fused deposition modeling technology. The filaments were based on poly(vinyl alcohol), a water-soluble semi-crystalline polymer known for its superior printability. The two PVP-based polymers were also added to the filament-forming mixture to introduce the additional functionalities into the printed matrices. Kollidon® VA64 was supposed to modify the physicochemical properties—the molecular arrangement in particular (analyzed using thermal analysis and X-ray diffractometry)—and Kollidon® CL-M was added to modify drug dissolution due to the improved tablet disintegration. We performed deep micro-computed tomography (μ-CT) analysis as the first attempt to analyze how the design of a printed object (degree of an infill) affects its reproducibility during printing. It was also used to analyze the structure of the printed dosage forms to support the dissolution data. To clearly understand the advantages of extrusion and printing processes, drug dissolution from printed formulations was compared with tablets having similar composition, obtained by the compression of either raw powders or milled filament.

2. Materials and Methods

2.1. Materials

Itraconazole (ITR, 1-(butan-2-yl)-4-{4-[4-(4-{[(2R,4S)-2-(2,4-dichlorophenyl)-2-[(1H-1,2,4-triazol-1-yl)methyl]-1,3-dioxolan-4-yl]methoxy}phenyl)piperazin-1-yl]phenyl}-4,5-dihydro-1H-1,2,4-triazol-5-one, 99.8%, Henan Tianfu Chemical Co., Ltd., Zhengzhou, China) served as a model drug. Poly(vinyl alcohol) (PVA, Parteck® MXP, Merck®- KGaA, Darmstadt, Germany), copovidone (K/VA, Kollidon® VA64, BASF®, Ludwigshafen, Germany), crospovidone (K/CL, Kollidon® CL-M, BASF®, Ludwigshafen, Germany) were utilized as the matrix-forming polymers to prepare both filaments and 3D printed tablets. Talc (Fagron®, Kraków, Poland) and magnesium stearate (Avantor® Performance Materials, Gliwice, Poland) were added to tablets prepared by compression in tablet press. Hydrochloric acid (Merck® KGaA, Darmstadt, Germany) and potassium chloride (Avantor® Performance Materials, Gliwice, Poland) were used as dissolution media ingredients. Water used in all experiments was produced by Elix 15UV Essential reversed osmosis system (Merck® KGaA, Darmstadt, Germany).

2.2. Preparation of Drug-Loaded Filaments

Filaments were extruded using a 40D, 12-mm co-rotating twin-screw extruder (RES-2P/12A Explorer, Zamak Mercator®, Skawina, Poland) equipped with a gravimetric feeder MCPOWDER® (Movacolor®, Sneek, The Netherlands) and an air-cooled conveying belt (Zamak Mercator®, Skawina, Poland). The mixtures of itraconazole and matrix-forming polymers, of the composition presented in Table 1, and the total mass equal to 200 g were extruded through a 1.75 mm die at 160 °C. The feeding rate was set to approximately 70 g/h, which resulted in the linear filament extrusion speed of 25 m/h. The barrel temperature varied from 40 to 190 °C. The optimized temperature profile and screw configuration are presented in Figure 1.

Table 1. Composition of the filaments.

Formulation	Itraconazole	Poly(vinyl alcohol)	Copovidone	Crospovidone
PVA		80%	-	-
PVA_K/VA	20%	56%	24%	-
PVA_K/CL		76%	-	4%

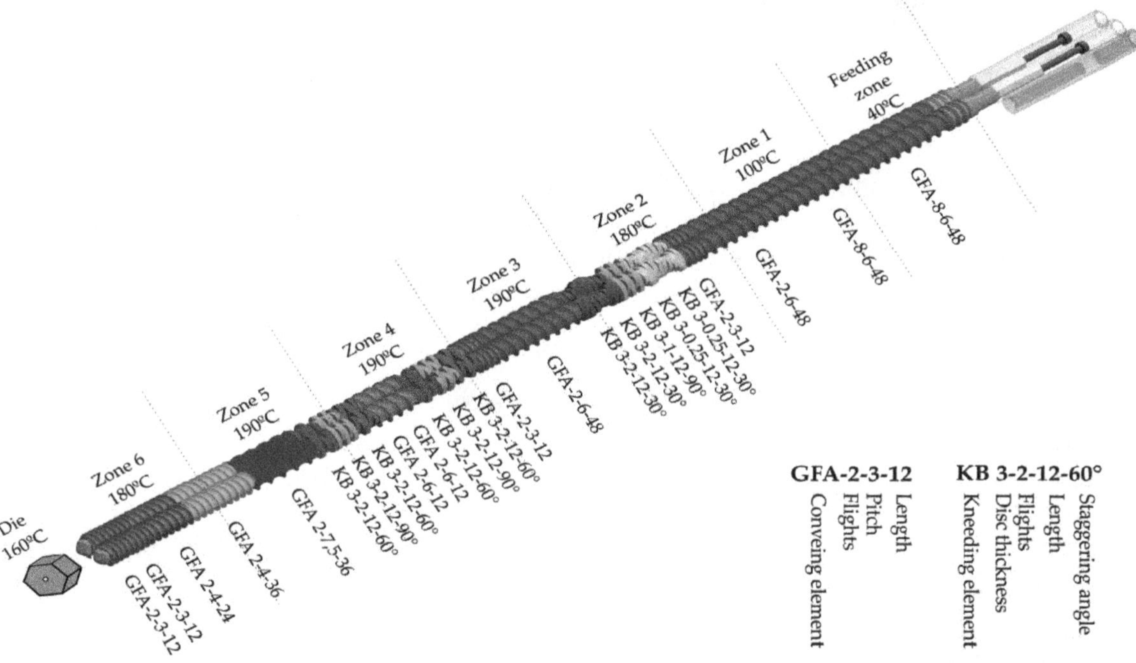

Figure 1. Screw configuration and temperature profile.

2.3. Evaluation of Filament Properties

The diameter uniformity of the obtained filament was evaluated using a Mitutoyo® micrometer screw (Kawasaki, Japan). Six randomly selected points were measured. Mechanical properties were assessed in stretching test performed with an EZ-SX tensile tester (Shimadzu®, Kioto, Japan). The measurements were performed six times for each type of filament. Randomly selected pieces of filament, 100 mm in length, were placed in the tensile tester's jaws and stretched up to breakage. Hardness and elasticity of the filaments were determined based on the measurements of tensile strength and Young's modulus.

2.4. Determination of Itraconazole Content in the Obtained Filament

Six randomly selected and accurately weighed pieces of filament were placed in conical flasks filled with 25 mL of a mixture of methanol and 0.1 M HCl of pH 1.2 (1:1 v/v) and shaken for 24 h using a Memmert® water bath (WNB 22, Schwabach, Germany). The drug concentration was assayed at $\lambda = 255$ nm using a Shimadzu® UV-1800 spectrophotometer (Kioto, Japan). The specificity of the analytical method was verified. There was no sign of interference between the drug and excipients at the analytical wavelength.

2.5. Preparation of 3D Printed Tablets

The Blender® 2.79b software was used to design the models of the oblong tablets (Blender Foundation, Amsterdam, The Netherlands). The basic model was 20 mm long and 10 mm wide. The model height varied from 2.4 to 3.65 mm, which was related to the number of 3D printed layers. Voxelizer® slicing software (version 1.4.18, ZMorph®, Wroclaw, Poland) was applied to define the height and the width of the single layer path. The 3D model was imported in stl format and divided into layers before printing. The thickness of the first layer was equal to 0.2 mm to improve the adhesion of the print to the printer bed, whereas the height of the subsequent layers was 0.15 mm. The path width was equal to the diameter of the printing nozzle, i.e., 0.4 mm. One outline and rectilinear infill (density of 20%, 35%, and 60%) were designed for the printing process. Each tablet was composed of 50 mg of ITR and 200 mg of polymer carriers (Table 1). The tablets were printed by an FDM ZMorph® 2.0 S personal fabricator (Wroclaw, Poland) equipped with a 1.75 mm commercially available printhead. Printing temperature was 205 °C. The tablets were printed with a 10–15 mm/s printing speed. The temperature of building platform was 40 °C.

2.6. Preparation of Tablets by Filament Compression (HME Tablets)

For comparison purposes, filament milled in a Tube Mill 100 control (IKA®, Staufen, Germany) and raw compounds were compressed in a Korsch® EK0 single-punch tablet press (Berlin, Germany). The composition of the tablets was similar to 3D printed tablets; each tablet was composed of 50 mg of ITR and 200 mg of polymer mixture. Additionally, the blends contained 12.5 mg of a talc and magnesium stearate mixture (9:1 w/w), which played the role of glidant and lubricant, respectively.

2.7. Preparation of Directly Compressed Tablets (DC Tablets)

Powder blends composed of 3DP tablet ingredients with the addition of the talc and magnesium stearate mixture (9:1 w/w) were compressed using Korsch® EK0 single-punch tablet press (Berlin, Germany) for comparison purposes, to investigate the impact of technological processes on the ITR dissolution profile.

2.8. Micro-Computed Tomography

Micro-computed tomography (µ-CT) analysis was performed using a SkyScan® 1172 microtomograph (Bruker®, Billerica, MA, USA). It was applied to examine the structure of the 3DP tablets with 20%, 35%, and 60% of infill and to verify the repeatability of printing process (the data collected for three tablets with 35% of infill were compared). The image pixel size was 6.9 µm for measurements of all samples. A cone beam reconstruction software program (Nrecon SkyScan®, Bruker®, Billerica, MA, USA) based on the Feldkamp algorithm was used for the reconstruction of the projections. A CT-Analyser® (SkyScan®, Bruker®, Billerica, MA, USA) was used for binarization purposes. The procedure was based on density distribution histograms collected for the whole sample volume. A CT-Analyser® was also used for the characterization of the morphological features of the tablets, their volume, and surface. CTVox® software (Bruker®, Billerica, MA, USA) was applied to present the 3D results.

2.9. Differential Scanning Calorimetry (DSC)

Thermodynamic properties of neat ITR, PVA, K/VA, K/CL, and their mixtures in the form of filaments and 3DP tablets were examined using a DSC 1 STAR^e System (Mettler-Toledo®, Greifensee,

Switzerland) equipped with an HSS8 ceramic sensor with 120 thermocouples and liquid nitrogen cooling station. Zinc and indium standards were used for the temperature and enthalpy calibration. The samples were measured in an aluminum, pinned crucible (40 mL). The samples were heated with a rate of 10 K/min. The experiments were performed in nitrogen atmosphere with a gas flow of 60 mL/min.

2.10. X-Ray Powder Diffraction (XRD)

A Rigaku Denki® D/MAX Rapid II-R (Tokyo, Japan) equipped with a rotating Ag anode and an image plate detector in the Debye–Scherrer geometry was used for the X-ray diffraction measurements. Graphite (002) crystal was used to monochromatize the incident radiation ($\lambda_{K\alpha}$ = 0.5608 Å). The width of the X-ray beam at the sample was 0.3 mm. The samples were pulverized before the experiment and measured at room temperature, in glass capillaries with a diameter of 1.5 mm and wall thickness of 0.01 mm. The background intensity from empty capillary was subtracted. The obtained two-dimensional diffraction patterns were converted into one-dimensional functions of intensity versus the scattering vector.

2.11. Dissolution Studies

The dissolution of ITR from tablets was determined in 1000 mL of 0.1 M HCl with the addition of KCl, in the pharmacopeial paddle apparatus (Vision® G2 Elite 8, Hanson Research®, Chatsworth, CA, USA) equipped with a VisionG2 AutoPlus autosampler. Stainless steel, spring-like sinkers were used to prevent tablet floating. The samples were filtered and analyzed on-line at 255 nm at predetermined periods using a UV-1800 spectrophotometer (Shimadzu®, Kioto, Japan) equipped with flow-through cuvettes. Three repetitions for each sample were carried out. The results represent the averaged results and the standard deviations (mean ± SD).

2.12. Solubility Study

An excess of physical mixture (PM), extrudate (HME), and printed systems (3DP) were dispersed in 20 mL of 0.1 MHCl and shaken at ambient temperature using a KS 130 basic orbital shaker (IKA®, Staufen im Breisgau, Germany). After 48h, the samples were filtered through a 0.45 μm Chromafil® Xtra CA-45/25 membrane filter and analyzed spectrophotometrically at λ = 255 nm (UV-1800 Shimadzu®, Kioto, Japan). The reported data represent the averages from three series of measurements with standard deviations (SD).

3. Results

3.1. Evaluation of the Filaments

All prepared filaments were made using a PVA as a filament-forming polymer, a semi-crystalline polymer of molecular weight equal to 32 kDa with 87–89% hydrolysis grade, having a glass transition temperature, melting point, and degradation temperature of 40–45 °C, 170 °C, and ≥250 °C, respectively [66]. The obtained itraconazole-loaded filaments were opaque and creamy in color. The diameter of the filaments was kept at a constant level; however, in the case of the PVA_K/CL filament, the diameter variations were higher than 0.05 mm, which is considered as a maximum acceptable deviation from the declared diameter [71]. The itraconazole content and its uniformity were satisfactory. All the API-loaded filaments were tested for their tensile strength and elasticity, which were found to be critical quality attributes in term of printability. The results are presented in Table 2. It was found that the addition of copovidone and crosslinked PVP resulted in a decrease in the tensile strength and Young's modulus of the filaments. All the prepared filaments were able to be printed with a ZMorph® 2.0 S 3D printer immediately after extrusion and after storage in zipper storage bags.

Table 2. Hot-melt extruded filament characteristics.

Filament Composition	Diameter ± SD (mm)	Itraconazole Content ± SD (%)	Tensile Strength ± SD (MPa)	Young's Modulus ± SD (MPa)
PVA	1.70 ± 0.02	19.67 ± 0.43	49.0 ± 10.3	2641.1 ± 144.4
PVA_K/CL	1.68 ± 0.07	19.60 ± 0.34	52.6 ± 19.8	2771.1 ± 347.2
PVA_K/VA	1.69 ± 0.05	19.20 ± 0.33	28.2 ± 7.1	2042.1 ± 256.3

In Figure 2, the differences in the mechanical characteristics are presented. The Young's modulus corresponds to the slope of the curve in the elastic behavior region.

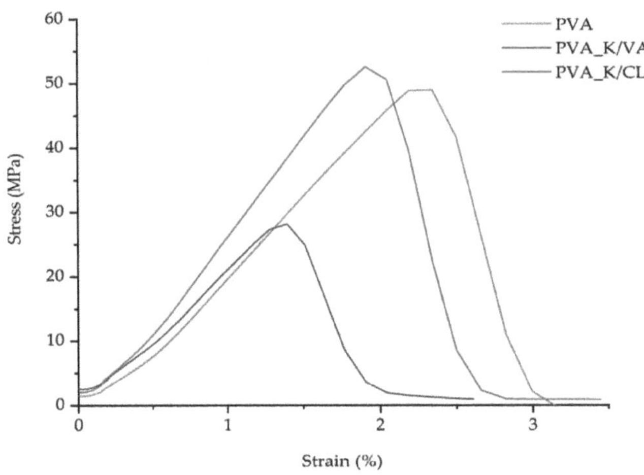

Figure 2. Comparison of the mechanical strength and resilience of the filaments.

3.2. Thermal and Structural Properties of the Filaments and 3DP Tablets

To investigate how the employed polymers modify the thermal properties of neat ITR, the systems, prepared in the form of both filaments and 3DP tablets, were measured (after pulverization) by means of DSC. The samples were examined in the temperature range from 273 to 453 K at a heating rate of 10 K/min. In Figure 3, the obtained DSC traces are compared to the thermogram of the neat, quench-cooled ITR. Because the used PVA polymer has a lower glass transition temperature than ITR (Table 3) (T_g of neat PVA and ITR are equal to 313 and 332 K, respectively), the plasticization effect was observed. Interestingly, the DSC thermograms of the same compositions with different forms, filament or 3DP, differ from each other. As can be seen in Figure 3, the thermograms of the 3DP tablets are characterized by: (i) a shift in glass transition temperature towards lower values when compared with filament and (ii) the appearance of an additional, very broad endothermal event in the vicinity of 320 to 420 K. The observed differences suggest that the 3DP tablets also contain water in addition to API and polymers. Water exerts a plasticization effect on the samples and evaporates at temperatures from in the range of 320 to 420 K.

When the neat ITR is heated above its glass transition temperature, on the DSC thermogram, one can distinguish two endothermal processes associated with the liquid crystal (LC) phase transitions. The thermal event located at 348 K reflects transition from smectic (Sm) to nematic (N) LC alignment, while at 364 K, ITR loses the nematic order and becomes an isotropic (I) liquid. The performed experiments reveal that the employed polymers shift to lower temperatures for both Sm-N and N-I phase transition. The determined, based on calorimetric studies, values of T_g, $T_{Sm\text{-}N}$, and $T_{N\text{-}I}$ for all investigated systems are compared in Table 3. It is worth noting that in one of the examined systems (PVA_K/VA), regardless of the applied technological process, the lack of the nematic phase was observed (i.e., the N-I endothermal event was not registered by means of DSC).

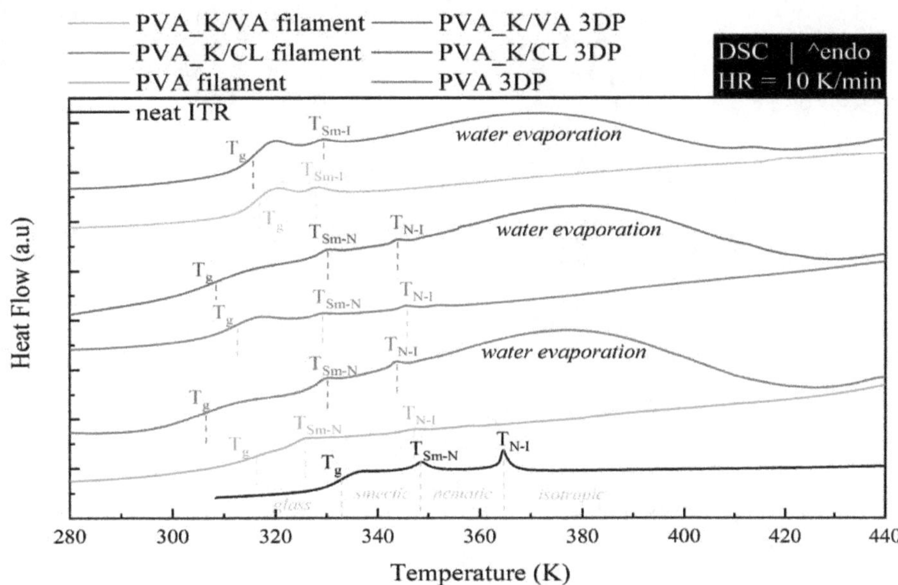

Figure 3. DSC thermograms of neat ITR and its mixtures with PVA, PVA_K/VA, and PVA_K/CL prepared in two forms: filament and 3DP tablet.

Table 3. Comparison of values of T_g, $T_{Sm\text{-}N}$, and $T_{N\text{-}I}$ of neat ITR and its mixtures with PVA, PVA_K/VA, and PVA_K/CL which were prepared in two forms: filament and 3DP tablet.

Sample	T_g (K)	$T_{Sm\text{-}N}$ (K)	$T_{N\text{-}I}$ (K)
Neat ITR	332	348	364
PVA filament	315	326	347
PVA 3DP tablet	306	330	344
PVA_K/CL filament	312	329	346
PVA_K/CL 3DP tablet	308	330	344
PVA_K/VA filament	317	328 ($T_{Sm\text{-}I}$)	
PVA_K/VA 3DP tablet	315	330 ($T_{Sm\text{-}I}$)	

In order to investigate whether the employed polymers indeed modify the ITR's LC alignment, both the neat ITR as well as the pulverized 3DP tablets were measured by wide-angle X-ray diffraction (XRD) technique. The comparison of the scattering patterns collected at room temperature for neat ITR and pulverized tablets containing either PVA, PVA_K/VA, or PVA_K/CL is presented in Figure 4. The presented XRD patterns demonstrate that the polymers affect the LC order in ITR. As can be seen, samples containing PVA or PVA_K/CL reveal less intense peaks at around 0.22, 0.45, and 0.68 $Å^{-1}$, which are indicators of smectic layering [72]. In the case of the system containing K/VA, the reduction in the intensity of the peaks at 0.22 and 0.68 $Å^{-1}$ is combined with the disappearance of the peak at 0.45 $Å^{-1}$. These results indicate that the layered structure in ITR is medicated by the employed additives.

3.3. Micro-Computed Tomography Studies of Tablets

The dimensions and masses of 3DP tablets corresponded to predefined values. The average tablet mass ranged from 239.73 to 253.05 mg. Tablet length varied from 19.85 to 20.15 mm, whereas height ranged from 1.78 to 3.65 mm. The real layer height was from 0.142 to 0.158 mm and was calculated by dividing the tablet height by the number of layers, given the fact that the first layer was 0.2 mm (Table 4). Digital photos of 3D printed tablets can be found in the Supplementary Materials associated with this article (Figures S1–S3, Supplementary Materials).

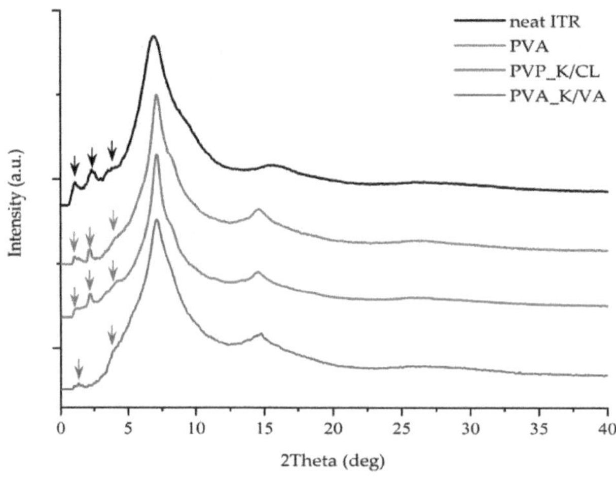

Figure 4. XRD diffraction patterns of neat ITR and its mixtures with PVA, PVA_K/VA, and PVA_K/CL in an initial form of 3DP tablet.

Table 4. Parameters of 3D printed tablets.

Polymers	Infill (%)	Mass (mg)	Width (mm)	Length (mm)	Height (mm)	Number of Layers	Real Layer Height (mm)
PVA	35	252.82 ± 4.16	10.18 ± 0.03	20.15 ± 0.03	2.34 ± 0.03	16	0.142
PVA_K/VA	35	253.05 ± 3.67	10.08 ± 0.01	20.09 ± 0.01	2.89 ± 0.05	20	0.142
PVA_K/CL	35	250.12 ± 4.52	9.98 ± 0.02	19.85 ± 0.12	2.67 ± 0.03	17	0.154
PVA_K/CL	20	244.12 ± 5.77	9.96 ± 0.03	19.86 ± 0.09	3.65 ± 0.03	24	0.150
PVA_K/CL	60	239.73 ± 3.01	9.99 ± 0.05	20.05 ± 0.03	1.78 ± 0.02	11	0.158

Based on the 3D tablet images obtained from Voxelizer slicing software (Figure 5) and predefined settings of the path size, the theoretical volume of 3DP PVA_K/CL tablets was calculated. The values varied from 184.4 mm^3 for T_20 tablets to 195.6 mm^3 for T_60 and 195.9 mm^3 for T_35 tablets.

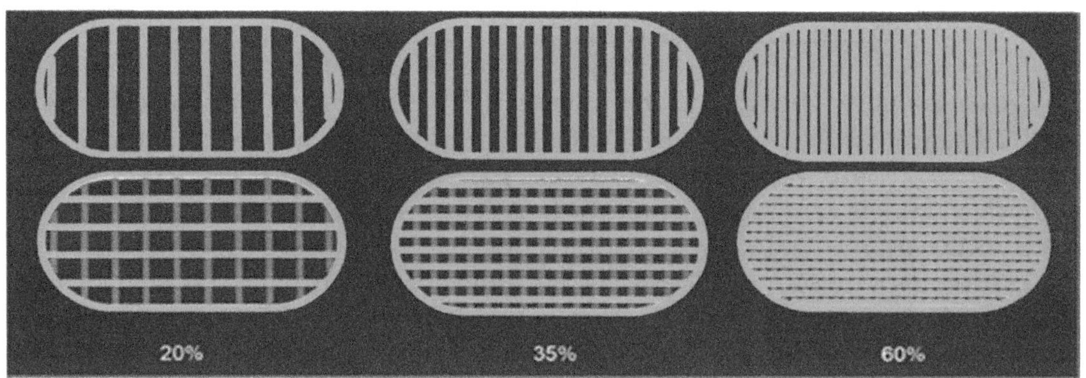

Figure 5. Images of PVA_K/CL tablet layers obtained from Voxelizer software.

The morphology of the PVA_K/CL printed tablets was verified by the μCT scans. Tablets with 20% of infill had the highest object volume (236 mm^3) and the highest open pore volume (485 mm^3). Medium pore size (structure separation) was 1.11 mm, whereas the average structure thickness was 0.25 mm. Tablets with 60% of infill were characterized by the lowest values of object volume (202 mm^3) and pore volume (134 mm^3) as well as structure separation (0.19 mm) and pore size (0.25 mm). Aforementioned parameters for tablets with 35% of infill can be placed between T_20 and T_60 values (Table 5, Figure 6).

Table 5. Comparison of μCT scan data of 3DP PVA_K/CL tablets with 20% (T_20), 35% (T_35), and 60% (T_60) infill ratio.

Description	Unit	T_20	T_35	T_60
Object volume	mm^3	236	220	202
Percent object volume	%	33	41	60
Structure thickness	mm	0.25	0.20	0.19
Structure separation	mm	1.11	0.62	0.25
Volume of open pore space	mm^3	485	312	134
Open porosity	%	67.2	58.5	39.9

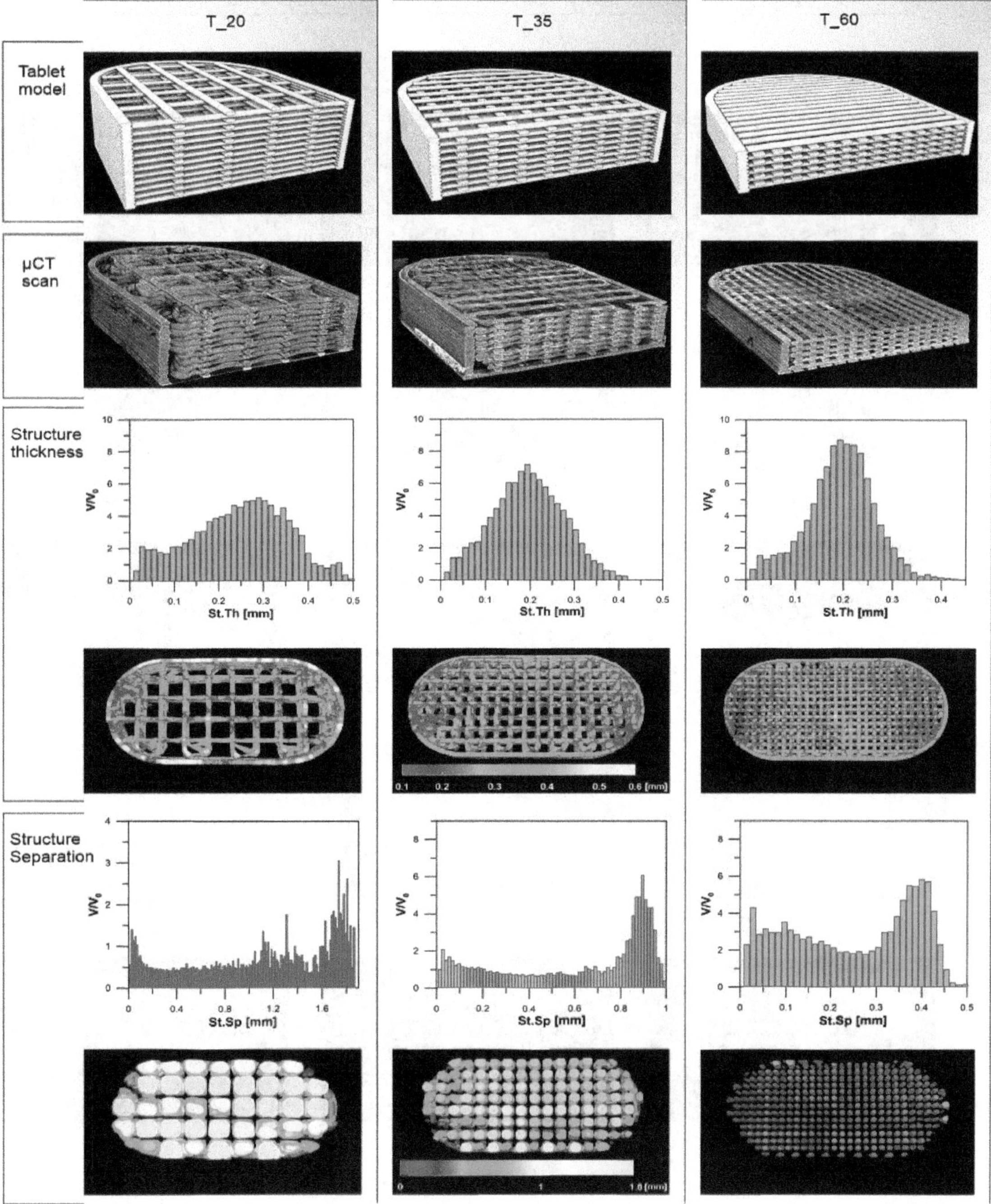

Figure 6. 3D tablet models, μ-CT scan images of 3DP tablets, and structure thickness and structure separation of 3DP tablets.

Parameters of tablets with 35% of infill are similar and no important differences between the three analyzed tablets can be distinguished (Table 6, Figure 7).

Table 6. Comparison of μCT scan data of 3DP PVA_K/CL tablets with 35% of infill ratio.

Description	Unit	T_35_1	T_35_2	T_35_3
Object volume	mm^3	220	224	213
Percent object volume	%	41	42	39
Structure thickness	mm	0.20	0.19	0.17
Structure separation	mm	0.62	0.62	0.62
Volume of open pore space	mm^3	312	307	327
Open porosity	%	58.5	57.7	60.4

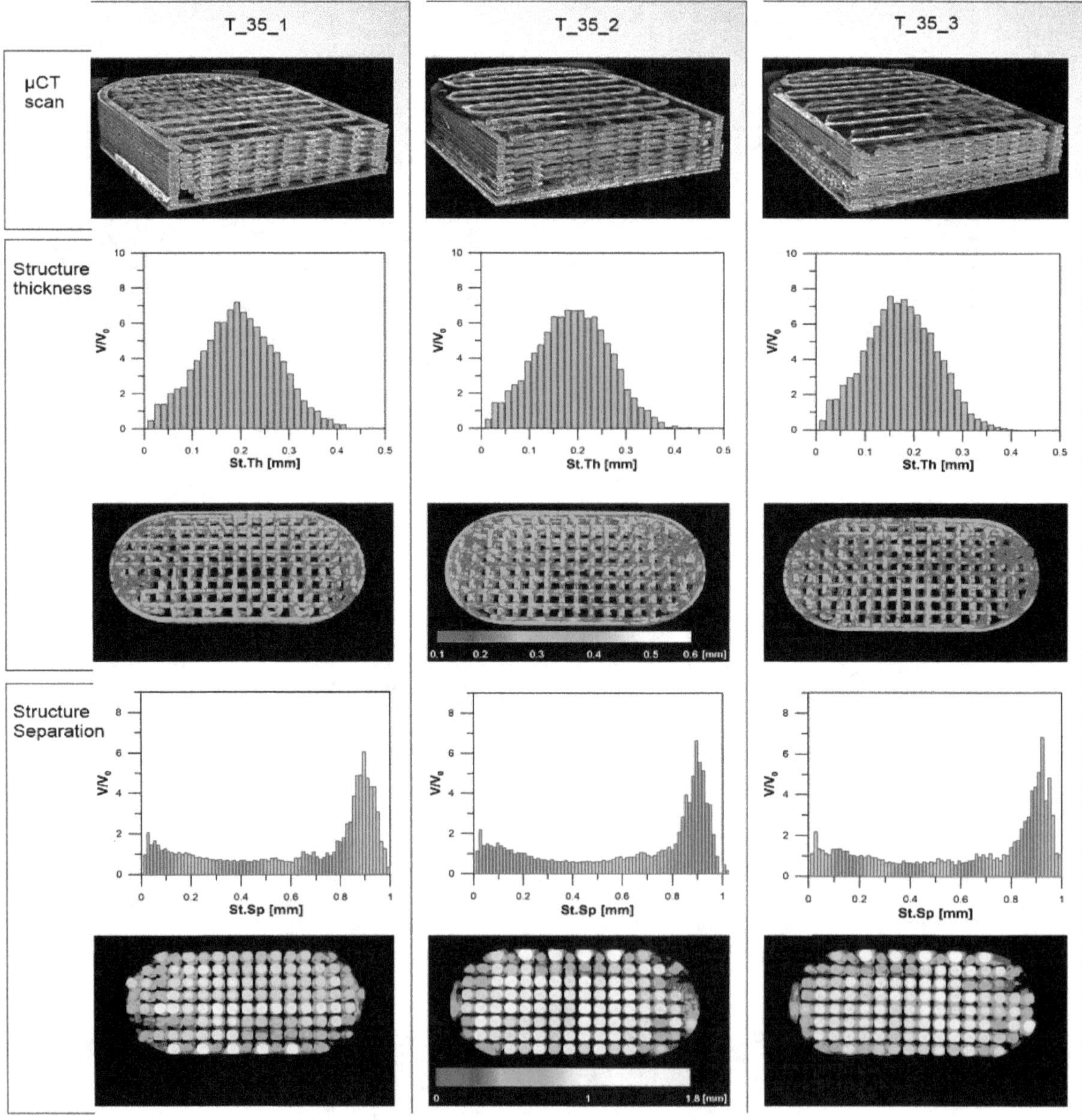

Figure 7. Comparison of 3DP tablets with 35% of infill.

3.4. Dissolution Studies

Itraconazole dissolution from 3D printed tablets with 35% infill was compared with the dissolution profiles obtained for the tablets made from milled extrudate (HME tablets) and directly compressed tablets (DC tablets) to evaluate the impact of the excipients and hot-melt extrusion on the dissolution of the API. Determined itraconazole solubility limits were equal to 5.8, 22.2, and 29.3 μg/mL for physical mixture, extrudate, and 3D printed matrix, respectively. The solubility limits were calculated as the percentage of ITR dose in tablets (11.6%, 44.4%, and 58.6% for physical mixture, extrudate, and 3D printed tablet, respectively) and are marked in Figure 8 to make the interpretation of the dissolution easier. It was found that the performed technological processes, namely hot-melt extrusion and 3D printing, affected the dissolution profile of itraconazole. The highest amount of the drug was dissolved from 3D printed tablets. The amount of ITR released from milled extrudate was significantly lower, while the smallest amount was released from directly compressed tablets (Figure 8). After 2 h of the dissolution test, 75.8%, 51.3%, and 11.0% of the itraconazole was released from the PVA-based 3D printed, hot-melt extruded, and directly compressed tablets, respectively. This relationship was confirmed for all the prepared formulations. It must be highlighted that in the case of all 3D printed formulations, i.e., PVA, PVA_K/VA, and PVA_K/CL, the amount of dissolved itraconazole was far above the solubility limit and the supersaturation lasted as long as the dissolution test was performed.

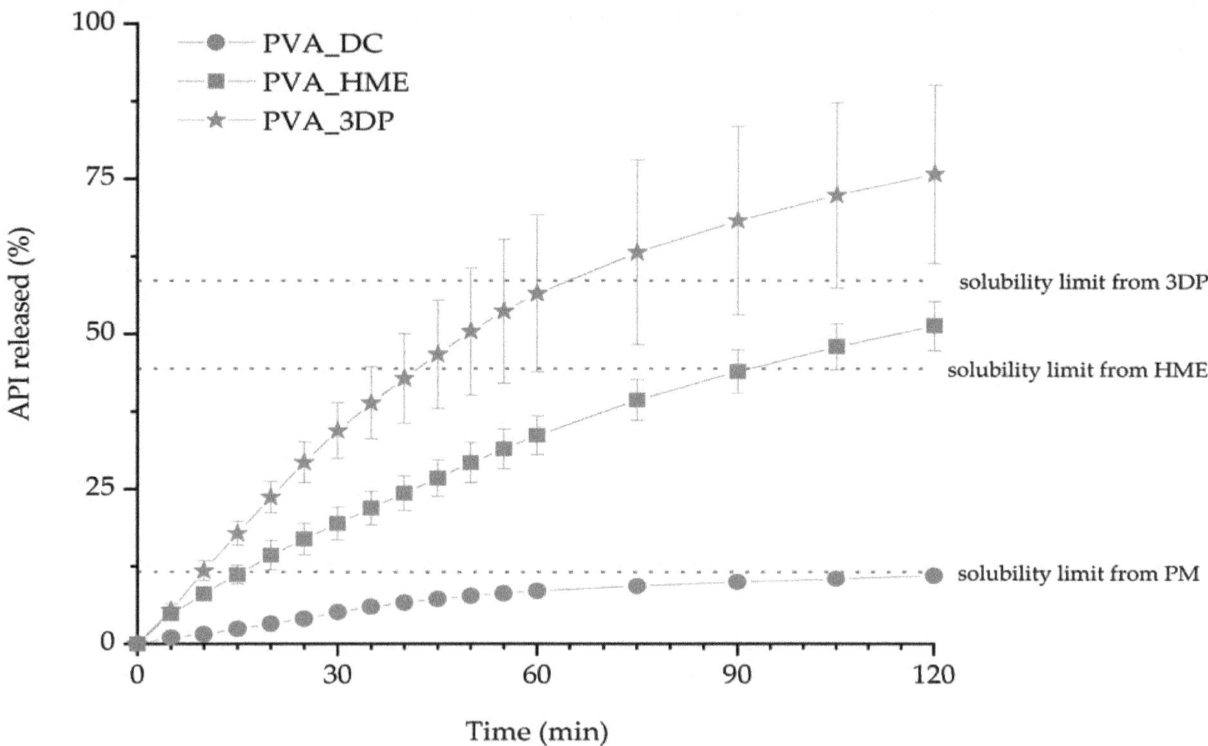

Figure 8. The influence of the technological process on the release profiles of itraconazole from PVA-based tablets (infill density equal to 35%).

The impact of copovidone and crospovidone addition to the PVA formulation on the release profile was also evaluated (Figure 9). The best dissolution profile was noticed for PVA_K/CL 3D printed tablets. After 45 min, 91.5% of the API was dissolved from PVA_K/CL 3D printed tablets, while only 64.3% and 46.7% of the drug was released from 3D printed tablets with Kollidon® VA64 and PVA-based tablets, respectively.

The impact of the infill density on the dissolution characteristics was evaluated for the PVA_K/CL formulation (Figure 10) as it was selected as the most promising formulation from all the prepared 3D printed tablets. Three rectilinear infills with different densities, namely 20%, 35%, and 60%, were evaluated. The results confirmed that the lower infill density favored faster dissolution of the API. After 45 min of the dissolution test, 96.9%, 89.7%, and 80.9% of the itraconazole was released from 3D printed tablets with 20%, 35%, and 60% infill, respectively.

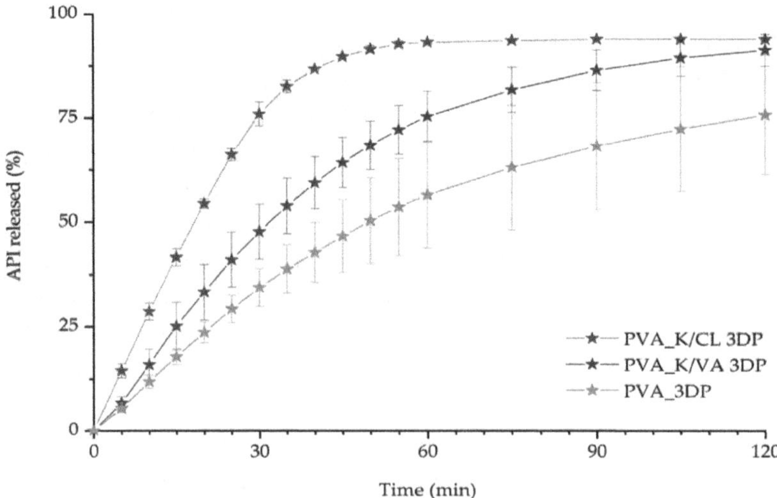

Figure 9. The influence of the excipients on dissolution profiles of itraconazole from 3DP tablets (infill density equal to 35%).

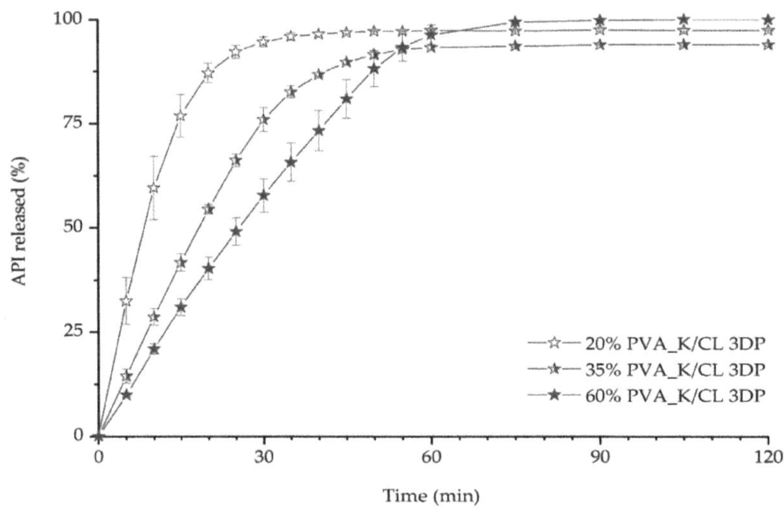

Figure 10. The influence of infill percentage on dissolution profiles of itraconazole from 3DP tablets.

4. Discussion

The filament extrusion went smoothly, and it can be carried out as a continuous manufacturing process. As a result of the optimization of the barrel temperature profile, generated torque, which may be considered as one of the major limitations during the extrusion, was as low as 2.82 ± 0.09 Nm during the filament extrusion process. All the prepared filaments were of satisfying quality and were printable using a ZMorph® 2.0 S 3D printer. PVA-based filaments were characterized by the most uniform diameter which may result from the simplest composition of the filament. Copovidone (K/VA) was added to the filament formulation to improve the solubility of the drug in the polymer matrix as it was shown by Włodarski et al. [65], while crosslinked PVP (K/CL) was added to improve disintegration and API dissolution from the extrudates and 3D printed tablets. The elasticity of the filaments was evaluated based on the Young's modulus values. The values obtained for itraconazole-loaded filaments were in the range 2042.1–2641.1 MPa and they were comparable to the results obtained by Feuerbach et al. for Resomer filaments [73]. The filament elasticity was not significantly affected by the addition of either copovidone or crospovidone to the formulation, while the values of the Young's modulus varied in the narrow range. However, it was found that the filament with the addition of copovidone was characterized by slightly higher elasticity than the one composed of only PVA or PVA-K/VA filaments. The obtained Young's modulus values for all prepared filaments suggest that they are suitable for fused deposition modeling 3D printing. The tensile strength was in the range from 28.2 to 52.6 MPa; the lowest value was obtained for the filament with the addition of Kollidon®VA64. Its introduction to the polymer matrix caused a more than 1.7-fold decrease in tensile strength in comparison with the itraconazole-loaded PVA filament. This may result from the Kollidon®VA64 extrudate's brittleness, which was confirmed by Fuenmayor et al. [74]; however, it was still durable enough to be printed.

A set of 10 × 20 mm^2 oblong tablets with different infill densities was printed with good repeatability. The tablets were uniform in shape and mass. The dimensions of the 3DP tablets were similar to predefined 3D objects. The adjustment of tablet height and, in consequence, the number of layers was related to the filament properties to obtain tablets with comparable mass (Table 4). The differences in tablet mass did not exceed 12.5 mg (±5%) from the theoretical value of 250 mg.

The theoretical tablets' volume was compared to the real object volume of 3DP PVA_K/CL tablets with infill of 20%, 35%, and 60% (Table 5), determined during the μCT scan. In the case of 20% of infill tablets (T_20), the real tablet volume was almost 1.3 times higher than calculated. This is related to the morphology of tablets with low infill density. The substantial distance between infill cross-points, in which two adjacent layers adhere, resulted in overhangs without support. It led to path disorder and an increase in vertical layer dimension. Therefore, subsequent cohesion in some spaces between cross-points was observed (Figure 6). In the case of T_35, the difference in tablet volume was smaller (1.12 times higher) whereas the volumes of T_60 tablets were similar (1.03 times higher). This improvement was related to the higher density of tablets' infill with increasing number of cross-points.

The phenomenon of path expansion between the cross-points can also be explained by the deviations of the structure thickness parameter in comparison with the theoretical value of 0.15 mm. This effect was observed for all degrees of infill; however, it was less pronounced in the systems with the higher infill density (Figure 6). The biggest difference was noticed in the case of T_20 tablets, for which the mean structure thickness was 100 μm higher than the theoretical layer height. For T_35 and T_60 tablets, the structure thickness was 40–50 μm higher. The differences in the structure thickness distribution are presented in Figure 6. The widest span of structure thickness was noticed for T_20 tablets and the structures with 0.25–0.35 mm thickness had the greatest volume within 3DP objects. On the contrary, the T_60 tablets exhibited the narrowest span, with structures of thickness varying between 0.15 and 0.25 mm highly represented within the object (Figure 6). Structure thickness distribution among a set of T_35 tested tablets was similar and showed good repeatability of printed dosage forms with 35% of infill (Table 6, Figure 7). Moreover, identical mean structure separation was observed within all T_35 tablets (Table 6) The porosity within T_35 tablets was similar, and histograms of structure separation distribution revealed that pores with size 0.8–1.0 mm are highly represented (Figure 7). Decreasing the tablet infill from 35% to 20% resulted in porosity changes. Pores with larger sizes, between 1.2 and 1.75 mm, are visible on the histograms and the total porosity increased from 58.5% to 67.2%. In the case of T_60 tablets, pore size did not exceed 0.5 mm and total porosity was almost 1.7 times smaller (39.9%) than T_20 (Figure 6). It should be emphasized that the volume of the open pore space within the 3DP T_20 tablet (485 mm^3) is twice as high as the volume of the solid part of the tablet (236 mm^3), whereas the volume of the open pore space of T_60 (134 mm^3) is 1.5 times smaller than the solid part of the tablet (202 mm^3). The tablet open space will promote the penetration of dissolution media through the tablet's internal structure and will have an impact on its disintegration and dissolution behavior. The influence of the internal structure of 3D printed objects on their properties was highlighted and widely discussed by Nazir et al. in the comprehensive review of the various 3D printed lattice and cellular structures, their advantages and limitations [75].

The results of the dissolution studies indicate that the 3D printing process improved itraconazole release when compared with tablets made by compression with either milled extrudate or a simple powder blend. This should be attributed to the developed internal structure and resulting extended surface area as well as the molecular rearrangement in the structure of API within the polymer matrix. Itraconazole release was faster from tablets containing added copovidone than PVA alone because the hot-melt extrusion and following 3D printing led to the formation of more disordered systems, which was confirmed by the lower intensity of the characteristic peaks in the XRD diffractograms and the lack of the nematic phase confirmed by DSC in the PVA_K/VA 3DP tablets. The release of itraconazole from filaments and 3D printed tablets containing only PVA was lower than from the corresponding systems containing the additive of PVP-based polymers since its structure was more ordered, as indicated by the presence of smectic and nematic domains. It is worth mentioning that the improved drug dissolution results from the applied technological processes, not just the addition of the polymers. The results of the dissolution from directly compressed tablets revealed that the presence of the polymers themselves did not enhance the dissolution of itraconazole as the amount of dissolved API did not exceed 12% of the initial dose.

The results indicated that the addition of the disintegrant, i.e., crospovidone, to the 3D printed tablets is beneficial in terms of ITR dissolution. The addition of the disintegrant to the formulation led to a higher increase in API dissolution than adding a copovidone to achieve molecularly disordered material. With the presented results, we have demonstrated that the PVA_K/CL formulation is the most promising in terms of immediate-release tablet preparation, as it is characterized by the best dissolution profile. Subsequent optimization was performed to evaluate the possibility of further improvement of itraconazole release. The optimization included changes in the infill density, as it was confirmed by many research groups that infill density significantly affects the dissolution rate of the API [76]. The tablets with infill density of 20%, 35%, and 60% were successfully 3D printed and tested. As predicted, lower infill density resulted in faster dissolution. However, the micro-computed tomography imaging revealed that during the printing of the tablets with 20% infill, there was an issue with maintaining the internal structure geometry, which also manifested in higher deviations in the amount of dissolved itraconazole in the first 20 min of the dissolution test (Figure 10). The tablets with 60% infill were characterized by the slowest itraconazole release. This is directly connected with the difficulty of water penetration into the tablet due to the smaller pores and channels in the internal structure. Therefore, we chose 35% infill as the best formulation to evaluate the tablet shape, dose, and internal structure reproducibility in the 3D printing process. In all cases of 3D printed tablets, long-lasting supersaturation of the itraconazole was achieved. It is well-known that the persisting state of supersaturation may lead to bioavailability improvements, which is especially beneficial in terms of poorly soluble drugs such as itraconazole [77].

5. Conclusions

Our study has shown the detailed methodology for the development of immediate-release 3D printed tablets with liquid crystal-forming itraconazole. The development stage included both the optimization of the formulation composition and the correlation between the geometry of the printed object, namely the degree of infill, with shape reproducibility and drug dissolution.

The use of well-printable PVA polymer alongside the functionalized excipients, i.e., polyvinylpyrrolidone derivatives, during the hot-melt extrusion process covered not only the optimization of the mechanical properties of the filament and its printability but also the function of the polymer matrix in terms of intended drug release profiles. The results of the dissolution study and physicochemical analysis indicated that improved disintegration obtained due to the use of Kollidon®CL-M was more beneficial than the molecular rearrangement and liquid crystal phase transitions. The lower infill density favored faster dissolution of the drug from printed tablets.

Micro-computed tomography was utilized to confirm that the design of printed objects was properly reconstructed. The comprehensive analysis revealed that the infill density, which is often considered as a way to control or improve drug dissolution, should be utilized with a deep understanding of its effect on the 3D printed objects' reproducibility. In the case of low infill densities, reproducibility issues, i.e., path disorder, increased layer dimension, and the path cohesion between cross-points, may occur. On the contrary, dense infill limits the surface area available for dissolution media and slows down the dissolution of the API.

In the case of the presented results, the most appropriate properties, i.e., good reproducibility during the object printing combined with superior drug dissolution, were achieved for the filament composed of 20% of itraconazole, 76% of PVA, and 4% of crospovidone acting as a disintegrant.

Author Contributions: Conceptualization, W.J., M.P. and R.J.; validation, J.S.-S.; investigation, W.J., J.P., M.K., J.K.-K., K.J., B.L. and A.W.; writing—original draft preparation, W.J.; writing—review and editing, J.P., M.K., J.S.-S., J.K.-K., M.P. and R.J.; visualization, W.J. and M.K.; supervision, R.J.; project administration, R.J. All authors have read and agreed to the published version of the manuscript.

References

1. Pandey, M.; Choudhury, H.; Fern, J.L.C.; Kee, A.T.K.; Kou, J.; Jing, J.L.J.; Her, H.C.; Yong, H.S.; Ming, H.C.; Bhattamisra, S.K.; et al. 3D printing for oral drug delivery: A new tool to customize drug delivery. *Drug Deliv. Transl. Res.* **2020**, *10*, 986–1001. [CrossRef] [PubMed]
2. Pereira, B.C.; Isreb, A.; Forbes, R.T.; Dores, F.; Habashy, R.; Petit, J.-B.; Alhnan, M.A.; Oga, E.F. 'Temporary Plasticiser': A novel solution to fabricate 3D printed patient-centred cardiovascular 'Polypill' architectures. *Eur. J. Pharm. Biopharm.* **2019**, *135*, 94–103. [CrossRef]
3. Solanki, N.G.; Tahsin, M.; Shah, A.V.; Serajuddin, A.T. Formulation of 3D Printed Tablet for Rapid Drug Release by Fused Deposition Modeling: Screening Polymers for Drug Release, Drug-Polymer Miscibility and Printability. *J. Pharm. Sci.* **2018**, *107*, 390–401. [CrossRef]
4. Jamróz, W.; Szafraniec, J.; Kurek, M.; Jachowicz, R. 3D Printing in Pharmaceutical and Medical Applications—Recent Achievements and Challenges. *Pharm. Res.* **2018**, *35*, 1–22. [CrossRef]
5. Tagami, T.; Nagata, N.; Hayashi, N.; Ogawa, E.; Fukushige, K.; Sakai, N.; Ozeki, T. Defined drug release from 3D-printed composite tablets consisting of drug-loaded polyvinylalcohol and a water-soluble or water-insoluble polymer filler. *Int. J. Pharm.* **2018**, *543*, 361–367. [CrossRef]
6. Korte, C.; Quodbach, J. 3D-Printed Network Structures as Controlled-Release Drug Delivery Systems: Dose Adjustment, API Release Analysis and Prediction. *AAPS PharmSciTech* **2018**, *19*, 3333–3342. [CrossRef] [PubMed]
7. Jamróz, W.; Kurek, M.; Szafraniec-Szczęsny, J.; Czech, A.; Gawlak, K.; Knapik-Kowalczuk, J.; Leszczyński, B.; Wróbel, A.; Paluch, M.; Jachowicz, R. Speed it up, slow it down ... An issue of bicalutamide release from 3D printed tablets. *Eur. J. Pharm. Sci.* **2020**, *143*, 105169. [CrossRef] [PubMed]
8. Allahham, N.; Fina, F.; Marcuta, C.; Kraschew, L.; Mohr, W.; Gaisford, S.; Basit, A.W.; Goyanes, A. Selective Laser Sintering 3D Printing of Orally Disintegrating Printlets Containing Ondansetron. *Pharmaceutics* **2020**, *12*, 110. [CrossRef] [PubMed]
9. Ong, J.J.; Awad, A.; Martorana, A.; Gaisford, S.; Stoyanov, E.; Basit, A.W.; Goyanes, A. 3D printed opioid medicines with alcohol-resistant and abuse-deterrent properties. *Int. J. Pharm.* **2020**, *579*, 119169. [CrossRef] [PubMed]
10. Martinez, P.R.; Goyanes, A.; Basit, A.W.; Gaisford, S. Influence of Geometry on the Drug Release Profiles of Stereolithographic (SLA) 3D-Printed Tablets. *AAPS PharmSciTech* **2018**, *19*, 3355–3361. [CrossRef] [PubMed]
11. Pere, C.P.P.; Economidou, S.N.; Lall, G.; Ziraud, C.; Boateng, J.S.; Alexander, B.D.; Lamprou, D.A.; Douroumis, D. 3D printed microneedles for insulin skin delivery. *Int. J. Pharm.* **2018**, *544*, 425–432. [CrossRef]
12. Healy, A.V.; Fuenmayor, E.; Doran, P.; Geever, L.M.; Higginbotham, C.L.; Lyons, J.G. Additive Manufacturing of Personalized Pharmaceutical Dosage Forms via Stereolithography. *Pharmaceutics* **2019**, *11*, 645. [CrossRef]
13. Karakurt, I.; Aydoğdu, A.; Çıkrıkcı, S.; Orozco, J.; Lin, L. Stereolithography (SLA) 3D printing of ascorbic acid loaded hydrogels: A controlled release study. *Int. J. Pharm.* **2020**, *584*, 119428. [CrossRef]
14. Uddin, J.; Scoutaris, N.; Economidou, S.N.; Giraud, C.; Chowdhry, B.Z.; Donnelly, R.F.; Douroumis, D. 3D printed microneedles for anticancer therapy of skin tumours. *Mater. Sci. Eng. C* **2020**, *107*, 110248. [CrossRef]
15. Fina, F.; Goyanes, A.; Madla, C.M.; Awad, A.; Trenfield, S.J.; Kuek, J.M.; Patel, P.; Gaisford, S.; Basit, A.W. 3D printing of drug-loaded gyroid lattices using selective laser sintering. *Int. J. Pharm.* **2018**, *547*, 44–52. [CrossRef]
16. Kadry, H.; Wadnap, S.; Xu, C.; Ahsan, F. Digital light processing (DLP) 3D-printing technology and photoreactive polymers in fabrication of modified-release tablets. *Eur. J. Pharm. Sci.* **2019**, *135*, 60–67. [CrossRef] [PubMed]

17. Yang, Y.; Zhou, Y.; Lin, X.; Yang, Q.; Yang, G. Printability of External and Internal Structures Based on Digital Light Processing 3D Printing Technique. *Pharmaceutics* **2020**, *12*, 207. [CrossRef] [PubMed]
18. Infanger, S.; Haemmerli, A.; Iliev, S.; Baier, A.; Stoyanov, E.; Quodbach, J. Powder bed 3D-printing of highly loaded drug delivery devices with hydroxypropyl cellulose as solid binder. *Int. J. Pharm.* **2019**, *555*, 198–206. [CrossRef]
19. Sen, K.; Manchanda, A.; Mehta, T.; Ma, A.W.; Chaudhuri, B. Formulation design for inkjet-based 3D printed tablets. *Int. J. Pharm.* **2020**, *584*, 119430. [CrossRef]
20. Goyanes, A.; Allahham, N.; Trenfield, S.J.; Stoyanov, E.; Gaisford, S.; Basit, A.W. Direct powder extrusion 3D printing: Fabrication of drug products using a novel single-step process. *Int. J. Pharm.* **2019**, *567*, 118471. [CrossRef]
21. Fanous, M.; Gold, S.; Muller, S.; Hirsch, S.; Ogorka, J.; Imanidis, G. Simplification of fused deposition modeling 3D-printing paradigm: Feasibility of 1-step direct powder printing for immediate release dosage form production. *Int. J. Pharm.* **2020**, *578*, 119124. [CrossRef]
22. Öblom, H.; Sjöholm, E.; Rautamo, M.; Sandler, N. Towards Printed Pediatric Medicines in Hospital Pharmacies: Comparison of 2D and 3D-Printed Orodispersible Warfarin Films with Conventional Oral Powders in Unit Dose Sachets. *Pharmaceutics* **2019**, *11*, 334. [CrossRef]
23. Cui, M.; Pan, H.; Fang, D.; Qiao, S.; Wang, S.; Pan, W. Fabrication of high drug loading levetiracetam tablets using semi-solid extrusion 3D printing. *J. Drug Deliv. Sci. Technol.* **2020**, *57*, 101683. [CrossRef]
24. Karavasili, C.; Gkaragkounis, A.; Moschakis, T.; Ritzoulis, C.; Fatouros, D.G. Pediatric-friendly chocolate-based dosage forms for the oral administration of both hydrophilic and lipophilic drugs fabricated with extrusion-based 3D printing. *Eur. J. Pharm. Sci.* **2020**, *147*, 105291. [CrossRef]
25. El Aita, I.; Breitkreutz, J.; Quodbach, J. Investigation of semi-solid formulations for 3D printing of drugs after prolonged storage to mimic real-life applications. *Eur. J. Pharm. Sci.* **2020**, *146*, 105266. [CrossRef]
26. Elbl, J.; Gajdziok, J.; Kolarczyk, J. 3D printing of multilayered orodispersible films with in-process drying. *Int. J. Pharm.* **2020**, *575*, 118883. [CrossRef]
27. Jamróz, W.; Kurek, M.; Czech, A.; Szafraniec, J.; Gawlak, K.; Jachowicz, R. 3D printing of tablets containing amorphous aripiprazole by filaments co-extrusion. *Eur. J. Pharm. Biopharm.* **2018**, *131*, 44–47. [CrossRef]
28. Gioumouxouzis, C.I.; Tzimtzimis, E.; Katsamenis, O.L.; Dourou, A.; Markopoulou, C.; Bouropoulos, N.; Tzetzis, D.; Fatouros, D.G. Fabrication of an osmotic 3D printed solid dosage form for controlled release of active pharmaceutical ingredients. *Eur. J. Pharm. Sci.* **2020**, *143*, 105176. [CrossRef]
29. Nazir, A.; Jeng, J.-Y. A high-speed additive manufacturing approach for achieving high printing speed and accuracy. *Proc. Inst. Mech. Eng. Part C J. Mech. Eng. Sci.* **2019**, *234*, 2741–2749. [CrossRef]
30. Shaw, L.L.; Islam, M.; Li, J.; Li, L.; Ayub, S.M.I. High-Speed Additive Manufacturing Through High-Aspect-Ratio Nozzles. *JOM* **2018**, *70*, 284–291. [CrossRef]
31. Wang, J.; Goyanes, A.; Gaisford, S.; Basit, A.W. Stereolithographic (SLA) 3D printing of oral modified-release dosage forms. *Int. J. Pharm.* **2016**, *503*, 207–212. [CrossRef]
32. Fina, F.; Goyanes, A.; Gaisford, S.; Basit, A.W. Selective laser sintering (SLS) 3D printing of medicines. *Int. J. Pharm.* **2017**, *529*, 285–293. [CrossRef]
33. Jamróz, W.; Kurek, M.; Łyszczarz, E.; Szafraniec, J.; Knapik-Kowalczuk, J.; Syrek, K.; Paluch, M.; Jachowicz, R. 3D printed orodispersible films with Aripiprazole. *Int. J. Pharm.* **2017**, *533*, 413–420. [CrossRef]
34. Speer, I.; Preis, M.; Breitkreutz, J. Novel Dissolution Method for Oral Film Preparations with Modified Release Properties. *AAPS PharmSciTech* **2018**, *20*, 7. [CrossRef]
35. Gioumouxouzis, C.I.; Baklavaridis, A.; Katsamenis, O.L.; Markopoulou, C.K.; Bouropoulos, N.; Tzetzis, D.; Fatouros, D.G. A 3D printed bilayer oral solid dosage form combining metformin for prolonged and glimepiride for immediate drug delivery. *Eur. J. Pharm. Sci.* **2018**, *120*, 40–52. [CrossRef]
36. Öblom, H.; Zhang, J.; Pimparade, M.; Speer, I.; Preis, M.; Repka, M.; Sandler, N. 3D-Printed Isoniazid Tablets for the Treatment and Prevention of Tuberculosis—Personalized Dosing and Drug Release. *AAPS PharmSciTech* **2019**, *20*, 1–13. [CrossRef]
37. Smith, D.; Kapoor, Y.; Hermans, A.; Nofsinger, R.; Kesisoglou, F.; Gustafson, T.P.; Procopio, A. 3D printed capsules for quantitative regional absorption studies in the GI tract. *Int. J. Pharm.* **2018**, *550*, 418–428. [CrossRef]

38. Melocchi, A.; Uboldi, M.; Parietti, F.; Cerea, M.; Foppoli, A.; Palugan, L.; Gazzaniga, A.; Maroni, A.; Zema, L. Lego-Inspired Capsular Devices for the Development of Personalized Dietary Supplements: Proof of Concept With Multimodal Release of Caffeine. *J. Pharm. Sci.* **2020**, *109*, 1990–1999. [CrossRef]
39. Fu, J.; Yu, X.; Jin, Y. 3D printing of vaginal rings with personalized shapes for controlled release of progesterone. *Int. J. Pharm.* **2018**, *539*, 75–82. [CrossRef]
40. Scoutaris, N.; Ross, S.A.; Douroumis, D. 3D Printed "Starmix" Drug Loaded Dosage Forms for Paediatric Applications. *Pharm. Res.* **2018**, *35*, 34. [CrossRef] [PubMed]
41. Kempin, W.; Domsta, V.; Brecht, I.; Semmling, B.; Tillmann, S.; Weitschies, W.; Seidlitz, A. Development of a dual extrusion printing technique for an acid- and thermo-labile drug. *Eur. J. Pharm. Sci.* **2018**, *123*, 191–198. [CrossRef]
42. Sadia, M.; Arafat, B.; Ahmed, W.; Forbes, R.T.; Alhnan, M.A. Channelled tablets: An innovative approach to accelerating drug release from 3D printed tablets. *J. Control. Release* **2018**, *269*, 355–363. [CrossRef]
43. Kimura, S.-I.; Ishikawa, T.; Iwao, Y.; Itai, S.; Kondo, H. Fabrication of Zero-Order Sustained-Release Floating Tablets via Fused Depositing Modeling 3D Printer. *Chem. Pharm. Bull.* **2019**, *67*, 992–999. [CrossRef]
44. Giri, B.R.; Song, E.S.; Kwon, J.; Lee, J.-H.; Park, J.-B.; Kim, D.S. Fabrication of Intragastric Floating, Controlled Release 3D Printed Theophylline Tablets Using Hot-Melt Extrusion and Fused Deposition Modeling. *Pharmaceutics* **2020**, *12*, 77. [CrossRef]
45. Melocchi, A.; Uboldi, M.; Inverardi, N.; Briatico-Vangosa, F.; Baldi, F.; Pandini, S.; Scalet, G.; Auricchio, F.; Cerea, M.; Foppoli, A.; et al. Expandable drug delivery system for gastric retention based on shape memory polymers: Development via 4D printing and extrusion. *Int. J. Pharm.* **2019**, *571*, 118700. [CrossRef]
46. Melocchi, A.; Inverardi, N.; Uboldi, M.; Baldi, F.; Maroni, A.; Pandini, S.; Briatico-Vangosa, F.; Zema, L.; Gazzaniga, A. Retentive device for intravesical drug delivery based on water-induced shape memory response of poly(vinyl alcohol): Design concept and 4D printing feasibility. *Int. J. Pharm.* **2019**, *559*, 299–311. [CrossRef]
47. Melocchi, A.; Parietti, F.; Maccagnan, S.; Ortenzi, M.A.; Antenucci, S.; Briatico-Vangosa, F.; Maroni, A.; Gazzaniga, A.; Zema, L. Industrial Development of a 3D-Printed Nutraceutical Delivery Platform in the Form of a Multicompartment HPC Capsule. *AAPS PharmSciTech* **2018**, *19*, 3343–3354. [CrossRef]
48. Jiang, H.; Yu, X.; Fang, R.; Xiao, Z.; Jin, Y. 3D printed mold-based capsaicin candy for the treatment of oral ulcer. *Int. J. Pharm.* **2019**, *568*, 118517. [CrossRef]
49. He, S.; Feng, S.; Nag, A.; Afsarimanesh, N.; Han, T.; Mukhopadhyay, S.C. Recent Progress in 3D Printed Mold-Based Sensors. *Sensors* **2020**, *20*, 703. [CrossRef]
50. Nag, A.; Feng, S.; Mukhopadhyay, S.; Kosel, J.; Inglis, D. 3D printed mould-based graphite/PDMS sensor for low-force applications. *Sens. Actuators A Phys.* **2018**, *280*, 525–534. [CrossRef]
51. Sarode, A.L.; Sandhu, H.; Shah, N.; Malick, W.; Zia, H. Hot melt extrusion (HME) for amorphous solid dispersions: Predictive tools for processing and impact of drug-polymer interactions on supersaturation. *Eur. J. Pharm. Sci.* **2013**, *48*, 371–384. [CrossRef] [PubMed]
52. Corcione, C.E.; Gervaso, F.; Scalera, F.; Montagna, F.; Maiullaro, T.; Sannino, A.; Maffezzoli, A. 3D printing of hydroxyapatite polymer-based composites for bone tissue engineering. *J. Polym. Eng.* **2017**, *37*, 741–746. [CrossRef]
53. Solanki, N.G.; Lam, K.; Tahsin, M.; Gumaste, S.G.; Shah, A.V.; Serajuddin, A.T. Effects of Surfactants on Itraconazole-HPMCAS Solid Dispersion Prepared by Hot-Melt Extrusion I: Miscibility and Drug Release. *J. Pharm. Sci.* **2019**, *108*, 1453–1465. [CrossRef]
54. Solanki, N.G.; Gumaste, S.G.; Shah, A.V.; Serajuddin, A.T. Effects of Surfactants on Itraconazole -Hydroxypropyl Methylcellulose Acetate Succinate Solid Dispersion Prepared by Hot Melt Extrusion. II: Rheological Analysis and Extrudability Testing. *J. Pharm. Sci.* **2019**, *108*, 3063–3073. [CrossRef]
55. Jennotte, O.; Koch, N.; Lechanteur, A.; Evrard, B. Three-dimensional printing technology as a promising tool in bioavailability enhancement of poorly water-soluble molecules: A review. *Int. J. Pharm.* **2020**, *580*, 119200. [CrossRef]
56. Albadarin, A.B.; Potter, C.B.; Davis, M.T.; Iqbal, J.; Korde, S.; Pagire, S.; Paradkar, A.; Walker, G.M. Development of stability-enhanced ternary solid dispersions via combinations of HPMCP and Soluplus® processed by hot melt extrusion. *Int. J. Pharm.* **2017**, *532*, 603–611. [CrossRef] [PubMed]
57. Zhang, S.; Lee, W.Y.T.; Chow, A.H.L. Crystallization of Itraconazole Polymorphs from Melt. *Cryst. Growth Des.* **2016**, *16*, 3791–3801. [CrossRef]

58. Heczko, D.; Kamińska, E.; Jurkiewicz, K.; Tarnacka, M.; Merkel, K.; Kamiński, K.; Paluch, M. The impact of various azole antifungals on the liquid crystalline ordering in itraconazole. *J. Mol. Liq.* **2020**, *307*, 112959. [CrossRef]
59. Zhong, Y.; Jing, G.; Tian, B.; Huang, H.; Zhang, Y.; Gou, J.; Tang, X.; He, H.; Wang, Y. Supersaturation induced by Itraconazole/Soluplus® micelles provided high GI absorption in vivo. *Asian J. Pharm. Sci.* **2016**, *11*, 255–264. [CrossRef]
60. Singh, A.; Bharati, A.; Frederiks, P.; Verkinderen, O.; Goderis, B.; Cardinaels, R.; Moldenaers, P.; Van Humbeeck, J.; Mooter, G.V.D. Effect of Compression on the Molecular Arrangement of Itraconazole-Soluplus Solid Dispersions: Induction of Liquid Crystals or Exacerbation of Phase Separation? *Mol. Pharm.* **2016**, *13*, 1879–1893. [CrossRef]
61. Solanki, N.; Gupta, S.S.; Serajuddin, A.T. Rheological analysis of itraconazole-polymer mixtures to determine optimal melt extrusion temperature for development of amorphous solid dispersion. *Eur. J. Pharm. Sci.* **2018**, *111*, 482–491. [CrossRef]
62. Miller, D.A.; DiNunzio, J.C.; Yang, W.; McGINITY, J.W.; Williams, R.O.; Williams, R.O. Targeted Intestinal Delivery of Supersaturated Itraconazole for Improved Oral Absorption. *Pharm. Res.* **2008**, *25*, 1450–1459. [CrossRef]
63. Meng, F.; Meckel, J.; Zhang, F. Investigation of itraconazole ternary amorphous solid dispersions based on povidone and Carbopol. *Eur. J. Pharm. Sci.* **2017**, *106*, 413–421. [CrossRef]
64. Parikh, T.; Serajuddin, A.T.M. Development of Fast-Dissolving Amorphous Solid Dispersion of Itraconazole by Melt Extrusion of its Mixture with Weak Organic Carboxylic Acid and Polymer. *Pharm. Res.* **2018**, *35*, 127. [CrossRef]
65. Wlodarski, K.; Zhang, F.; Liu, T.; Sawicki, W.; Kipping, T. Synergistic Effect of Polyvinyl Alcohol and Copovidone in Itraconazole Amorphous Solid Dispersions. *Pharm. Res.* **2018**, *35*, 16. [CrossRef] [PubMed]
66. Zheng, M.; Bauer, F.; Birk, G.; Lubda, D. Polyvinyl Alcohol in Hot Melt Extrusion to Improve the Solubility of Drugs. 2013. Available online: https://www.sigmaaldrich.com/content/dam/sigma-aldrich/0/content/pdf/PS-PVA-HME-Improve-Solubility-03-2017_EN_MS.pdf (accessed on 27 October 2020).
67. Malaquias, L.F.; Schulte, H.L.; Chaker, J.A.; Karan, K.; Durig, T.; Marreto, R.N.; Gratieri, T.; Gelfuso, G.M.; Cunha-Filho, M. Hot Melt Extrudates Formulated Using Design Space: One Simple Process for Both Palatability and Dissolution Rate Improvement. *J. Pharm. Sci.* **2018**, *107*, 286–296. [CrossRef]
68. Lang, B.; McGINITY, J.W.; Williams, R.O.; Williams, R.O. Dissolution Enhancement of Itraconazole by Hot-Melt Extrusion Alone and the Combination of Hot-Melt Extrusion and Rapid Freezing—Effect of Formulation and Processing Variables. *Mol. Pharm.* **2013**, *11*, 186–196. [CrossRef]
69. Feng, D.; Peng, T.; Huang, Z.; Singh, V.; Shi, Y.; Wen, T.; Lu, M.; Quan, G.; Pan, X.; Wu, C. Polymer-Surfactant System Based Amorphous Solid Dispersion: Precipitation Inhibition and Bioavailability Enhancement of Itraconazole. *Pharmaceutics* **2018**, *10*, 53. [CrossRef]
70. Solanki, N.G.; Kathawala, M.; Serajuddin, A.T. Effects of Surfactants on Itraconazole-Hydroxypropyl Methylcellulose Acetate Succinate Solid Dispersion Prepared by Hot Melt Extrusion III: Tableting of Extrudates and Drug Release From Tablets. *J. Pharm. Sci.* **2019**, *108*, 3859–3869. [CrossRef]
71. Ponsar, H.; Wiedey, R.; Quodbach, J. Hot-Melt Extrusion Process Fluctuations and Their Impact on Critical Quality Attributes of Filaments and 3D-Printed Dosage Forms. *Pharmaceutics* **2020**, *12*, 511. [CrossRef]
72. Knapik, J.; Jurkiewicz, K.; Kocot, A.; Paluch, M. Rheo-dielectric studies of the kinetics of shear-induced nematic alignment changes in itraconazole. *J. Mol. Liq.* **2020**, *302*, 112494. [CrossRef]
73. Feuerbach, T.; Callau-Mendoza, S.; Thommes, M. Development of filaments for fused deposition modeling 3D printing with medical grade poly(lactic-co-glycolic acid) copolymers. *Pharm. Dev. Technol.* **2018**, *24*, 487–493. [CrossRef] [PubMed]
74. Fuenmayor, E.; Forde, M.; Healy, A.V.; Gately, N.; Lyons, J.G.; McConville, C.; Major, I. Material Considerations for Fused-Filament Fabrication of Solid Dosage Forms. *Pharmaceutics* **2018**, *10*, 44. [CrossRef] [PubMed]
75. Nazir, A.; Abate, K.M.; Kumar, A.; Jeng, J.-Y. A state-of-the-art review on types, design, optimization, and additive manufacturing of cellular structures. *Int. J. Adv. Manuf. Technol.* **2019**, *104*, 3489–3510. [CrossRef]
76. Kyobula, M.; Adedeji, A.; Alexander, M.R.; Saleh, E.; Wildman, R.D.; Ashcroft, I.; Gellert, P.R.; Roberts, C.J. 3D inkjet printing of tablets exploiting bespoke complex geometries for controlled and tuneable drug release. *J. Control. Release* **2017**, *261*, 207–215. [CrossRef] [PubMed]
77. Park, H.; Ha, E.-S.; Kim, M.-S. Current Status of Supersaturable Self-Emulsifying Drug Delivery Systems. *Pharmaceutics* **2020**, *12*, 365. [CrossRef]

9

Drug Delivery Applications of Three-Dimensional Printed (3DP) Mesoporous Scaffolds

Tania Limongi [1,*], Francesca Susa [1], Marco Allione [2] and Enzo di Fabrizio [1]

1 Dipartimento di Scienza Applicata e Tecnologia, Politecnico di Torino, Corso Duca Degli Abruzzi 24, 10129 Torino, Italy; francesca.susa@polito.it (F.S.); enzo.difabrizio@polito.it (E.d.F.)
2 SMILEs Lab, PSE Division, King Abdullah University of Science and Technology, Thuwal 23955-6900, Saudi Arabia; marco.allione@kaust.edu.sa
* Correspondence: tania.limongi@polito.it

Abstract: Mesoporous materials are structures characterized by a well-ordered large pore system with uniform porous dimensions ranging between 2 and 50 nm. Typical samples are zeolite, carbon molecular sieves, porous metal oxides, organic and inorganic porous hybrid and pillared materials, silica clathrate and clathrate hydrates compounds. Improvement in biochemistry and materials science led to the design and implementation of different types of porous materials ranging from rigid to soft two-dimensional (2D) and three-dimensional (3D) skeletons. The present review focuses on the use of three-dimensional printed (3DP) mesoporous scaffolds suitable for a wide range of drug delivery applications, due to their intrinsic high surface area and high pore volume. In the first part, the importance of the porosity of materials employed for drug delivery application was discussed focusing on mesoporous materials. At the end of the introduction, hard and soft templating synthesis for the realization of ordered 2D/3D mesostructured porous materials were described. In the second part, 3DP fabrication techniques, including fused deposition modelling, material jetting as inkjet printing, electron beam melting, selective laser sintering, stereolithography and digital light processing, electrospinning, and two-photon polymerization were described. In the last section, through recent bibliographic research, a wide number of 3D printed mesoporous materials, for in vitro and in vivo drug delivery applications, most of which relate to bone cells and tissues, were presented and summarized in a table in which all the technical and bibliographical details were reported. This review highlights, to a very cross-sectional audience, how the interdisciplinarity of certain branches of knowledge, as those of materials science and nano-microfabrication are, represent a growing valuable aid in the advanced forum for the science and technology of pharmaceutics and biopharmaceutics.

Keywords: drug delivery; three-dimensional porous scaffolds; electron beam melting; selective laser sintering; stereolithography; electrospinning; two-photon polymerization; osteogenesis; antibiotics; anti-inflammatory

1. Introduction

Recently, one of the main thrusts of the micro and nano technologies application in the biomedical and clinical field has certainly been observed in the pharmaceutical drug delivery technologies optimization. Whether it is based on active or passive drug delivery, the way in which drugs are delivered substantially impact their efficacy and toxicity affecting their biocompatibility, pharmacokinetics, and pharmacodynamics. Drugs and active molecules can be introduced into the body via a number of administration routes such as buccal/sublingual, nasal, ocular, oral, pulmonary, anal/vaginal, transdermal and parenteral drug delivery [1–3]. Since a high percentage of the active pharmaceutical ingredients settled by the pharmaceutical production are precluded for a classical administration route, due to their low bioavailability [4], novel technologies assist modern drug delivery. As a result, an increase is observed in the effectiveness and reduction of side effects of the formulations in relation to patient compliance and costs reduction. In the past years, many drug delivery systems as organic and inorganic micro- and nanoparticulated systems as nanoparticles, micelles, liposomes, extracellular vesicles, nanotubes, metal–organic frameworks (MOF) and hydrogels have been used to deliver drugs at their therapeutic concentration to specific cell types and tissues [5–8]. Both material and design should be taken into account when optimizing a drug delivery carrier able to guarantee tuneable release (sustained, controlled, or pulsed), to act as a temporary reservoir, to increase the solubility of hydrophobic formulations, to float in the gastrointestinal tract and to protect the biological cargo from degradation [9].

Porous carriers have been successfully used as drug delivery matrices for their surface properties, high surface area and tuneable pore dimensions [10,11]. According to their pore sizes, porous materials are classified into three different categories, namely microporous, mesoporous, and macroporous [9,12]. Microporous materials such as MOFs and zeolites, are characterized by a well-interconnected network of pores less than 2 nm in size and high thermal stability and catalytic activity [13]. In macroporous materials, pores dimension ranges between 50 and 1000 nm [14] while in mesoporous materials pore size is between 2 to 50 nm [15]. In more details, mesoporous materials with a narrow pore dimension distribution and high surface area can be considered valuable candidates in drug delivery applications [16,17]. In the wide category of mesoporous, many materials are included such as mesoporous silica, hydroxyapatite and carbon, hydrogel and nanogel, metal and metal-doped nanoparticles. These materials have great versatility since their actions can be regulated by tuning the chemical environment optimizing the loading and consequent release of the chosen drug [18–20]. The drug incorporation into a mesoporous material is usually carried out by embedding the matrix in a concentrated solution of the drug and by a successive drying step. The size of the absorbable molecule (from small active molecules to proteins) is related to the dimension of the pore, and generally, a pore/drug size ratio >1 allows the adsorption of active molecules inside the pores. By using polymeric structure-directing agents, varying the chain length of surfactant or solubilizing supplementary substances into micelles, mesopores sizes can be adjusted from some nanometres to several tens of nanometers [21].

Recent advancement in micro/nano-fabrication techniques, materials science, chemistry and pharmacology has allowed the development of a number of mesoporous materials for drug delivery application characterized by evident structural advancement such as tuneable pore sizes, different grade of skeleton rigidity and two/three dimensional (2D–3D) architectures arrangement [22–26].

Hard (nanocasting) or soft templating approaches are applied to produce ordered mesostructured porous materials. The templated synthesis usually requires three successive steps: template preparation, template-directed synthesis and template removal. Hard templating leads to very robust structures containing several constituents as carbon, and metals (oxides, nitrides and sulphides) [27,28]. It is a synthetic method based on the deposition of the targeted materials into the narrowed spaces of the template, resulting in a reversed copy of the mold. The pores of these templates are soaked with a precursor of the looked-for product (e.g., a metal salt for metal oxides) which is in situ thermally transformed to the final product. When the template is removed, mesoporous material remains as the negative replica of the hard template [29].

Soft-templating techniques allow direct synthesis of porous materials through block copolymers including blocks of ionic and non-ionic oligomers, amphiphilic surfactants employed as structure-directing agents (SDAs) and through the addition of precursors as metal salts for metal oxide nanomaterials and organosilanes or triethoxysilane for SiO_2-based nanomaterials. Soft-templating techniques are those in which small sub-units self-assemble to define the final structure, which is an aggregate of these starting units, which are not embedded in other matrices or removed as in the techniques described above. Upon self-assembly in a solvent, a micellar structure is realized by the fact that the hydrophobic sides of the molecules of the amphiphilic surfactants point inward and the hydrophilic ones outward in case the solvent is polar, while the opposite occurs if the solvent is non-polar. After this step, micelles are functionalized on their external corona structure using functional groups, frequently polymeric oligomers. Finally, it is the cross-linking of these external terminations which assemble the micelles in a mesoporous superstructure [30].

Producing porous hierarchical materials by integrating macropores in mesoporous tools manifestly increases their practical drug delivery applicability since macropores increase mass transport decreasing diffusion restraints characterizing purely mesoporous materials, while the mesopores empower great surface area [31,32].

Many methodologies have been optimized to engineer the hierarchically structured mesoporous solutions. The dual-templating synthesis method, applying colloidal crystal (opal) hard-templating and soft-templating techniques, is employed for realizing, as schematized in Figure 1, 3D macro/mesoporous materials for a wide range of applications, including the drug delivery ones [33,34].

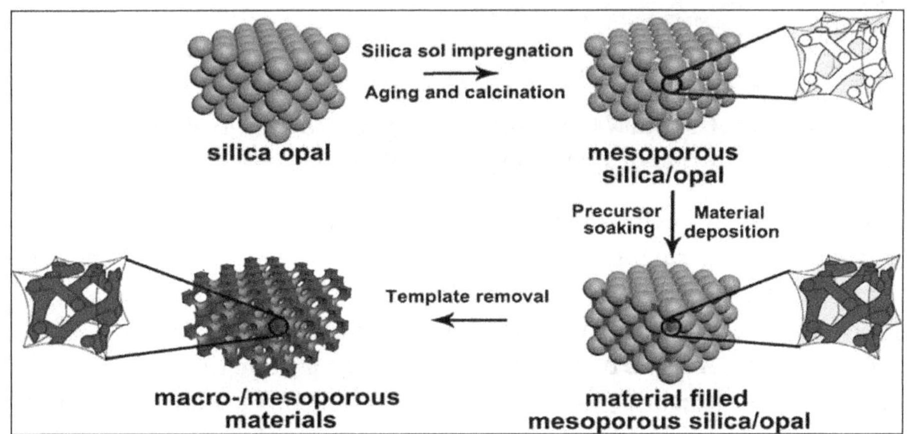

Figure 1. Schematic representation of 3D macro/mesoporous materials preparation reproduced with permission from [34], Chemistry of Materials, 2018.

2. 3D Printed (3DP) Mesoporous Scaffolds Fabrication Technique

The idea of realizing a macroscopic object via a bottom-up approach has been attractive for a long time but recently, the advancement of both the materials to be used and the techniques to be exploited have made possible the fabrication of 3D printers able to produce any shape in many different natural [35], synthetic, plastic and metallic materials, at variable size scales and with potentially very high accuracy in positioning [36–38]. This has pushed some researchers towards the idea to explore the possibility to use these techniques to realize solutions with different designs, characterized by being made of different types of mesoporous materials [21]. 3D porous substrates, used with or without further functionalization or engineering, are used more and more frequently in in vitro and in vivo drug delivery studies to assist cell growth or tissue regeneration ensuring the right degree of asepticity and differentiation [39–41].

2D and 3D printing tools are appealing for drug delivery applications since state-of-the-art equipment allows the deposition of liquid, gel, and solid constituents enclosing a wide range of pharmaceutics according to predefined schemes. The layer-by-layer assembling mode to print scaffold allows exact control of the design and of the geometry of the internal pores system, which consequently leads to tune the strength of the final products [42,43].

3DP technology can successfully assist engineers, pharmacologists and clinicians in the design and realization of 3D mesoporous scaffolds to be used for different medical applications such as tissue engineering and regenerative medicine implants characterized by the adjustable loading and unloading activity of pharmacologically active substances such as, antibiotics, growth and differentiation factors (Figure 2) [44].

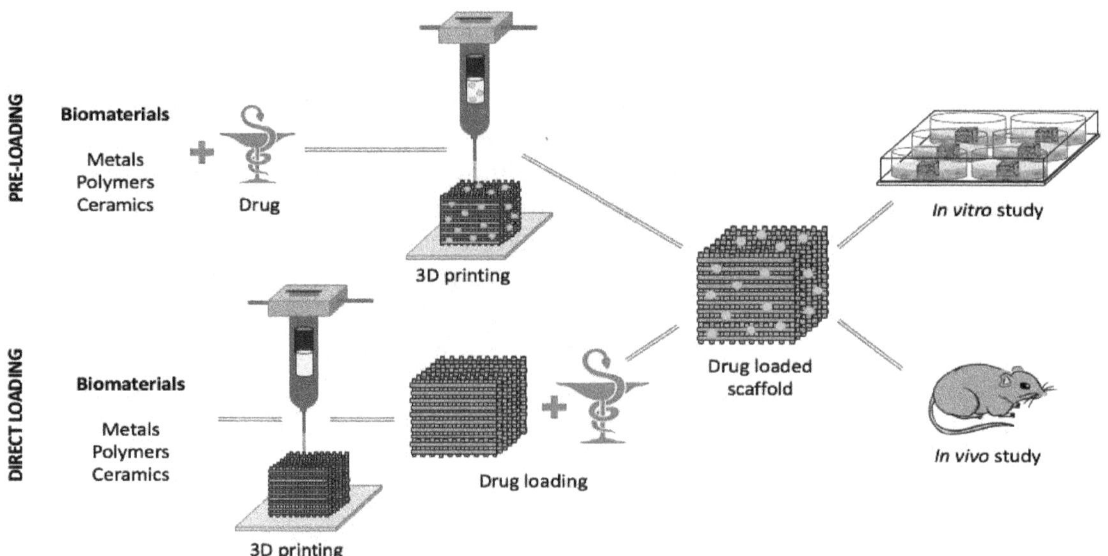

Figure 2. Schematic layout summarizing pre-loading and direct loading 3DP porous substrate fabrication for in vitro and in vivo drug delivery applications.

These active substances can be incorporated inside the mesoporous 3D structures in two different main steps: during the manufacturing process (pre-loading, PL) by mixing the substances with the printable material and then proceeding with the 3DP technique in mild conditions (i.e., electrospinning or inkjet printing), or at the end of the printing step (direct loading, DL), by soaking the 3D-printed scaffold in a solution of the molecule to be loaded as reported for bone morphogenetic protein-2 (BMP-2) mesoporous calcium silicate (MesoCS) 3D-printed scaffold [45]. PL methods are usually applied for the production of scaffolds able to locally deliver antibiotiotics [46], but unfortunately, antibiotics such as those of the cephalosporin family have significantly reduced efficiency when exposed to heat and, consequently, the DL method is definitely applied to sensitive molecules when the 3DP process is carried out at high temperatures or pressures [47].

There are many 3DP strategies available to the scientific community that allow the realization of mesoporous scaffolds under computer aids combining different processes and materials like carbon nanotubes, nanoparticles, nanofibers, polymers with active biomolecules with or without live cells. These 3DP fabrication techniques, as summarized in Figure 3, include fused deposition modeling (FDM), material jetting as inkjet printing (IP), electron beam melting (EBM), selective laser sintering (SLS), stereolithography (SLA) and digital light processing, electrospinning, and two-photon polymerization (TPP).

2.1. *Fused Deposition Modeling*

FDM is one of the most inexpensive nozzle-based deposition systems that allows direct printing of 3D CAD designed layer by layer objects. Thermoplastic degradable (polylactic acid, PLA, poly(ε-caprolactone), PCL, polyvinyl alcohol, PVA) and non-degradable (acrylo-nitrile butadiene styrene, ABS, ethylene vinyl acetate, EVA, poly methyl methacrylate, PMMA) polymer filament are pushed into the heater block to melt before extruding from a high-temperature nozzle solidifying onto the previous layer on the build plate [48].

The easiest method of loading target drugs into the thermoplastic polymer filament is the impregnation obtained leaving the just printed device in a concentrated drug solution (mostly ethanol or methanol) followed by a drying step [49,50].

2.2. *Inkjet Printing*

The inkjet-based non-contact printing technology reproduces digital patterns with tiny ink drops through thermal, piezoelectric and magnetic approaches. The thermal stimulation, reaching until

100–300 °C, nucleates a bubble and directly leads to droplet expulsion from the printhead. The size of droplets is related to the temperature gradient and ink viscosity employed. Likewise, the ink drop generation can be produced by the pulse strain and acoustic waves generated from a piezoelectric actuator and larger size ink droplets can be produced by means of electromagnetic filed [51–53].

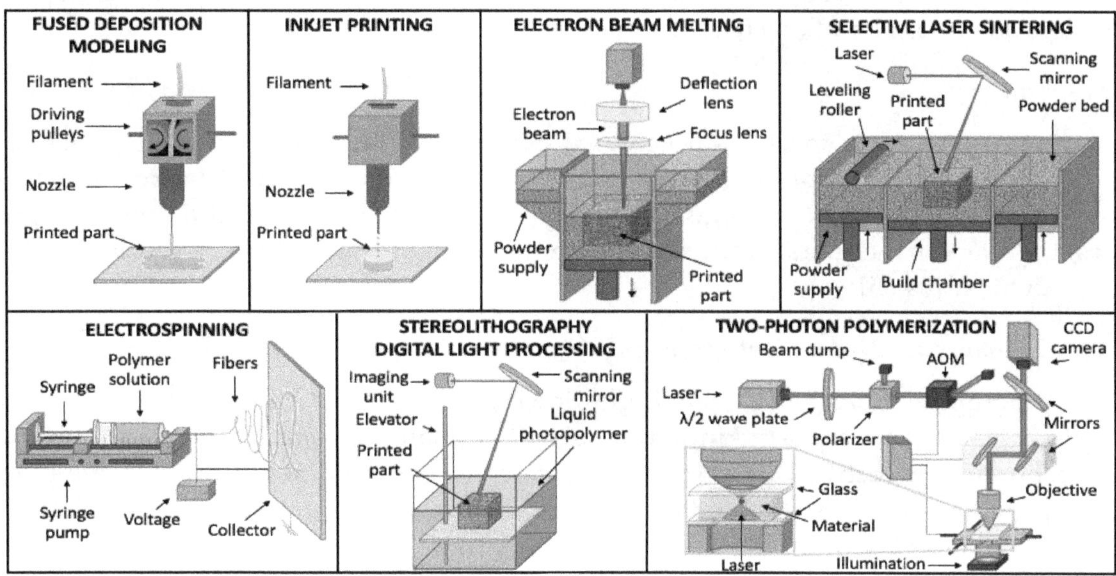

Figure 3. Schematic illustrations of the most diffused 3D printing fabrication techniques for porous scaffolds manufacturing: fused deposition modeling, inkjet printing, electron beam melting, selective laser sintering, stereolithography, electrospinning, two-photon polymerization.

2.3. Electron Beam Melting

EBM is a modern fast solution to manufacture metal parts on a layer-by-layer basis through an electron beam that, bombarding the metal powders, melts them, constructing 3D geometries. This technique compared with ones using a laser, are characterized by high energy utilization and material absorption rate, improved stability, and reduced maintenance fees [54]. Although this technique is successfully used for the realization of porous orthopedic and dental implants made of metallic biomedical alloys as Ti6Al4V [55], to date, there are no applications of EBM for the production of 3D printed mesoporous devices for drug delivery application. This is due to the fact that these kinds of scaffolds are characterized by large surface roughness since EBM microfabrication accuracy ranges from 0.3–0.4 mm.

2.4. Selective Laser Sintering

SLS operates without a mold through a computer-controlled laser beam, powder bed, a piston assuring a vertical movement, and a roller to spread continuously powder layers [55]. This technique allows the realization of polymeric, metallic, and ceramic parts. SLS implies solid and semisolid consolidation procedures at a sintering temperature usually lower than the melting point. In the semisolid process suitable for treating low melting point polymer, as PCL, polyglycolide, PLA and poly(L-lactic) acid (PLLA), partially melted powder particles produce a certain volume of the liquid phase, which glues other solid elements. Microsphere-based hydroxyapatite (HA)/PCL scaffolds realized by SLS, shows a highly ordered porous structure [56]. Polyamide/HA composite platforms with porosities ranging from 40% to 70% and with a maximum tensile strength of 21.4 MPa were obtained by SLS [55,57]. Although the low near-infrared laser absorptivity of oxide ceramics, the direct SLS of ceramics throughout powder coating adds to the low melting point or composites ceramics has been done [58]. Many sacrificial binders as waxes, thermoplastics, long-chain fatty acids or sometimes a combination of binders as thermoset/semi-crystalline PA-11 or wax/PMMA are used for the realization of porous 3D structured materials as graphite and composite ceramic Al_2O_3-ZrO_2-TiC [59–61]. A high-energy laser beam increasing the temperature on the surface promotes the particle interaction to each other before sintering together, while the material on the grain borderline continues to diffuse into the pores, stimulating densification activities. Since SLS is characterized by a high heating rate and short holding time, it results as an excellent alternative in producing scaffolds supported by low-dimensional nanomaterials such as graphene and carbon nanotubes [62].

2.5. *Electrospinning*

Nanodimensional high specific surface area devices can be fabricated with bioactive loaded polymer through the electrospinning technique [63]. In a conventional electrospinning system, generally comprising of a high-voltage power supply, syringe, pump and a collector, polymeric nanofibers, inorganic nanofibers, and composite nanofibers are ejected into a sequence of droplets forming steady fiber [64,65].

2.6. *Stereolithography and Digital Light Processing*

Stereolithographic (SLA) and Digital Light Processing 3DP allow the layer by layer realization of 3D mesoporous stuff by cross-linking photo-sensitive materials using laser light or digital light projection technique, respectively [66]. The curing stereolithographic step, both in single-photon and two-photon polymerization, is actuated by tuning the incidence, the intensity, and the duration of near-infrared, visible or UV light.

2.7. *Two-Photon Polymerization*

While single-photon polymerization requires one-photon absorption, in TPP, the molecule simultaneously absorbs two photons. By employing a focused femtosecond near-IR, TPP stereolithography, processing biocompatible synthetic or natural hydrogels or polymers, grants the ultra-fast production of 3D structures with submicron resolution [67].

3. Applications of 3DP Mesoporous Material for Drug Delivery

Doing a search on the Web of Science and on Pubmed at the beginning of June 2020, resulted that in the last decades a fair number of publications are strictly related to the specific topic covered in this review and, more in details, related to mesoporous 3D printed materials for drug delivery applications. As highlighted in Table 1, most of the results focalized on the application of these 3D porous materials for tissue engineering bone substitute realization. Their porosity, by mimicking the bone structure, allows nutrient transport, waste removal, cell migration, angiogenesis and differentiation phenomena, assisting bone regeneration in bone defects related to traumatic events or pathologies.

3.1. *Bone Regeneration*

3.1.1. Growth Factors and Peptides

Several FDA approved growth factors as BMP-2 have been used in clinics for bone and cartilage regeneration. In a mesoporous bioactive glass (MBG) covered silicate 1393 bioactive glass scaffolds candidate for bone repairing application, BMP-2 release was higher than that of DNA and dexamethasone. MBG successfully physically absorbed and released the active molecule without upsetting its pharmacological activity [68]. Fish hydrogel-based mesoporous strontium-doped calcium silicate scaffolds were proved to be efficient BMP-2 carriers for in vitro human Wharton jelly mesenchymal stem cell differentiation [69]. Customized 3D-printed osteoinductive implants were realized integrating porous silicon BMP-2 carriers within a 3D-printed PCL patient-specific implant [70]. FDM 3D MesoCS scaffolds combined with PCL were presented as odontoinductive biomaterial with efficient BMP-2 delivery capability [71]. In vitro tested BMP-2 pre-loaded mesoporous calcium silicate/PCL scaffolds, even if not suitable for clinical applications, exhibited high biocompatibility and sustained drug delivery pattern compared to the ones directly immersed with BMP-2 after the FDM fabrication [45].

As some authors reported some relevant side-effect related to the use of BMP-2 [72], 3D dipyridamole-coated hydroxyapatite (HA)/beta-tri-calcium phosphate (β-TCP) scaffolds were successfully used to promote bone regeneration in critical bone defects as well as BMP-2 [73].

Since vascularization is a key step of the osteogenesis process, 3DP dimethyloxallyl glycine loaded MBGs and poly(3-hydroxybutyrate-*co*-3-hydroxyhexanoate) polymers scaffolds and results showed that dimethyloxallyl glycine was effectively released improving angiogenesis and osteregeneration in the bone faults [74]. Vascular endothelial growth factor (VEGF), was well encapsulated in chitosan/dextran sulfate microparticles and mixed into a calcium phosphate paste for the 3D plotting of growth factor loaded calcium-phosphate-based scaffolds applicable for bone tissue engineering [75].

Materials for tissue regeneration can be functionalized with engineered peptides able to regulate bone healing and regeneration. In vitro tests with naringin and calcitonin gene-related peptide-loaded 3DP MBG/sodium alginate/gelatin scaffolds showed that their high porosity assure efficient sustained drug delivery [76]. Peptide osteostatin and Zn^{2+} ions loaded meso-macroporous 3D scaffolds based on MBGs, exhibited a synergistic effect improving human mesenchymal stem cell growth, promoting their osteogenic differentiation [77]. SLS 3DP poly(3-hydroxybutyrate) scaffolds, when post-printing loaded with osteogenic growth peptide, exhibited the ability to support cell growth and tissue restoration [78].

3.1.2. Anti-Inflammatory and Antibiotics

Since any bone loss such as that following trauma, bone diseases and surgery, potentially provides suitable conditions for the onset of chronic infections or biofilm, it is highly desired the realization of anti-inflammatory and antibiotic-eluting scaffolds for sustained release without side effect in osteointegration, osteogenesis and osteoconduction processes. Dexamethasone loaded mesoporous $CaSiO_3$/calcium sulfate hemihydrate (MCS/CSH) cement scaffolds have been realized by 3D printing. Compared to the tissue culture plates control, MCS/CSH scaffolds exhibited a good in vitro OCT-1 cells response, an extra balanced degradation rate and capacities to slowly release the uploaded drug in targeted sites [79].

3DP high porosity dual-drug delivery layered MBG/sodium-alginate (SA)–SA scaffolds were successfully fabricated enriching the printing step with SA cross-linking. They resulted able to stimulate proliferation and osteogenic differentiation of human bone marrow-derived mesenchymal stem cells, furthermore, bovine serum albumin (BSA) and ibuprofen were successfully loaded in SA layer and the MBG of MBG/SA layer, respectively, resulting in a quite fast BSA release due to the macroporous network of SA, and in a constant release of ibuprofen due to the retention effect of the mesoporous channels of MBG [80].

It is well-known that inflammation phenomena thwart bone regeneration in transplanted loci and the local effect of short-term corticosteroid administration increase the effectiveness of bone tissue engineering [81]. Dexamethasone-loaded polydopamine-functionalized MBG was incorporated into polyglycolic acid/poly-1-lactic acid (PGPL) to fabricate a 3D mesoporous scaffold via laser additive manufacturing able to stimulate cell differentiation, biomineralization [82]. Loaded dexamethasone electrospun fibrous scaffolds of PCL-gelatin, incorporating MBG nanoparticles (MBGn), were presented excellent valid 3D platforms for bone tissue engineering [83].

In the case of dexamethasone-loaded 3DP strontium-containing MBG scaffolds the mesoporous matrix with enhanced mechanical strength to ensure great bone-growing bioactivity together with marked drug delivery capability [84]. 3DP scaffolds realized by using MBG and concentrated alginate pastes efficiently delivered dexamethasone in an in vitro test with human bone marrow-derived mesenchymal stem cells thanks to their matrix characterized by a well-ordered network of nano-channels and micro and macro-pores [85]. Poly(1,8-octanediol-*co*-citrate) and β-tricalcium phosphate (β-$Ca_3(PO_4)_2$), together with ibuprofen-loaded SiO_2 were made-up by micro-droplet jetting

3DP technique. Their hierarchically macro/mesoporous extremely interconnected pore matrix made them a valid antimicrobial bioengineered solution for bone regeneration [86,87].

The antimicrobials local application usually provides higher drug delivery than those attained with the intravenous application [88,89] and many 3DP macro/meso-porous composite scaffolds, are at the moment used to support a reproducible safe a better and well-regulated in situ antibiotics delivery. Some doxorubicin-loaded 3DP magnetic Fe_3O_4 nanoparticles containing mesoporous bioactive glass/polycaprolactone composite scaffolds enhanced osteogenic activity also assured sustained local anticancer delivery coupled with magnetic hyperthermia treatment [90].

Multidrug-loaded scaffold undoubtedly improves the applicability of 3D rapid prototype implants to ward off biofilm growth and drug resistance. Antibiotics are usually locally delivered via PMMA bone cement spacers [91,92] compatible with a restricted number of antibiotics and characterized by having low release profiles. Mesoporous bioactive glass/metal-organic framework and macro/meso-porous composite bioactive ceramics bound with poly (3-hydroxybutyrate-*co*-3-hydroxyhexanoate) scaffolds loaded with high dosages of isoniazid and/or rifampin, anti- tuberculosis drugs, had good biocompatibility and bioactivity when tested for long-term therapy after osteoarticular tuberculosis debridement surgery. Hierarchical 3DP multidrug scaffolds built with nanocomposite bioceramic and PVA were coated of gelatin-glutaraldehyde (Gel-Glu). Levofloxacin was loaded into the mesopores of the bioceramic part, vancomycin was packed into the biopolymer portion while rifampin in the external layer of Gel-Glu. The early delivery of rifampin followed by a sustained release of vancomycin and levofloxacin, represented an excellent and encouraging alternative for bone infection management [93]. 3DP rifampin- and vancomycin-loaded calcium phosphate scaffolds, used in a mouse model implant-associated staphylococcus aureus bone infection, proved that the concomitant local delivery of rifampin and vancomycin significantly improves the outcomes of the implant compared to PMMA spacers which cannot carry rifampin [94]. Gelatine and Si-doped hydroxyapatite porous 3D scaffolds were successfully loaded with vancomycin since they were rapidly prototyped fabricated at room temperature and apart from by increasing in vitro pre-osteoblastic MC3T3-E1 cell differentiation they also inhibit bacterial growth [95].

3.1.3. Metallic Ions and Trace Elements

Recently, many metallic ions such as zinc, copper, silver, cerium, strontium and cobalt, were combined with bioactive glasses to improve osteogenesis and angiogenesis [96–98]. Silver, among all, is the one that stands out for its strong antibacterial qualities. Silver/graphene oxide homogeneous nanocomposites were modified on 3DP β-tricalcium phosphate bioceramic scaffolds leading to a bifunctional scaffold with, just test in vitro, antibacterial and osteogenic activity were realized and in vitro tested [99].

In addition to the direct effect that a drug-loaded on a scaffold can have at the implantation site, several authors highlighted that also the integration of trace elements such as strontium, zinc, magnesium, calcium, copper, boron and cerium in 3DP mesoporous bioactive glass scaffolds enhance in vitro and in vivo osteogenic and differentiation activity [100–102].

3.2. Other Applications

Apart from the numerous applications in the bone regeneration field, mesoporous 3DP scaffolds including also mesoporous elastomer characterized by ordered and aligned nanofibrillar architecture that can be rapidly managed into multifaceted objects are starting to be more and more widespread even in other branches of biomedical research and medical clinic [103].

Coaxial electrospinned silk fibroin-based scaffolds are successfully tested as a potential brain-derived neurotrophic factor and VEGF delivery carrier in nerve repair and reconstruction applications [104].

Anti-HIV-1 drugs, including emtricitabine, tenofovir disoproxil fumarate and efavirenz were successfully loaded in a 24-layered rectangular prism-shaped 3DP controlled release fixed-dose combination tablets able to control the intestinal release of the active molecules [105].

Table 1. Applications of 3DP porous materials for tissue engineering and bone substitute realization.

Material	3D Printing Method	Drug	Drug Loading Method	Application	Reference
Mesoporous strontium substitution calcium silicate/recycled fish gelatin 3D cell-laden scaffold.	IP	BMP-2	DL	Bone tissue engineering. In vitro	[69]
PCL 3DP patient-specific implant, with degradable porous silicon-based carriers.	SLA		DL	Bone graft for critical size bone defects. In vitro	[70]
Mesoporous calcium silicate 3DP scaffold.	FDM		DL	Bone regeneration. In vitro	[45]
Hierarchical 3D multidrug scaffolds based on nanocomposite bioceramic and PVA with an external coating of gelatin-glutaraldehyde.	IP	Dipyridamole and BMP-2	DL	Bone tissue engineering. In vivo (mice)	[73]
Scaffold is composed of MBG and poly(3-hydroxybutyrate-*co*-3-hydroxyhexanoate) polymers.	IP	Dimethyloxallyl glycine	PL	Angiogenesis and osteogenesis for bone tissue engineering. In vivo (rats)	[74]
MBG with sodium alginate and gelatin.	IP	Naringin and calcitonin gene-related peptide	DL	Bone repair. In vitro	[76]
MBG.	IP	Peptide osteostatin and Zn^{2+} ions	DL	Bone grafts with enhanced osteogenic capacity. In vitro	[77]
Poly(3-hydroxybutyrate) scaffold.	SLS	Osteogenic growth peptide and its C-terminal sequence (10–14)	DL	Bone tissue engineering. In vitro	[78]
Calcium phosphate cement scaffolds by 3D plotting with growth factors encapsulating chitosan/dextran sulfate microparticles mixed into the paste.	IP	BSA and VEGF	PL	Encapsulate growth factors in a cement. In vitro	[75]
Layered MBG/SA.	IP	BSA and ibuprofen	PL	Stimulate human bone mesenchymal stem cells (hBMSCs) adhesion, proliferation and osteogenic differentiation. In vitro	[80]
Integrate MBG with 3D printing basic 1393 bioactive glass scaffolds.	IP	Dexamethasone and BMP-2	DL	Bone repair and relative bone disease treatment. In vivo (rats)	[68]

Table 1. *Cont.*

Material	3D Printing Method	Drug	Drug Loading Method	Application	Reference
MBG is functionalized with polydopamine and PGPL.	SLS	Dexamethasone	PL	Osteogenic differentiation and biomineralization. In vitro	[82]
Calcium sulfate hemihydrate cement is incorporated in mesoporous calcium silicate.	IP		PL	Bone tissue engineering. In vitro	[79]
Electrospun fibrous scaffolds of PCL-gelatin incorporating mesoporous bioactive glass nanoparticles.	ES		PL	Bone regeneration. In vivo (rats)	[83]
MBG with strontium.	IP		PL	Bone regeneration. In vitro	[84]
Hierarchical scaffolds of MBG and concentrated alginate pastes.	IP		PL	Bone tissue engineering. In vitro	[85]
3D magnetic Fe_3O_4 nanoparticles containing MBG/PCL composite scaffolds.	IP	Doxorubicin	PL	Osteogenic activity, local anticancer drug delivery and magnetic hyperthermia. In vitro	[90]
Hollow mesoporous structure of silica (SiO_2) microspheres loaded in a Poly(1,8-octanediol-*co*-citrate) and β-tricalcium phosphate scaffold.	IP	Ibuprofen	PL	Bone regeneration of infected bone defects. In vitro	[86]
Poly(1,8-octanediol-*co*-citrate) and β-tricalcium phosphate scaffold.	IP		PL	Bone defect repair. In vitro	[87]
MBG with MOFs and PCL.	IP	Isoniazid	PL	Osteoarticular tuberculosis treatment. In vitro	[106]
Carboxylic MBG and methyl-functionalized mesoporous silica nanoparticles.	IP	Isoniazid and rifampin	PL	Filler after surgical treatment of osteoarticular tuberculosis. In vivo (rabbits)	[107]
Hierarchical 3D multidrug scaffolds based on nanocomposite bioceramic and PVA with an external coating of Gel-Glu.	IP	Rifampin, levofloxacin and vancomycin	PL	Destroy Gram-positive and Gram-negative bacteria biofilms for local bone infection therapy. In vitro	[93]
3D printed calcium phosphate scaffolds.	IP	Rifampin and vancomycin	PL	Treat an implant-associated Staphylococcus aureus bone infection. In vivo (mice)	[94]
Porous 3-D scaffolds consisting of gelatine and Si-doped hydroxyapatite.	IP	Vancomycin	PL	Pre-osteoblastic MC3T3-E1 cell differentiation. In vitro	[95]

Table 1. *Cont.*

Material	3D Printing Method	Drug	Drug Loading Method	Application	Reference
β-tricalcium phosphate bioceramic scaffolds with a homogeneous nanocomposite made of silver nanoparticles and graphene oxide.	IP	Silver nanoparticles and graphene oxide	PL	Bone grafts with good antibacterial performance. In vitro	[99]
Borosilicate MBG.	IP	Boron and silicon ions	PL	Repair bone defects. In vivo (rats)	[100]
3D porous composite scaffolds made of cerium oxide, mesoporous calcium silicate and PCL.	IP	Cerium ions	PL	Bone regeneration. In vitro	[101]
MBG with strontium.	IP	Strontium ions	PL	Bone regeneration. In vivo (rats)	[102]
MBG modified β-tricalcium phosphate.	IP	Calcium, phosphorus and silicon ions	PL	Angiogenesis and osteogenesis for bone tissue engineering. In vivo (rabbits)	[108]
Mesoporous calcium silicate 3D-printed scaffold.	IP	BMP-2	PL	Odontoinductive biomaterial in regenerative endodontics. In vitro	[71]
Silk fibroin porous scaffold.	ES	Brain-derived neurotrophic factor and VEGF	PL	Cavernous nerve regeneration. In vivo (rats)	[104]
Nanostructured ordered mesoporous elastomers composed of molecular double networks (poly(ethylene oxide)–poly(propylene oxide)–poly(ethylene oxide) pluronic copolymers, and PMMA.	IP	Ibuprofen and vancomycin	DL	Biomedical and engineering applications as the need for high mechanical performance coexisting with precise nano-microstructural features. In vitro	[103]
Humic acid-polyquaternium 10 tablet.	IP	Efavirenz, tenofovir disoproxil fumarate and emtricitabine	PL	Anti-HIV-1 controlled drug delivery. In vivo (pigs)	[105]
Mesoporous iron oxide nanoraspberry inside microneedles.	DLP	Minoxdil	DL	Treatment of androgenetic alopecia. In vivo (mice)	[109]
Porous poly(ethylene glycol) dimethacrylate devices.	TPP	Rhodamine B as model drug	PL	Different biomedical applications. In vitro	[110]

4. Conclusions

For many years, 3D devices have been assisting research in very different areas, ranging from simple cell cultures to tissue engineering and drug delivery applications. 2D cell culture represents a chief tool in molecular and cellular biology due to its fast, ease, reproducibility and cheap distinctive characteristic. However, it is now universally accepted that 2D cell culture methods understate the live cells in vivo setting unlike reported for last-generation 3D biomaterials which, on the contrary, are able to mimic in a much more realistic way the environment required for a whole range of biomedical and clinical applications. The development of three-dimensional supports has even greater resonance in tissue engineering and regenerative medicine applications since, in those cases, the function of tissues or organs must be restored ensuring the spatial and functional interconnection between different cell types, in order to guarantee the exchange of gas, nutrients or drugs and the elimination of waste products. In this review, we wanted to highlight how these characteristics can be optimized by merging together the need to provide solid supports capable of assisting cell growth at the level of tissue and organ and, at the same time, the right degree of porosity of the materials that in the specific case of 3D biomaterials offers a whole series of drug delivery capabilities worthy of study and implementation. The way an active molecule is carried to a specific region or cellular type can impact on its interaction efficacy. Each drug has a therapeutic window in which health benefits must be maximized and side effects minimized. This need has materialized in the ever-stricter demand of a multidisciplinary approach for the implementation of new materials and methods for an effective in vitro and in vivo drug delivery. Materials science, chemistry and micro/nanofabrication offer both original and effective solutions applicable in research and clinical areas. The rapid and often inexpensive fabrication of 3DP structures enhances the performance of devices no longer used only as structural supports for tissue regeneration and differentiation thanks to the optimization of their intrinsic and tuneable porosity. 3DP mesoporous devices allow an effective drug delivery of personalized therapy, customizable both from the geometric point of view and from the point of view of pharmacological requests for each individual patient. With the topics covered in this review, we want to highlight how 3D printing techniques allow the production of CAD designing structures that fully correspond to the request of each patient in response to needs following trauma or pathologies. The future implementation of new biodegradable biopolymers and of multi-step etching processes for post-printing functionalization/modification, will also allow more efficient drug delivery application of scaffolds as the 3D EBM produced ones, by conferring them the not-yet optimized degree of mesoporosity.

Author Contributions: T.L., F.S., M.A. and E.d.F. conceived the review, analyzed the data of literature and wrote the paper. All authors have read and agreed to the published version of the manuscript.

References

1. Anselmo, A.C.; Gokarn, Y.; Mitragotri, S. Non-invasive delivery strategies for biologics. *Nat. Rev. Drug Discov.* **2019**, *18*, 19–40. [CrossRef]
2. Thabet, Y.; Klingmann, V.; Breitkreutz, J. Drug Formulations: Standards and Novel Strategies for Drug Administration in Pediatrics. *J. Clin. Pharmacol.* **2018**, *58*, S26–S35. [CrossRef]
3. Moon, C.; Smyth, H.D.C.; Watts, A.B.; Williams, R.O. Delivery Technologies for Orally Inhaled Products: An Update. *AAPS PharmSciTech* **2019**, *20*, 117. [CrossRef] [PubMed]
4. Santos, A.; Veiga, F.; Figueiras, A. Dendrimers as Pharmaceutical Excipients: Synthesis, Properties, Toxicity and Biomedical Applications. *Materials* **2019**, *13*, 65. [CrossRef] [PubMed]
5. Palazzolo, S.; Bayda, S.; Hadla, M.; Caligiuri, I.; Corona, G.; Toffoli, G.; Rizzolio, F. The Clinical Translation of Organic Nanomaterials for Cancer Therapy: A Focus on Polymeric Nanoparticles, Micelles, Liposomes and Exosomes. *Curr. Med. Chem.* **2018**, *25*, 4224–4268. [CrossRef] [PubMed]
6. Limongi, T.; Rocchi, A.; Cesca, F.; Tan, H.; Miele, E.; Giugni, A.; Orlando, M.; Perrone Donnorso, M.; Perozziello, G.; Benfenati, F.; et al. Delivery of Brain-Derived Neurotrophic Factor by 3D Biocompatible Polymeric Scaffolds for Neural Tissue Engineering and Neuronal Regeneration. *Mol. Neurobiol.* **2018**, *55*, 8788–8798. [CrossRef] [PubMed]

7. Abu, B.; Mohd Salman, K.; Muhammad Zafar, I.; Mohd Sajid, K. Tumor-Targeted Drug Delivery by Nanocomposites. *Curr. Drug Metab.* **2020**, *21*, 1–15. [CrossRef]
8. Dianzani, C.; Foglietta, F.; Ferrara, B.; Rosa, A.C.; Muntoni, E.; Gasco, P.; Della Pepa, C.; Canaparo, R.; Serpe, L. Solid lipid nanoparticles delivering anti-inflammatory drugs to treat inflammatory bowel disease: Effects in an in vivo model. *World J. Gastroenterol.* **2017**, *23*, 4200–4210. [CrossRef] [PubMed]
9. Arruebo, M. Drug delivery from structured porous inorganic materials. *WIREs Nanomed. Nanobiotechnol.* **2012**, *4*, 16–30. [CrossRef]
10. Choi, Y.; Kim, J.; Yu, S.; Hong, S. pH- and temperature-responsive radially porous silica nanoparticles with high-capacity drug loading for controlled drug delivery. *Nanotechnology* **2020**, *31*, 335103. [CrossRef]
11. Hongfei, L.; Jie, Z.; Pengyue, B.; Yueping, D.; Jiapeng, W.; Yi, D.; Yang, Q.; Ying, X. Establishment and In Vitro Evaluation of Porous Ion-responsive Targeted Drug Delivery System. *Protein Pept. Lett.* **2020**, *27*, 1–12. [CrossRef]
12. Ahuja, G.; Pathak, K. Porous carriers for controlled/modulated drug delivery. *Indian J. Pharm. Sci.* **2009**, *71*, 599–607. [CrossRef] [PubMed]
13. Chowdhury, A.H.; Salam, N.; Debnath, R.; Islam, S.M.; Saha, T. Chapter 8—Design and Fabrication of Porous Nanostructures and Their Applications. In *Nanomaterials Synthesis*; Beeran Pottathara, Y., Thomas, S., Kalarikkal, N., Grohens, Y., Kokol, V., Eds.; Elsevier: Amsterdam, The Netherlands, 2019; pp. 265–294. [CrossRef]
14. Solano, V.; Vega-Baudrit, J. Micro, Meso and Macro Porous Materials on Medicine. *J. Biomater. Nanobiotechnol.* **2015**, *6*, 247–256. [CrossRef]
15. Seaton, N.A. Determination of the connectivity of porous solids from nitrogen sorption measurements. *Chem. Eng. Sci.* **1991**, *46*, 1895–1909. [CrossRef]
16. Aquib, M.; Farooq, M.A.; Banerjee, P.; Akhtar, F.; Filli, M.S.; Boakye-Yiadom, K.O.; Kesse, S.; Raza, F.; Maviah, M.B.J.; Mavlyanova, R.; et al. Targeted and stimuli–responsive mesoporous silica nanoparticles for drug delivery and theranostic use. *J. Biomed. Mater. Res. Part A* **2019**, *107*, 2643–2666. [CrossRef] [PubMed]
17. Guimarães, R.S.; Rodrigues, C.F.; Moreira, A.F.; Correia, I.J. Overview of stimuli-responsive mesoporous organosilica nanocarriers for drug delivery. *Pharmacol. Res.* **2020**, *155*, 104742. [CrossRef]
18. Yu, Q.; Deng, T.; Lin, F.-C.; Zhang, B.; Zink, J.I. Supramolecular Assemblies of Heterogeneous Mesoporous Silica Nanoparticles to Co-deliver Antimicrobial Peptides and Antibiotics for Synergistic Eradication of Pathogenic Biofilms. *ACS Nano* **2020**, *14*, 5926–5937. [CrossRef]
19. Quinlan, E.; López-Noriega, A.; Thompson, E.M.; Hibbitts, A.; Cryan, S.A.; O'Brien, F.J. Controlled release of vascular endothelial growth factor from spray-dried alginate microparticles in collagen–hydroxyapatite scaffolds for promoting vascularization and bone repair. *J. Tissue Eng. Regen. Med.* **2017**, *11*, 1097–1109. [CrossRef]
20. Laurenti, M.; Lamberti, A.; Genchi, G.G.; Roppolo, I.; Canavese, G.; Vitale-Brovarone, C.; Ciofani, G.; Cauda, V. Graphene Oxide Finely Tunes the Bioactivity and Drug Delivery of Mesoporous ZnO Scaffolds. *ACS Appl. Mater. Interfaces* **2019**, *11*, 449–456. [CrossRef]
21. Vallet-Regí, M.; Balas, F.; Arcos, D. Mesoporous Materials for Drug Delivery. *Angew. Chem. Int. Ed.* **2007**, *46*, 7548–7558. [CrossRef]
22. Sengottuvelan, A.; Mederer, M.; Boccaccini, A.R. Preparation and characterization of mesoporous calcium-doped silica-coated TiO2 scaffolds and their drug releasing behavior. *Int. J. Appl. Ceram. Technol.* **2018**, *15*, 892–902. [CrossRef]
23. Sun, Y.; Han, X.; Wang, X.; Zhu, B.; Li, B.; Chen, Z.; Ma, G.; Wan, M. Sustained Release of IGF-1 by 3D Mesoporous Scaffolds Promoting Cardiac Stem Cell Migration and Proliferation. *Cell. Physiol. Biochem.* **2018**, *49*, 2358–2370. [CrossRef] [PubMed]
24. Boccardi, E.; Philippart, A.; Juhasz-Bortuzzo, J.A.; Beltrán, A.M.; Novajra, G.; Vitale-Brovarone, C.; Spiecker, E.; Boccaccini, A.R. Uniform Surface Modification of 3D Bioglass(®)-Based Scaffolds with Mesoporous Silica Particles (MCM-41) for Enhancing Drug Delivery Capability. *Front. Bioeng. Biotechnol.* **2015**, *3*, 177. [CrossRef] [PubMed]
25. Davis, M.E. Ordered porous materials for emerging applications. *Nature* **2002**, *417*, 813–821. [CrossRef]
26. Marcos-Hernández, M.; Villagrán, D. 11-Mesoporous Composite Nanomaterials for Dye Removal and Other Applications. In *Composite Nanoadsorbents*; Kyzas, G.Z., Mitropoulos, A.C., Eds.; Elsevier: Amsterdam, The Netherlands, 2019; pp. 265–293. [CrossRef]

27. Pellicer, E.; Cabo, M.; Solsona, P.; Suriñach, S.; Baró, M.; Sort, J. Nanocasting of Mesoporous In-TM (TM = Co, Fe, Mn) Oxides: Towards 3D Diluted-Oxide Magnetic Semiconductor Architectures. *Adv. Funct. Mater.* **2013**, *23*, 900–911. [CrossRef]
28. Yonemoto, B.T.; Hutchings, G.S.; Jiao, F. A General Synthetic Approach for Ordered Mesoporous Metal Sulfides. *J. Am. Chem. Soc.* **2014**, *136*, 8895–8898. [CrossRef]
29. Savic, S.; Vojisavljević, K.; Počuča-Nešić, M.; Živojević, K.; Mladenovic, M.; Knezevic, N. Hard Template Synthesis of Nanomaterials Based on Mesoporous Silica. *Metall. Mater. Eng.* **2018**, *24*. [CrossRef]
30. Zhao, T.; Elzatahry, A.; Li, X.; Zhao, D. Single-micelle-directed synthesis of mesoporous materials. *Nat. Rev. Mater.* **2019**, *4*, 775–791. [CrossRef]
31. Lokupitiya, H.N.; Jones, A.; Reid, B.; Guldin, S.; Stefik, M. Ordered Mesoporous to Macroporous Oxides with Tunable Isomorphic Architectures: Solution Criteria for Persistent Micelle Templates. *Chem. Mater.* **2016**, *28*, 1653–1667. [CrossRef]
32. Zuo, X.; Xia, Y.; Ji, Q.; Gao, X.; Yin, S.; Wang, M.; Wang, X.; Qiu, B.; Wei, A.; Sun, Z.; et al. Self-Templating Construction of 3D Hierarchical Macro-/Mesoporous Silicon from 0D Silica Nanoparticles. *ACS Nano* **2017**, *11*, 889–899. [CrossRef]
33. Manzano, M.; Colilla, M.; Vallet-Regí, M. Drug delivery from ordered mesoporous matrices. *Expert Opin. Drug Deliv.* **2009**, *6*, 1383–1400. [CrossRef] [PubMed]
34. Sun, T.; Shan, N.; Xu, L.; Wang, J.; Chen, J.; Zakhidov, A.A.; Baughman, R.H. General Synthesis of 3D Ordered Macro-/Mesoporous Materials by Templating Mesoporous Silica Confined in Opals. *Chem. Mater.* **2018**, *30*, 1617–1624. [CrossRef]
35. Kang, Y.G.; Wei, J.; Shin, J.W.; Wu, Y.R.; Su, J.; Park, Y.S.; Shin, J.-W. Enhanced biocompatibility and osteogenic potential of mesoporous magnesium silicate/polycaprolactone/wheat protein composite scaffolds. *Int. J. Nanomed.* **2018**, *13*, 1107–1117. [CrossRef] [PubMed]
36. Wijk, A.; van Wijk, I. *3D Printing with Biomaterials: Towards a Sustainable and Circular Economy*; IOS Press: Amsterdam, The Netherlands, 2015; pp. 1–85. [CrossRef]
37. Erokhin, K.S.; Gordeev, E.G.; Ananikov, V.P. Revealing interactions of layered polymeric materials at solid-liquid interface for building solvent compatibility charts for 3D printing applications. *Sci. Rep.* **2019**, *9*, 20177. [CrossRef]
38. Salea, A.; Prathumwan, R.; Junpha, J.; Subannajui, K. Metal oxide semiconductor 3D printing: Preparation of copper(ii) oxide by fused deposition modelling for multi-functional semiconducting applications. *J. Mater. Chem. C* **2017**, *5*, 4614–4620. [CrossRef]
39. Zhang, S.; Xing, M.; Li, B. Recent advances in musculoskeletal local drug delivery. *Acta Biomater.* **2019**, *93*, 135–151. [CrossRef]
40. Trofimov, A.D.; Ivanova, A.A.; Zyuzin, M.V.; Timin, A.S. Porous Inorganic Carriers Based on Silica, Calcium Carbonate and Calcium Phosphate for Controlled/Modulated Drug Delivery: Fresh Outlook and Future Perspectives. *Pharmaceutics* **2018**, *10*, 167. [CrossRef]
41. Liang, F.; Qin, L.; Xu, J.; Li, S.; Luo, C.; Huang, H.; Ma, D.; Li, Z.; Xu, J. A hydroxyl-functionalized 3D porous gadolinium-organic framework platform for drug delivery, imaging and gas separation. *J. Solid State Chem.* **2020**, *289*, 121544. [CrossRef]
42. Rawtani, D.; Agrawal, Y.K. Emerging Strategies and Applications of Layer-by-Layer Self-Assembly. *Nanobiomedicine* **2014**, *1*, 8. [CrossRef]
43. Vanderburgh, J.; Sterling, J.A.; Guelcher, S.A. 3D Printing of Tissue Engineered Constructs for In Vitro Modeling of Disease Progression and Drug Screening. *Ann. Biomed. Eng.* **2017**, *45*, 164–179. [CrossRef]
44. Charbe, N.B.; McCarron, P.A.; Lane, M.E.; Tambuwala, M.M. Application of three-dimensional printing for colon targeted drug delivery systems. *Int. J. Pharm. Investig.* **2017**, *7*, 47–59. [CrossRef] [PubMed]
45. Huang, K.-H.; Lin, Y.-H.; Shie, M.-Y.; Lin, C.-P. Effects of bone morphogenic protein-2 loaded on the 3D-printed MesoCS scaffolds. *J. Formos. Med. Assoc.* **2018**, *117*, 879–887. [CrossRef] [PubMed]
46. Shim, J.-H.; Kim, M.-J.; Park, J.Y.; Pati, R.G.; Yun, Y.-P.; Kim, S.E.; Song, H.-R.; Cho, D.-W. Three-dimensional printing of antibiotics-loaded poly-ε-caprolactone/poly(lactic-co-glycolic acid) scaffolds for treatment of chronic osteomyelitis. *Tissue Eng. Regen. Med.* **2015**, *12*, 283–293. [CrossRef]
47. Visscher, L.E.; Dang, H.P.; Knackstedt, M.A.; Hutmacher, D.W.; Tran, P.A. 3D printed Polycaprolactone scaffolds with dual macro-microporosity for applications in local delivery of antibiotics. *Mater. Sci. Eng. C Mater. Biol. Appl.* **2018**, *87*, 78–89. [CrossRef] [PubMed]

48. Long, J.; Gholizadeh, H.; Lu, J.; Bunt, C.; Seyfoddin, A. Review: Application of Fused Deposition Modelling (FDM) Method of 3D Printing in Drug Delivery. *Curr. Pharm. Des.* **2016**, *22*, 433–439. [CrossRef]
49. Goole, J.; Amighi, K. 3D printing in pharmaceutics: A new tool for designing customized drug delivery systems. *Int. J. Pharm.* **2016**, *499*, 376–394. [CrossRef]
50. Goyanes, A.; Buanz, A.B.M.; Hatton, G.B.; Gaisford, S.; Basit, A.W. 3D printing of modified-release aminosalicylate (4-ASA and 5-ASA) tablets. *Eur. J. Pharm. Biopharm.* **2015**, *89*, 157–162. [CrossRef]
51. Cui, X.; Boland, T.; D'Lima, D.D.; Lotz, M.K. Thermal Inkjet Printing in Tissue Engineering and Regenerative Medicine. *Recent Pat. Drug Deliv. Formul.* **2012**, *6*, 149–155. [CrossRef]
52. Boehm, R.D.; Miller, P.R.; Daniels, J.; Stafslien, S.; Narayan, R.J. Inkjet printing for pharmaceutical applications. *Mater. Today* **2014**, *17*, 247–252. [CrossRef]
53. Mathew, E.; Pitzanti, G.; Larrañeta, E.; Lamprou, D.A. 3D Printing of Pharmaceuticals and Drug Delivery Devices. *Pharmaceutics* **2020**, *12*, 266. [CrossRef]
54. Ni, J.; Ling, H.; Zhang, S.; Wang, Z.; Peng, Z.; Benyshek, C.; Zan, R.; Miri, A.K.; Li, Z.; Zhang, X.; et al. Three-dimensional printing of metals for biomedical applications. *Mater. Today Bio* **2019**, *3*, 100024. [CrossRef] [PubMed]
55. Yang, Y.; Wang, G.; Liang, H.; Gao, C.; Peng, S.; Shen, L.; Shuai, C. Additive manufacturing of bone scaffolds. *Int. J. Bioprint.* **2019**, *2019*, 5. [CrossRef] [PubMed]
56. Du, Y.; Liu, H.; Yang, Q.; Wang, S.; Wang, J.; Ma, J.; Noh, I.; Mikos, A.G.; Zhang, S. Selective laser sintering scaffold with hierarchical architecture and gradient composition for osteochondral repair in rabbits. *Biomaterials* **2017**, *137*, 37–48. [CrossRef] [PubMed]
57. Kumaresan, T.; Gandhinathan, R.; Murugan, R.; Muthusamy, A.; Kamarajan, B. Design, analysis and fabrication of polyamide/ hydroxyapatite porous structured scaffold using selective laser sintering method for bio-medical applications. *J. Mech. Sci. Technol.* **2016**, *30*, 5305–5312. [CrossRef]
58. Gan, M.X.; Wong, C.H. Properties of selective laser melted spodumene glass-ceramic. *J. Eur. Ceram. Soc.* **2017**, *37*, 4147–4154. [CrossRef]
59. Bai, P.K.; Cheng, J.; Liu, B. Selective laser sintering of polymer-coated Al2O3/ZrO2/TiC ceramic powder. *Trans. Nonferrous Metals Soc. China* **2005**, *15*, 261–265.
60. Deckers Jan, P.; Shahzad, K.; Cardon, L.; Rombouts, M.; Vleugels, J.; Kruth, J.-P. Shaping ceramics through indirect selective laser sintering. *Rapid Prototyp. J.* **2016**, *22*, 544–558. [CrossRef]
61. Chang, S.; Li, L.; Lu, L.; Fuh, J.Y.H. Selective Laser Sintering of Porous Silica Enabled by Carbon Additive. *Materials* **2017**, *10*, 1313. [CrossRef]
62. Gao, C.; Feng, P.; Peng, S.; Shuai, C. Carbon nanotube, graphene and boron nitride nanotube reinforced bioactive ceramics for bone repair. *Acta Biomater.* **2017**, *61*, 1–20. [CrossRef]
63. Moulton, S.E.; Wallace, G.G. 3-dimensional (3D) fabricated polymer based drug delivery systems. *J. Controll. Release* **2014**, *193*, 27–34. [CrossRef]
64. Partheniadis, I.; Nikolakakis, I.; Laidmäe, I.; Heinämäki, J. A Mini-Review: Needleless Electrospinning of Nanofibers for Pharmaceutical and Biomedical Applications. *Processes* **2020**, *8*, 673. [CrossRef]
65. Contreras-Cáceres, R.; Cabeza, L.; Perazzoli, G.; Díaz, A.; López-Romero, J.M.; Melguizo, C.; Prados, J. Electrospun Nanofibers: Recent Applications in Drug Delivery and Cancer Therapy. *Nanomaterials* **2019**, *9*, 656. [CrossRef] [PubMed]
66. Melchels, F.P.W.; Feijen, J.; Grijpma, D.W. A review on stereolithography and its applications in biomedical engineering. *Biomaterials* **2010**, *31*, 6121–6130. [CrossRef] [PubMed]
67. Pereira, R.F.; Bártolo, P.J. 3D Photo-Fabrication for Tissue Engineering and Drug Delivery. *Engineering* **2015**, *1*, 90–112. [CrossRef]
68. Wang, H.; Deng, Z.; Chen, J.; Qi, X.; Pang, L.; Lin, B.; Adib, Y.T.Y.; Miao, N.; Wang, D.; Zhang, Y.; et al. A novel vehicle-like drug delivery 3D printing scaffold and its applications for a rat femoral bone repairing in vitro and in vivo. *Int. J. Biol. Sci.* **2020**, *16*, 1821–1832. [CrossRef]
69. Yu, C.-T.; Wang, F.-M.; Liu, Y.-T.; Ng, H.Y.; Jhong, Y.-R.; Hung, C.-H.; Chen, Y.-W. Effect of Bone Morphogenic Protein-2-Loaded Mesoporous Strontium Substitution Calcium Silicate/Recycled Fish Gelatin 3D Cell-Laden Scaffold for Bone Tissue Engineering. *Processes* **2020**, *8*, 493. [CrossRef]
70. Rosenberg, M.; Shilo, D.; Galperin, L.; Capucha, T.; Tarabieh, K.; Rachmiel, A.; Segal, E. Bone Morphogenic Protein 2-Loaded Porous Silicon Carriers for Osteoinductive Implants. *Pharmaceutics* **2019**, *11*, 602. [CrossRef]

71. Huang, K.-H.; Chen, Y.-W.; Wang, C.-Y.; Lin, Y.-H.; Wu, Y.-H.A.; Shie, M.-Y.; Lin, C.-P. Enhanced Capability of Bone Morphogenetic Protein 2–loaded Mesoporous Calcium Silicate Scaffolds to Induce Odontogenic Differentiation of Human Dental Pulp Cells. *J. Endod.* **2018**, *44*, 1677–1685. [CrossRef]
72. James, A.W.; LaChaud, G.; Shen, J.; Asatrian, G.; Nguyen, V.; Zhang, X.; Ting, K.; Soo, C. A Review of the Clinical Side Effects of Bone Morphogenetic Protein-2. *Tissue Eng. Part B Rev.* **2016**, *22*, 284–297. [CrossRef]
73. Ishack, S.; Mediero, A.; Wilder, T.; Ricci, J.L.; Cronstein, B.N. Bone regeneration in critical bone defects using three-dimensionally printed β-tricalcium phosphate/hydroxyapatite scaffolds is enhanced by coating scaffolds with either dipyridamole or BMP-2. *J. Biomed. Mater. Res. B Appl. Biomater.* **2017**, *105*, 366–375. [CrossRef]
74. Min, Z.; Shichang, Z.; Chen, X.; Yufang, Z.; Changqing, Z. 3D-printed dimethyloxallyl glycine delivery scaffolds to improve angiogenesis and osteogenesis. *Biomater. Sci.* **2015**, *3*, 1236–1244. [CrossRef] [PubMed]
75. Akkineni, A.R.; Luo, Y.; Schumacher, M.; Nies, B.; Lode, A.; Gelinsky, M. 3D plotting of growth factor loaded calcium phosphate cement scaffolds. *Acta Biomater.* **2015**, *27*, 264–274. [CrossRef] [PubMed]
76. Wu, J.; Miao, G.; Zheng, Z.; Li, Z.; Ren, W.; Wu, C.; Li, Y.; Huang, Z.; Yang, L.; Guo, L. 3D printing mesoporous bioactive glass/sodium alginate/gelatin sustained release scaffolds for bone repair. *J. Biomater. Appl.* **2018**, *33*, 755–765. [CrossRef] [PubMed]
77. Heras, C.; Sanchez-Salcedo, S.; Lozano, D.; Peña, J.; Esbrit, P.; Vallet-Regi, M.; Salinas, A.J. Osteostatin potentiates the bioactivity of mesoporous glass scaffolds containing Zn^{2+} ions in human mesenchymal stem cells. *Acta Biomater.* **2019**, *89*, 359–371. [CrossRef] [PubMed]
78. Saska, S.; Pires, L.C.; Cominotte, M.A.; Mendes, L.S.; de Oliveira, M.F.; Maia, I.A.; da Silva, J.V.L.; Ribeiro, S.J.L.; Cirelli, J.A. Three-dimensional printing and in vitro evaluation of poly(3-hydroxybutyrate) scaffolds functionalized with osteogenic growth peptide for tissue engineering. *Mater. Sci. Eng. C* **2018**, *89*, 265–273. [CrossRef] [PubMed]
79. Pei, P.; Wei, D.; Zhu, M.; Du, X.; Zhu, Y. The effect of calcium sulfate incorporation on physiochemical and biological properties of 3D-printed mesoporous calcium silicate cement scaffolds. *Microporous Mesoporous Mater.* **2017**, *241*, 11–20. [CrossRef]
80. Fu, S.; Du, X.; Zhu, M.; Tian, Z.; Wei, D.; Zhu, Y. 3D printing of layered mesoporous bioactive glass/sodium alginate-sodium alginate scaffolds with controllable dual-drug release behaviors. *Biomed. Mater.* **2019**, *14*, 065011. [CrossRef]
81. Chihara, T.; Zhang, Y.; Li, X.; Shinohara, A.; Kagami, H. Effect of short-term betamethasone administration on the regeneration process of tissue-engineered bone. *Histol. Histopathol.* **2020**, *35*, 709–717. [CrossRef]
82. Xu, Y.; Hu, Y.; Feng, P.; Yang, W.; Shuai, C. Drug loading/release and bioactivity research of a mesoporous bioactive glass/polymer scaffold. *Ceram. Int.* **2019**, *45*, 18003–18013. [CrossRef]
83. El-Fiqi, A.; Kim, J.-H.; Kim, H.-W. Osteoinductive Fibrous Scaffolds of Biopolymer/Mesoporous Bioactive Glass Nanocarriers with Excellent Bioactivity and Long-Term Delivery of Osteogenic Drug. *ACS Appl. Mater. Interfaces* **2015**, *7*, 1140–1152. [CrossRef]
84. Zhang, J.; Zhao, S.; Zhu, Y.; Huang, Y.; Zhu, M.; Tao, C.; Zhang, C. Three-dimensional printing of strontium-containing mesoporous bioactive glass scaffolds for bone regeneration. *Acta Biomater.* **2014**, *10*, 2269–2281. [CrossRef]
85. Luo, Y.; Wu, C.; Lode, A.; Gelinsky, M. Hierarchical mesoporous bioactive glass/alginate composite scaffolds fabricated by three-dimensional plotting for bone tissue engineering. *Biofabrication* **2012**, *5*, 015005. [CrossRef] [PubMed]
86. Chen, F.; Song, Z.; Gao, L.; Hong, H.; Liu, C. Hierarchically macroporous/mesoporous POC composite scaffolds with IBU-loaded hollow SiO2 microspheres for repairing infected bone defects. *J. Mater. Chem. B* **2016**, *4*, 4198–4205. [CrossRef] [PubMed]
87. Gao, L.; Li, C.; Chen, F.; Liu, C. Fabrication and characterization of toughness-enhanced scaffolds comprising β -TCP/POC using the freeform fabrication system with micro-droplet jetting. *Biomed. Mater.* **2015**, *10*, 035009. [CrossRef]
88. Kluin, O.S.; van der Mei, H.C.; Busscher, H.J.; Neut, D. Biodegradable vs non-biodegradable antibiotic delivery devices in the treatment of osteomyelitis. *Expert Opin. Drug Deliv.* **2013**, *10*, 341–351. [CrossRef]
89. Kamboj, N.; Rodriguez, M.; Rahmani Ahranjani, R.; Prashanth, K.G.; Hussainova, I. Bioceramic scaffolds by additive manufacturing for controlled delivery of the antibiotic vancomycin. *Proc. Est. Acad. Sci.* **2019**, *68*, 185–190. [CrossRef]

90. Zhang, J.; Zhao, S.; Zhu, M.; Zhu, Y.; Zhang, Y.; Liu, Z.; Zhang, C. 3D-printed magnetic Fe3O4/MBG/PCL composite scaffolds with multifunctionality of bone regeneration, local anticancer drug delivery and hyperthermia. *J. Mater. Chem. B* **2014**, *2*, 7583–7595. [CrossRef] [PubMed]
91. Jaeblon, T. Polymethylmethacrylate: Properties and Contemporary Uses in Orthopaedics. *J. Am. Acad. Orthop. Surg.* **2010**, *18*, 297–305. [CrossRef] [PubMed]
92. Darouiche, R.O. Treatment of infections associated with surgical implants. *N. Engl. J. Med.* **2004**, *350*, 1422–1429. [CrossRef]
93. García-Alvarez, R.; Izquierdo-Barba, I.; Vallet-Regí, M. 3D scaffold with effective multidrug sequential release against bacteria biofilm. *Acta Biomater.* **2017**, *49*, 113–126. [CrossRef]
94. Inzana, J.A.; Trombetta, R.P.; Schwarz, E.M.; Kates, S.L.; Awad, H.A. 3D printed bioceramics for dual antibiotic delivery to treat implant-associated bone infection. *Eur. Cell Mater.* **2015**, *30*, 232–247. [CrossRef]
95. Martínez-Vázquez, F.J.; Cabañas, M.V.; Paris, J.L.; Lozano, D.; Vallet-Regí, M. Fabrication of novel Si-doped hydroxyapatite/gelatine scaffolds by rapid prototyping for drug delivery and bone regeneration. *Acta Biomater.* **2015**, *15*, 200–209. [CrossRef] [PubMed]
96. Philippart, A.; Gómez-Cerezo, N.; Arcos, D.; Salinas, A.J.; Boccardi, E.; Vallet-Regi, M.; Boccaccini, A.R. Novel ion-doped mesoporous glasses for bone tissue engineering: Study of their structural characteristics influenced by the presence of phosphorous oxide. *Non-Cryst. Solids* **2017**, *455*, 90–97. [CrossRef]
97. Hoppe, A.; Güldal, N.S.; Boccaccini, A.R. A review of the biological response to ionic dissolution products from bioactive glasses and glass-ceramics. *Biomaterials* **2011**, *32*, 2757–2774. [CrossRef]
98. Kaya, S.; Cresswell, M.; Boccaccini, A.R. Mesoporous silica-based bioactive glasses for antibiotic-free antibacterial applications. *Mater. Sci. Eng. C* **2018**, *83*, 99–107. [CrossRef]
99. Zhang, Y.; Zhai, D.; Xu, M.; Yao, Q.; Zhu, H.; Chang, J.; Wu, C. 3D-printed bioceramic scaffolds with antibacterial and osteogenic activity. *Biofabrication* **2017**, *9*, 025037. [CrossRef]
100. Qi, X.; Wang, H.; Zhang, Y.; Pang, L.; Xiao, W.; Jia, W.; Zhao, S.; Wang, D.; Huang, W.; Wang, Q. Mesoporous bioactive glass-coated 3D printed borosilicate bioactive glass scaffolds for improving repair of bone defects. *Int. J. Biol. Sci.* **2018**, *14*, 471–484. [CrossRef]
101. Zhu, M.; Zhang, J.; Zhao, S.; Zhu, Y. Three-dimensional printing of cerium-incorporated mesoporous calcium-silicate scaffolds for bone repair. *J. Mater. Sci.* **2016**, *51*, 836–844. [CrossRef]
102. Zhao, S.; Zhang, J.; Zhu, M.; Zhang, Y.; Liu, Z.; Tao, C.; Zhu, Y.; Zhang, C. Three-dimensional printed strontium-containing mesoporous bioactive glass scaffolds for repairing rat critical-sized calvarial defects. *Acta Biomater.* **2015**, *12*, 270–280. [CrossRef]
103. Rajasekharan, A.K.; Gyllensten, C.; Blomstrand, E.; Liebi, M.; Andersson, M. Tough Ordered Mesoporous Elastomeric Biomaterials Formed at Ambient Conditions. *ACS Nano* **2020**, *14*, 241–254. [CrossRef]
104. Zhang, Y.; Huang, J.; Huang, L.; Liu, Q.; Shao, H.; Hu, X.; Song, L. Silk Fibroin-Based Scaffolds with Controlled Delivery Order of VEGF and BDNF for Cavernous Nerve Regeneration. *ACS Biomater. Sci. Eng.* **2016**, *2*, 2018–2025. [CrossRef]
105. Siyawamwaya, M.; du Toit, L.C.; Kumar, P.; Choonara, Y.E.; Kondiah, P.P.P.D.; Pillay, V. 3D printed, controlled release, tritherapeutic tablet matrix for advanced anti-HIV-1 drug delivery. *Eur. J. Pharm. Biopharm.* **2019**, *138*, 99–110. [CrossRef]
106. Pei, P.; Tian, Z.; Zhu, Y. 3D printed mesoporous bioactive glass/metal-organic framework scaffolds with antitubercular drug delivery. *Microporous Mesoporous Mater.* **2018**, *272*, 24–30. [CrossRef]
107. Zhu, M.; Li, K.; Zhu, Y.; Zhang, J.; Ye, X. 3D-printed hierarchical scaffold for localized isoniazid/rifampin drug delivery and osteoarticular tuberculosis therapy. *Acta Biomater.* **2015**, *16*, 145–155. [CrossRef] [PubMed]
108. Zhang, Y.; Xia, L.; Zhai, D.; Shi, M.; Luo, Y.; Feng, C.; Fang, B.; Yin, J.; Chang, J.; Wu, C. Mesoporous bioactive glass nanolayer-functionalized 3D-printed scaffolds for accelerating osteogenesis and angiogenesis. *Nanoscale* **2015**, *7*, 19207–19221. [CrossRef]
109. Fang, J.-H.; Liu, C.-H.; Hsu, R.-S.; Chen, Y.-Y.; Chiang, W.-H.; Wang, H.-M.D.; Hu, S.-H. Transdermal Composite Microneedle Composed of Mesoporous Iron Oxide Nanoraspberry and PVA for Androgenetic Alopecia Treatment. *Polymers* **2020**, *12*, 1392. [CrossRef]
110. Do, A.-V.; Worthington, K.S.; Tucker, B.A.; Salem, A.K. Controlled drug delivery from 3D printed two-photon polymerized poly(ethylene glycol) dimethacrylate devices. *Int. J. Pharm.* **2018**, *552*, 217–224. [CrossRef]

10

Loading Graphene Quantum Dots into Optical-Magneto Nanoparticles for Real-Time Tracking *In Vivo*

Yu Wang [1,2], Nan Xu [1,2], Yongkai He [1,2,3], Jingyun Wang [4], Dan Wang [1,2], Qin Gao [1,2], Siyu Xie [1,2], Yage Li [1,2], Ranran Zhang [3,*] and Qiang Cai [1,2,3,*]

1 State key Laboratory of New Ceramics and Fine Processing, School of Materials Science and Engineering, Tsinghua University, Beijing 100084, China
2 Key Laboratory of Advanced Materials of Ministry of Education of China, Tsinghua University, Beijing 100084, China
3 Tsinghua Shenzhen International Graduate School, Tsinghua University, Shenzhen 518055, China
4 Shenzhen Geim Graphene Center, Tsinghua-Berkeley Shenzhen Institute, Tsinghua University, Shenzhen 518055, China
* Correspondence: biomnano@163.com (R.Z.); caiqiang@mail.tsinghua.edu.cn (Q.C.);

Abstract: Fluorescence imaging offers a new approach to visualize real-time details on a cellular level *in vitro* and *in vivo* without radioactive damage. Poor light stability of organic fluorescent dyes makes long-term imaging difficult. Due to their outstanding optical properties and unique structural features, graphene quantum dots (GQDs) are promising in the field of imaging for real-time tracking *in vivo*. At present, GQDs are mainly loaded on the surface of nanoparticles. In this study, we developed an efficient and convenient one-pot method to load GQDs into nanoparticles, leading to longer metabolic processes in blood and increased delivery of GQDs to tumors. Optical-magneto ferroferric oxide@polypyrrole (Fe_3O_4@PPy) core-shell nanoparticles were chosen for their potential use in cancer therapy. The *in vivo* results demonstrated that by loading GQDs, it was possible to monitor the distribution and metabolism of nanoparticles. This study provided new insights into the application of GQDs in long-term *in vivo* real-time tracking.

Keywords: GQDs; real-time tracking; optical-magneto nanoparticles; *in vivo*

1. Introduction

Cancer is known to be one of the leading causes of death in almost every country of the world [1]. The ideal therapy for cancer is to deliver suitable treatment (chemotherapeutic drugs, genetic drugs, nanoparticles, etc.) to the right place at the right time. Various delivery systems are designed to track the release and infiltration process of nanoparticles or drugs at the tumor site, guiding local treatment and monitoring the effects after treatment [2–4]. Due to low temporal or spatial resolution, the contemporary methods available are unable to track the kinetics of drugs or nanoparticles *in vivo* for a sustained period of time [5]. Optical imaging presents non-ionizing, non-invasive, and non-destructive features with high precision and efficiency [6]. Small molecule organic dyes, including near-infrared fluorescent dyes sulfo-cyanine7 (Cy7), indocyanine green (ICG), Dye800 and green fluorescent dyes fluorescein isothiocyanate (FITC), are employed as imaging probes for their excellent luminescence, while properties such as poor light stability severely limit their biomedical applications [7,8]. Semiconductor quantum dots have excellent luminescence and light stability, and are considered as alternatives to organic dyes. However, high toxicity and poor water solubility would hinder their application in biomedical fields. Moreover, the relatively large size of semiconductor quantum dots and the scintillating fluorescence are both obstacles to successful imaging at the molecular level [9]. Therefore, the development of new fluorescent materials is of great significance to biomedical imaging.

Graphene quantum dots (GQDs) have drawn more attention in recent years due to their outstanding properties, including excellent light stability and water solubility. Other noteworthy properties of GQDs include their ultra-small size, highly adjustable photoluminescence, as well as excellent multiphoton excitation, high luminosity, and chemical inertness [10,11]. Moreover, various nanomaterials including GQDs and GQD-based nanomaterials are reported to yield reactive oxygen species (ROS) in cells, leading to the promise of photodynamic therapy for cancer [12,13]. GQDs have shown even more promising applications in fluorescence imaging, imaging-guided surgery and biosensing [6,14]. Studies pay close attention to the biocompatibility of GQDs when they are applied in biomedical fields. *In vitro* studies illustrate that GQDs show excellent biocompatibility when co-incubated with various cells; *in vivo* studies also demonstrate the biocompatibility of GQDs [15]. N-doped graphene quantum dots exhibit low cytotoxicity when concentrations are under 200 μg/mL [16]. These studies indicate the promising biomedical applications of GQDs and GQD-based materials.

To achieve multiple functions, it is common to combine GQDs with other nanomaterials. There are many studies on the combination of GQDs and nanomaterials by dipping or sticking GQDs on the surface of nanoparticles for drug delivery and imaging [17–19]. Our study proposed an efficient and convenient one-pot approach to load GQDs into Fe_3O_4@PPy nanoparticles, which could avoid complicated binders and be easily extended to other nanoparticles. Fe_3O_4@PPy nanoparticles were chosen as model nanoparticles since they were proven to be excellent tumor diagnosis and treatment platforms, performing multiple diagnostic functions (such as magnetic resonance imaging and photoacoustic imaging), and have been utilized in various therapies (magnetic hyperthermia and photothermal therapy) [20]. Combination of the GQDs and magnetic nanoparticles enabled the function of real-time tracking in the optical-magneto nanoparticles. Moreover, when loading GQDs into PPy-coated Fe_3O_4 nanoparticles, longer metabolic processing in the blood and increased delivery of GQDs were achieved, laying the foundation for the application of GQDs *in vivo*.

2. Materials and Methods

2.1. Preparation and Characterization

Polyvinyl alcohol (Sinopharm Chemical Reagent Co., Ltd, Shanghai, China) (PVA, 7.5 g) was dissolved in 100 mL of deionized water. Next, 0.1 g of ferroferric oxide (Sinopharm Chemical Reagent Co., Ltd, Shanghai, China) was dissolved in 10 mL of deionized water and then mixed with 40 mL of PVA solution, followed by 30 minutes of stirring. GQDs (0.15 g) were dissolved in 5 mL of deionized water, then mixed with the above solution and stirred for 30 minutes for uniform dispersion. The synthesis of used OH–GQDs was carried out according to a previous work of Wang et al. [21]. Subsequently, 0.2 mL of pyrrole liquid was slowly added to the above mixed solution and stirred for 10 min. Then, 0.1 g of ferric chloride hexahydrate (Sinopharm Chemical Reagent Co., Ltd, Shanghai, China) was added and stirred at room temperature for three hours. Eventually, the solution was centrifuged five times, washed, and finally dried at 70 °C. The obtained nanoparticles were referred to as GQD-NPs. The as-prepared GQD-NPs were characterized and analyzed by a high resolution transmission electron microscope (HRTEM; JEM-2010F, JEOL, Tokyo, Japan), X-ray diffraction (XRD, Bruker D8 Advance X-ray diffractometer, Bruker, Karlsruhe, Germany), Raman spectroscopy analysis (HORIBA, Montpellier, France), and X-ray photoelectron spectroscopy (XPS; Escalab 250Xi, Thermo Scientific, Waltham, MA USA). Fluorescent spectra were measured at room temperature with a fluorescence spectrometer (FLSP920, Edinburgh Instruments, Edinburgh, UK). Magnetic properties were detected by a vibrating sample magnetometer (Lake Shore VSM 7307, Lakeshore, Columbus, OH, USA).

2.2. Cell Toxicity

Murine fibrosarcoma L929 cells were purchased from Peking Union Medical College and cultured in RPMI 1640 basic medium (Gibco, Carlsbad, CA, USA) supplied with 10% fetal bovine serum (Gibco, Carlsbad, CA, USA) and 1% penicillin–streptomycin (Gibco, Carlsbad, CA, USA). Cells were seeded in 96-well plates at 5×10^3 cells per well for 24 h. Then, GQD-NPs with gradient concentrations (50 μg/mL, 100 μg/mL, 160 μg/mL, 250 μg/mL, 500 μg/mL, and 1000 μg/mL) were added into each well. The doses of GQD-NPs were selected according to previous studies [3,22–24]. After incubation for 24 h or 48 h, cell viability was measured using a cell counting kit-8 (CCK-8; Dojindo, Kyushu, Japan) following the manufacturer's instructions. The cell viability values were all normalized to control groups (untreated cells after incubation for 24 h or 48 h). The experiments were conducted in triplicate and the data were expressed as means ± standard deviation. Student's t-test was used to determine the level of significance. Differences with $p < 0.05$ and $p < 0.01$ were considered statistically significant and highly significant, respectively.

2.3. In Vivo Tracking

Animal experiments were conducted under the guidance of the Animal Testing Center of Tsinghua University in accordance with strict animal ethical standards. The BALB/c female mice (5–6 weeks old and 16–18 g) used in our experiments were purchased from Beijing Weitong Lihua Experimental Animal Technology Co., Ltd. (Beijing, China). To establish the tumor model, 0.2 mL human breast cancer cell line MCF-7 cell suspension (5×10^6 cells) was injected subcutaneously into the hind limb of the nude mice. After the tumor grew to 75–100 mm^3, the nude mice were used in the animal experiments. Each mouse was injected with 0.15 mL of 1 mg mL^{-1} solution intravenously. Subsequently, the mice were anesthetized at 6 h, 24 h, 48 h and then placed in supine position. For image acquisition, the Cellvizio®dual band imaging system (Mauna Kea Technologies, Paris, France) was used to obtain real-time images of the blood vessels (imaged by tail vein injection of Evans blue under 660 nm excitation), and GQD-NPs (imaged under 488 nm excitation) at the tumor site.

3. Results and Discussion

The structure of the obtained samples could be clearly seen in the HRTEM image (Figure 1a) since the outside layer and inside nanoparticles had different contrasts. The HRTEM image (shown in Figure 1b,c) further illustrated the amorphous coating of the polymer and the inside nanoparticles with a clear lattice structure. The energy dispersive spectroscopy (EDS) map (Figure 1d–i) demonstrated that the inside nanoparticles mainly consisted of Fe and O, and the outer layer mainly contained C and N. GQDs were hardly identified in the HRTEM and EDS images (Figure S1).

X-ray diffraction was employed to further validate the content of the nanocomposites. Peaks in Figure 2a were ascribed to Fe_3O_4 [3]. The Raman spectrum of the GQD-NPs was shown in Figure 2b. The D peak at 1372 cm^{-1} was generally considered to be the disordered vibration peak of GQDs, caused by lattice vibrations leaving the center of the Brillouin zone, which characterized the defects or edges of the GQDs. The peak present at 1582 cm^{-1} was the G peak, which was a characteristic peak of GQDs. The G peak was higher than the D peak, indicating the more edged structure of the GQDs [21]. The XPS spectra of GQD-NPs were shown in Figure 2c–g. From Figure 2c, it could be seen that the nanocomposites consisted of C, N, O and Fe. The C=C peak of C1s in Figure 2d indicated that there were a large number of conjugated structures in the nanocomposites. The appearance of the C–O peak revealed that there were both amino groups and hydroxyl groups on the surface of GQDs. In the spectrum of O1s in Figure 2e, the C–O and O–H peaks further confirmed the presence of hydroxyl groups on the surface of GQDs. The peak of N–H in Figure 2f was presumed to be the N–H in the nitrogen-containing ring in PPy. The Fe2p in Figure 2g illustrated the presence of Fe_3O_4. The XPS spectra further demonstrated that there were Fe_3O_4, PPy and GQDs in the nanocomposites [3,21,25]. Studies have shown that excellent fluorescent luminescence performance is one of the most outstanding properties of graphene quantum dots [11,26,27]. Therefore, after loading the GQDs, the optical performance of the nanocomposite would be of concern. As shown in Figure 2h, the GQD-NPs presented an absorption peak under the excitation wavelength of 490 nm, which was the characteristic peak of the GQDs. In Figure 2i, the GQD-NPs retained a slightly decreased saturation magnetization compared to bare Fe_3O_4, allowing them to perform as a contrast agent for magnetic resonance imaging.

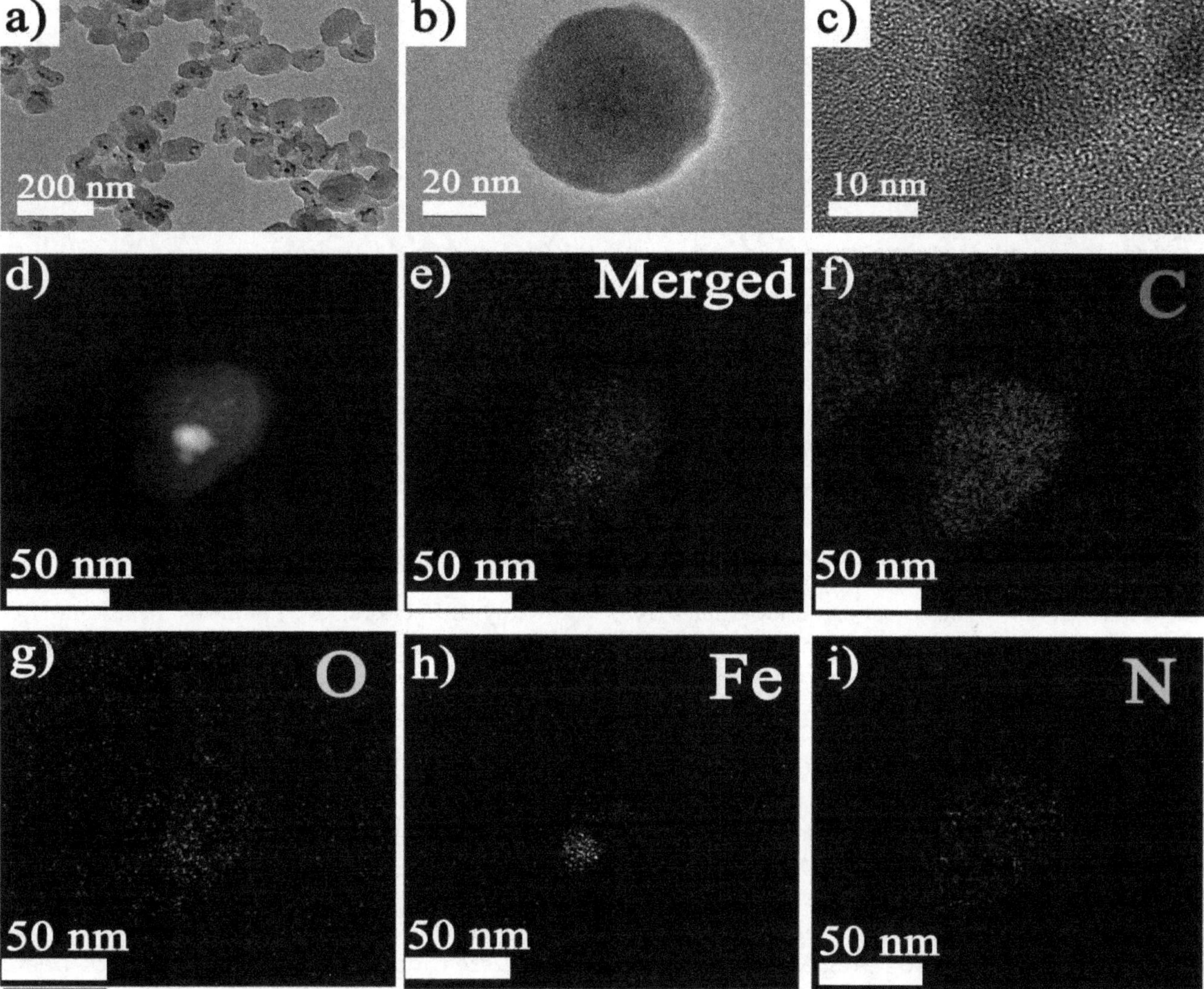

Figure 1. Morphology and elemental analysis of graphene quantum dots (GQDs) loaded nanoparticles: (**a~c**) high resolution tranmission electron microscopy (HRTEM) images at different magnifications (bright field image); (**d~i**) energy dispersive spectroscopy (EDS) analysis of the nanocomposite; (**d**) graph representation, (**e**) EDS analysis of the nanocomposite (merged), (**f**) EDS C elemental map, (**g**) EDS O elemental map, (**h**) EDS Fe elemental map, (**i**) EDS N elemental map.

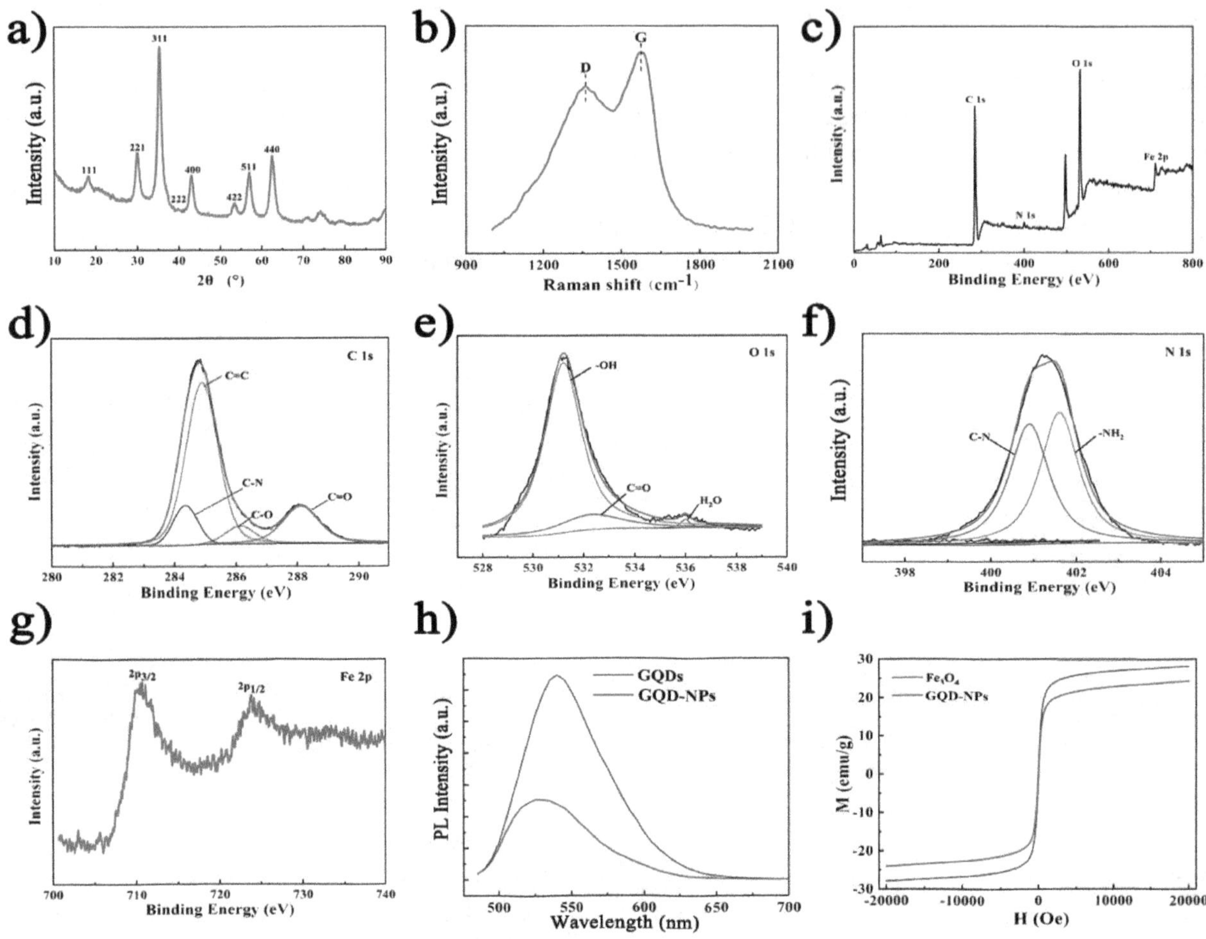

Figure 2. Properties of GQD-nanoparticles (NPs): (**a**) X-ray diffraction (XRD) patterns; (**b**) Raman spectrum, the ordered G band and disordered D band were indicated; (**c**) X-ray photoelectron spectrum (XPS); (**d–g**) XPS analysis of C, O, N and Fe, respectively; (**h**) Photoluminescence (PL) spectra with the pulsed laser excitations at 490 nm; (**i**) Magnetizing curve, magnetization (M), magnetic field strength (H).

The viability of L929 cells incubated with gradient concentrations of GQD-NPs (50 μg/mL, 100 μg/mL, 160 μg/mL, 250 μg/mL, 500 μg/mL, and 1000 μg/mL) for 24 h or 48 h was detected by CCK8. As shown in Figure 3, after co-incubation for 24 h, there were significant differences between the groups whose concentrations of GQD-NPs were higher than 50 μg/mL and the control group; after co-incubation for 48 h, high significant differences were found between all the groups treated with GQD-NPs and the control group. The outcome illustrated that GQD-NPs exhibited excellent biocompatibility when the concentration was lower than 250 μg/mL. This particular outcome was in line with previous studies which investigated the cell toxicity of GQDs [28] or Fe_3O_4@PPy [22].

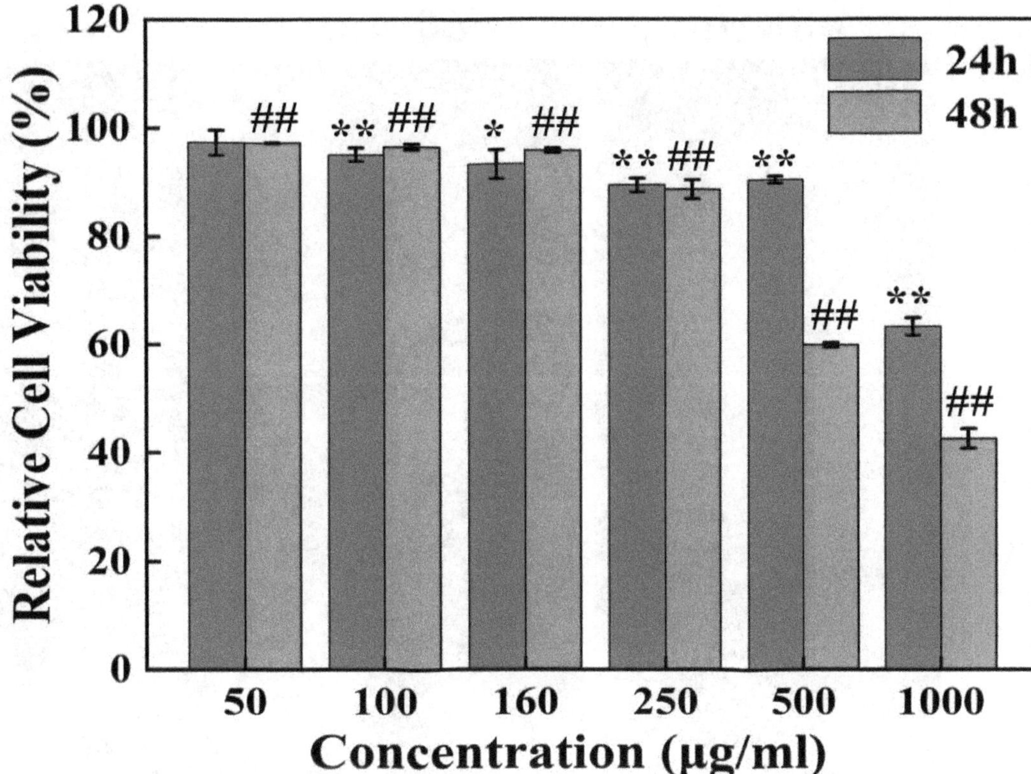

Figure 3. Cell viability of L929 cells incubated with GQD-NPs. The experiments were carried out in triplicate. Data were presented as mean ± standard deviation (SD) ($n = 3$). The cell viability values were all normalized to control groups (untreated cells after incubation for 24 h or 48 h). Asterisk (*) and double asterisks (**) refer to statistical significance of $p < 0.05$ and $p < 0.01$, respectively, compared with control groups between the cell viability values after co-incubation for 24 h; double pounds (##) refer to a statistical significance of $p < 0.01$ compared with control groups between the cell viability values after co-incubation for 48 h.

Evans blue dye strongly binds to hemoglobin in blood, and is therefore widely used to track the presence of blood vessels [29]. As seen in Figure 4, prior to injection, a clear vascular system was displayed at the tumor site under excitation with the 660 nm laser. A few green fluorescence lights were seen under 488 nm, since some substances in the visible light band would also emit green fluorescence under visible-light excitation. GQDs were employed in the tracking of nanoparticles *in vivo*. When the GQD-NPs were injected for six hours, green fluorescence indicated the presence of GQD-NPs, while the blood vessels at the tumor site were still clearly visible (red). In the merged image, it could be seen that a large number of GQD-NPs apeared in the tumor blood vessels, and a small amount of GQD-NPs penetrated into the surrounding tissues through the tumor blood vessel wall. When the GQD-NPs were injected for 24 h, the blood vessels at the tumor site were still clearly visible (red), and there were still many GQD-NPs within the tumor blood vessels (green). As time passed (from 6 h to 24 h), a large amount of GQD-NPs passed through the tumor vessel wall and penetrated into the surrounding tissues as for the enhanced permeability and retention (EPR) effect, achieving enrichment in the tumor tissues. When the GQD-NPs were injected for 48 h, there were still fluorescence signals of the GQD-NPs (green) in the tumor tissues and the blood vessels, but the fluorescence signals in the tumor tissues were significantly weakened (relative to 24 h). This indicated that more GQD-NPs had been metabolized. Thus, reduced enrichment of the GQD-NPs at the tumor site was found. The results illustrated that by loading GQDs into nanoparticles, the dynamic changes of nanoparticles could be tracked *in vivo*.

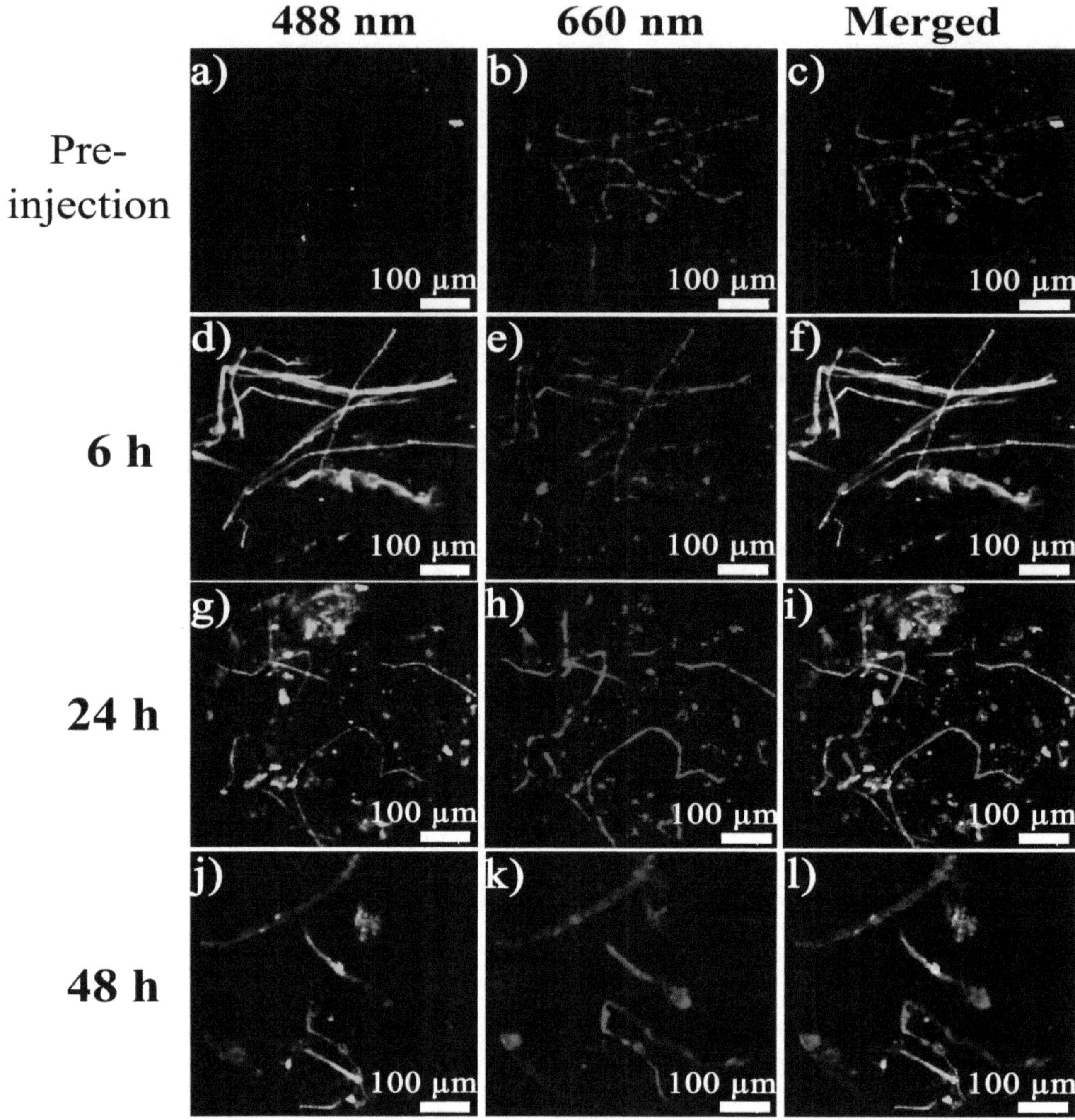

Figure 4. Fibered confocal fluorescence microscopic (FCFM) images of GQD-NPs (imaged under 488 nm excitation, green) and blood vessels (imaged by tail vein injection of Evans blue under 660 nm excitation, red) in tumor tissues over time.

4. Conclusions

The one-pot method of loading graphene quantum dots (GQDs) was proposed as a means to modify nanoparticles for fluorescent imaging. GQDs were loaded into the optical-magneto Fe_3O_4@PPy nanoparticles instead of on the surface. The morphology, components, optical and magnetic properties, biocompatibility and biomedical application of the GQD-loaded optical-magneto nanoparticles were investigated. The GQD-loaded optical-magneto nanoparticles performed as an excellent tacking agent, highlighting the potential application of GQDs in tracking the real-time distribution and metabolism of nanoparticles *in vivo*.

Author Contributions: Conceptualization, writing—review and editing, R.Z. and Q.C.; Writing—original draft preparation, Y.W.; Material preparation and characterization Y.W., Y.H.; Cell experiment, N.X., In vivo experiment D.W., Q.G.; Figures, J.W.; Data analysis S.X., Y.L.

Acknowledgments: We gratefully acknowledge the measurement support from State key Laboratory of New Ceramics and Fine Processing, School of Materials Science and Engineering, Tsinghua University, Beijing 100084, China.

References

1. Bray, F.; Ferlay, J.; Soerjomataram, I.; Siegel, R.L.; Torre, L.A.; Jemal, A. Global Cancer Statistics 2018: Globocan Estimates of Incidence and Mortality Worldwide for 36 Cancers in 185 Countries. *Ca A Cancer J. Clin.* **2018**, *68*, 394–424. [CrossRef] [PubMed]
2. Wang, Q.; Zhao, X.; Yan, H.; Kang, F.; Li, Z.; Qiao, Y.; Li, D. A Cross-Talk Egfr/Vegfr-Targeted Bispecific Nanoprobe for Magnetic Resonance/Near-Infrared Fluorescence Imaging of Colorectal Cancer. *Mrs Commun.* **2018**, *8*, 1008–1017. [CrossRef]
3. Yan, H.; Zhao, L.; Shang, W.; Liu, Z.; Xie, W.; Qiang, C.; Xiong, Z.; Zhang, R.; Li, B.; Sun, X.; et al. General Synthesis of High-Performing Magneto-Conjugated Polymer Core-Shell Nanoparticles for Multifunctional Theranostics. *Nano Res.* **2017**, *10*, 704–717. [CrossRef]
4. Wang, C.; Xu, H.; Liang, C.; Liu, Y.; Li, Z.; Yang, G.; Cheng, L.; Li, Y.; Liu, Z. Iron Oxide @ Polypyrrole Nanoparticles as a Multifunctional Drug Carrier for Remotely Controlled Cancer Therapy with Snergistic Antitumor Effect. *Acs Nano* **2013**, *7*, 6782–6795. [CrossRef] [PubMed]
5. Ogata, G.; Ishii, Y.; Asai, K.; Sano, Y.; Nin, F.; Yoshida, T.; Higuchi, T.; Sawamura, S.; Ota, T.; Hori, K.; et al. AMicrosensing System for the *in vivo* Real-Time Detection of Local Drug Kinetics. *Nat. Biomed. Eng.* **2017**, *1*, 654–666. [CrossRef] [PubMed]
6. Cai, Y.; Wei, Z.; Song, C.; Tang, C.; Han, W.; Dong, X. Optical Nano-Agents in the Second Near-Infrared Window for Biomedical Applications. *Chem. Soc. Rev.* **2019**, *48*, 22–37. [CrossRef] [PubMed]
7. Resch-Genger, U.; Grabolle, M.; Cavaliere-Jaricot, S.; Nitschke, R.; Nann, T. Quantum Dots Versus Organic Dyes as Fluorescent Labels. *Nat. Methods* **2008**, *5*, 763–775. [CrossRef]
8. Wang, J.; Qiu, J. A Review of Organic Nanomaterials in Photothermal Cancer Therapy. *Cancer Res. Front.* **2016**, *2*, 67–84. [CrossRef]
9. Ponomarenko, L.A.; Schedin, F.; Katsnelson, M.I.; Yang, R.; Hill, E.W.; Novoselov, K.S.; Geim, A.K. Chaotic Dirac Billiard in Graphene Quantum Dots. *Science* **2008**, *320*, 356–358. [CrossRef]
10. Liu, R.; Wu, D.; Feng, X.; Mullen, K. Bottom-Up Fabrication of Photoluminescent Graphene Quantum Dots with Uniform Morphology. *J. Am. Chem. Soc.* **2011**, *133*, 15221–15223. [CrossRef]
11. Yan, Y.; Gong, J.; Chen, J.; Zeng, Z.; Huang, W.; Pu, K.; Liu, J.; Chen, P. Recent Advances on Graphene Quantum Dots: From Chemistry and Physics to Applications. *Adv. Mater.* **2019**, *31*, 1808283. [CrossRef]
12. Tabish, T.A.; Scotton, C.J.; J Ferguson, D.C.; Lin, L.; der Veen, A.V.; Lowry, S.; Ali, M.; Jabeen, F.; Ali, M.; Winyard, P.G.; et al. Biocompatibility and Toxicity of Graphene Quantum Dots for Potential Application in Photodynamic Therapy. *Nanomedicine* **2018**, *13*, 1923–1937. [CrossRef] [PubMed]
13. Saquib, Q.; Faisal, M.; Al-Khedhairy, A.A.; Alatar, A.A. *Cellular and Molecular Toxicology of Nanoparticles*; Springer: Cham, Switzerland, 2018; Volume 1048.
14. Iannazzo, D.; Pistone, A.; Celesti, C.; Triolo, C.; Patané, S.; Giofré, S.; Romeo, R.; Ziccarelli, I.; Mancuso, R.; Gabriele, B.; et al. A Smart Nanovector for Cancer Targeted Drug Delivery Based on Graphene Quantum Dots. *Nanomaterials* **2019**, *9*, 282. [CrossRef] [PubMed]
15. Zhang, X.; Wei, C.; Li, Y.; Yu, D. Shining Luminescent Graphene Quantum Dots: Synthesis, Physicochemical Properties, and Biomedical Applications. *Trac Trends Anal. Chem.* **2019**, *116*, 109–121. [CrossRef]
16. Şenel, B.; Demir, N.; Büyükköroğlu, G.; Yıldız, M. Graphene Quantum Dots: Synthesis, Characterization, Cell Viability, Genotoxicity for Biomedical Applications. *Saudi Pharm. J.* **2019**. [CrossRef]
17. Chen, T.; Yu, H.; Yang, N.; Wang, M.; Ding, C.; Fu, J. Graphene Quantum Dot-Capped Mesoporous Silica Nanoparticles through an Acid-Cleavable Acetal Bond for Intracellular Drug Delivery and Imaging. *J. Mater. Chem. B* **2014**, *2*, 4979. [CrossRef]

18. Su, X.; Chan, C.; Shi, J.; Tsang, M.; Pan, Y.; Cheng, C.; Gerile, O.; Yang, M. A Graphene Quantum Dot@Fe_3O_4@SiO_2 Based Nanoprobe for Drug Delivery Sensing and Dual-Modal Fluorescence and Mri Imaging in Cancer Cells. *Biosens. Bioelectron.* **2017**, *92*, 489–495. [CrossRef]
19. Wang, X.; Sun, X.; Lao, J.; He, H.; Cheng, T.; Wang, M.; Wang, S.; Huang, F. Multifunctional Graphene Quantum Dots for Simultaneous Targeted Cellular Imaging and Drug Delivery. *Colloids Surf. B Biointerfaces* **2014**, *122*, 638–644. [CrossRef]
20. Tian, Q.; Wang, Q.; Yao, K.X.; Teng, B.; Zhang, J.; Yang, S.; Han, Y. Multifunctional Polypyrrole@Fe_3O_4 Nanoparticles for Dual-Modal Imaging and In Vivo Photothermal Cancer Therapy. *Small* **2014**, *10*, 1063–1068. [CrossRef]
21. Wang, L.; Wang, Y.; Xu, T.; Liao, H.; Yao, C.; Liu, Y.; Li, Z.; Chen, Z.; Pan, D.; Sun, L.; et al. Gram-Scale Synthesis of Single-Crystalline Graphene Quantum Dots with Superior Optical Properties. *Nat. Commun.* **2014**, *5*, 5357. [CrossRef]
22. Feng, W.; Zhou, X.; Nie, W.; Chen, L.; Qiu, K.; Zhang, Y.; He, C. Au/Polypyrrole@Fe_3O_4 Nanocomposites for Mr/Ct Dual-Modal Imaging Guided-Photothermal Therapy: An *in vitro* Study. *ACS Appl. Mater. Inter.* **2015**, *7*, 4354–4367. [CrossRef] [PubMed]
23. Yan, H.; Shang, W.; Sun, X.; Zhao, L.; Wang, J.; Xiong, Z.; Yuan, J.; Zhang, R.; Huang, Q.; Wang, K.; et al. "All-in-One" Nanoparticles for Trimodality Imaging-Guided Intracellular Photo-Magnetic Hyperthermia Therapy Under Intravenous Administration. *Adv. Funct. Mater.* **2018**, *28*, 1705710. [CrossRef]
24. Yao, W.; Ni, T.; Chen, S.; Li, H.; Lu, Y. Graphene/Fe_3O_4@Polypyrrole Nanocomposites as a Synergistic Adsorbent for Cr(Vi) Ion Removal. *Compos. Sci. Technol.* **2014**, *99*, 15–22. [CrossRef]
25. Wang, J.; Yan, H.; Liu, Z.; Wang, Z.; Gao, H.; Zhang, Z.; Wang, B.; Xu, N.; Zhang, S.; Liu, X. Langmuir–Blodgett Self-Assembly of Ultrathin Graphene Quantum Dot Films with Modulated Optical Properties. *Nanoscale* **2018**, *10*, 19612–19620. [CrossRef] [PubMed]
26. Iannazzo, D.; Ziccarelli, I.; Pistone, A. Graphene Quantum Dots: Multifunctional Nanoplatforms for Anticancer Therapy. *J. Mater. Chem. B* **2017**, *5*, 6471–6489. [CrossRef]
27. Bacon, M.; Bradley, S.J.; Nann, T. Graphene Quantum Dots. *Part. Part. Syst. Charact.* **2014**, *31*, 415–428. [CrossRef]
28. Chong, Y.; Ma, Y.; Shen, H.; Tu, X.; Zhou, X.; Xu, J.; Dai, J.; Fan, S.; Zhang, Z. The In Vitro and In Vitro Toxicity of Graphene Quantum Dots. *Biomaterials* **2014**, *35*, 5041–5048. [CrossRef]
29. Han, Z.; Shang, W.; Liang, X.; Yan, H.; Hu, M.; Peng, L.; Jiang, H.; Fang, C.; Wang, K.; Tian, J. An Innovation for Treating Orthotopic Pancreatic Cancer by Preoperative Screening and Imaging-Guided Surgery. *Mol. Imaging Biol.* **2019**, *21*, 67–77. [CrossRef]

11

Prototype Gastro-Resistant Soft Gelatin Films and Capsules—Imaging and Performance In Vitro

Bartosz Maciejewski [1], Vishnu Arumughan [2], Anette Larsson [2] and Małgorzata Sznitowska [1,*]

1. Department of Pharmaceutical Technology, Medical University of Gdansk, 80-416 Gdansk, Poland; bartosz.maciejewski@gumed.edu.pl
2. Department of Chemistry and Chemical Engineering, Chalmers University of Technology, 412 96 Gothenburg, Sweden; vishnu.arumughan@chalmers.se (V.A.); anette.larsson@chalmers.se (A.L.)

* Correspondence: msznito@gumed.edu.pl or malgorzata.sznitowska@gumed.edu.pl

Abstract: The following study is a continuation of the previous work on preparation of gastro-resistant films by incorporation of cellulose acetate phthalate (CAP) into the soft gelatin film. An extended investigation on the previously described binary Gelatin-CAP and ternary Gelatin-CAP-carrageenan polymer films was performed. The results suggest that the critical feature behind formation of the acid-resistant films is a spinodal decomposition in the film-forming mixture. In the obtained films, upon submersion in an acidic medium, gelatin swells and dissolves, exposing a CAP-based acid-insoluble skeleton, partially coated by a residue of other ingredients. The dissolution-hindering effect appears to be stronger when iota-carrageenan is added to the film-forming mixture. The drug release study performed in enhancer cells confirmed that diclofenac sodium is not released in the acidic medium, however, at pH 6.8 the drug release occurs. The capsules prepared with a simple lab-scale process appear to be resistant to disintegration of the shell structure in acid, although imperfections of the sealing have been noticed.

Keywords: gelatin; gastro-resistant; films; capsules; structure; drug release

---

1. Introduction

Gastro-resistant formulations are an example of the most common type of modified drug release systems. Gastro-resistant forms of drug administration allow to:

(1) minimize adverse effects such as nausea and bleeding associated with irritation of gastric mucosa that may be caused by some active substances;
(2) deliver drug intended for local action in intestines;
(3) protect the drug substance from degradation in an acidic environment of the stomach [1].

Gastro-resistant soft gelatin capsules can prove their usefulness in oral administration of drugs of irritating or acid-labile nature, often displaying at the same time enhanced bioavailability in a liquid form, which can be considered an advantage to coated tablets [2]. The most obvious examples of the substances that need to be formulated in gastro-resistant dosage forms are non-steroidal anti-inflammatory drugs (NSAIDs), which are irritating to gastric mucosa.

The products in the form of gastro-resistant capsules usually are designed as conventional hard capsule shells filled with the enteric-coated pellets or minitablets. Manufacturing of gastro-resistant soft capsules, however, is a challenge. Due to the liquid fill, modification of the drug release rate from soft capsules can be achieved only by modification of the capsule shell to make it resistant to acidic pH. This issue can be approached by-coating of standard capsules with acid-resistant polymers such as methacrylic acid—methyl acrylate copolymers (e.g., Eudragit L or S®) [3]. A less popular alternative is incorporation of gastro-resistant polymers in the shell material used to form the capsules [4]. Both approaches are technologically perplexing at some points, although modification of the shell material can be considered more beneficial from both economic and technological point of view. However, it is not yet utilized in commercial products. It is substantial to take into consideration that any changes in the composition of the film-forming mixture can result in significant alteration of the overall physicochemical properties of the prepared films, that can lead to the loss of their potential to be formed into capsules in a conventional manufacturing process.

A very important issue associated with the development of a new capsule shell composition is to identify the physiochemical phenomena that can be utilized in designing and manufacturing of modified release gelatin-based films. In our previous work, selection of the most effective modification of the shell material composition was performed, and their microstructure and barrier properties were described [5,6]. However, there are still a few unexplained issues in the description of the phenomena that lead to formation of the films, as well as the changes that the films undergo when exposed to various conditions. Therefore, in the present work, a more detailed investigation of the events associated with the formation of the gastro-resistant film was performed and further, the structural changes upon submersion of such films in acidic dissolution fluid is performed. For the purpose of better characterization of the films and film formation processes, several modern techniques may be employed. In the present research, a scanning electron microscopy (SEM), confocal laser scanning microscopy (CLSM), confocal Raman microscopy and quartz crystal microbalance with dissipation monitoring (QCM-D) were used. Additionally, the barrier properties of the films against oxygen were evaluated.

In comparison to tablets or hard capsules, the transfer of a new technology for soft capsules from the lab to the production site is much more complicated, and a scale-up procedure may be complicated and time-consuming. One of the main issues when soft capsules are developed is a poor access to a lab-scale equipment that could allow to assess the utility of the modified films for capsule formation. The most problematic is the fact that, at a commercial scale, specific rheological and mechanical properties of the film-forming material are required [7–9]. The fact that the shell-forming material has to be tested on a large scale, significantly increases the cost of technology development. In our present work, the lab-scale production process of the soft capsules is presented, utilizing a simple mold for suppositories, what allowed to evaluate the shell compatibility with the filling material.

2. Materials and Methods

2.1. Materials

Components of films and capsules: gelatin type B, bovine hide, 220 bloom (Sigma Aldrich, Saint Louis, MO, USA), glycerol 99.5% w/w (Chempur, Piekary Slaskie, Poland), Aquacoat®CPD (FMC Biopolymer, Philadelphia, PA, USA), aqueous dispersion of cellulose acetate phthalate (CAP), iota-carrageenan (Sigma Aldrich, Saint Louis, MO, USA), medium-chain triglycerides (MCT)—Miglyol 812 N (Caelo, Hilden, Germany), polyethylene glycol 400 (PEG 400)—Kollisolv PEG E400 (Sigma Aldrich, Saint Louis, MO, USA), cetearyl alcohol—TEGO Alkanol 1618 (Evonik, Essen, Germany). Diclofenac sodium was a gift from Polpharma Pharmaceutical Works (Starogard Gdanski, Poland).

Analysis: QCM-D: branched polyethyleneimine Mw 25,000 (Sigma Aldrich, Saint Louis, MO, USA), formaldehyde 37% (Sigma Aldrich, Saint Louis, MO, USA), ethanol 95% (Sigma Aldrich, Saint Louis, MO, USA). Disintegration and dissolution media (0.1 M HCl and phosphate buffer pH 6.8) were prepared according to the European Pharmacopeia 10th edition.

2.2. Capsule Formation

Schematic presentation of the capsule formation process is shown in Figure 1.

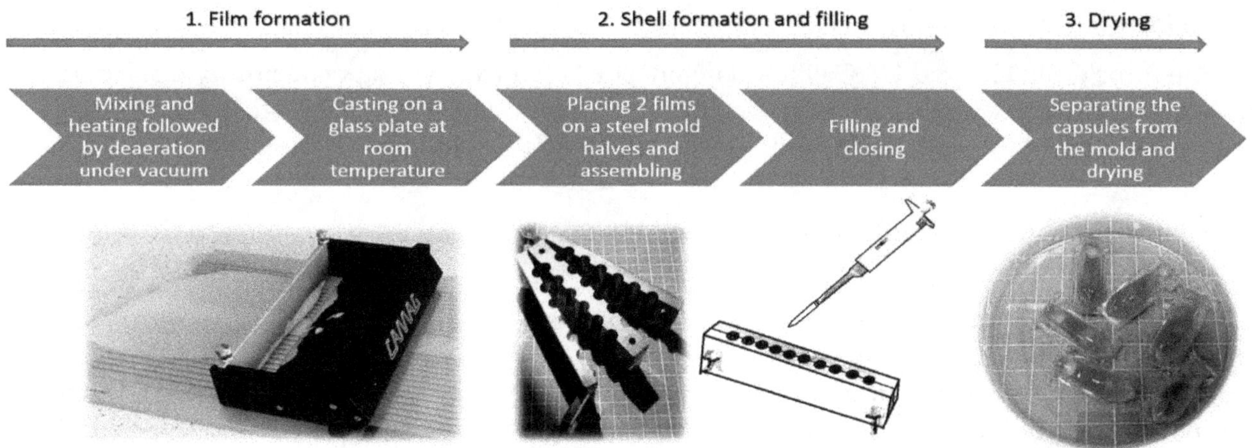

Figure 1. Capsule formation scheme.

The preparation method of the film-forming mixtures and films was described in detail in the previously published work [5,6]. Shortly, the mixture of components (Table 1) was stirred at 80 °C for 2 h, which was followed by deaeration under vacuum. Afterwards the mixture was casted on a glass plate using a plate coating device (Camag TLC Plate Coater, Camag, Muttenz, Switzerland) with a height of fluid layer of 1500 μm. After drying the thickness of the film was around 600 μm.

Table 1. Compositions of the films.

Composition Symbol	Mixture Components (g/100 g)				
	Gelatin	Aquacoat CPD	Iota-Carrageenan	Water	Glycerol
GEL [1]	41.2	–	–	40.0	18.8
GA [2]	30.9	34.4	–	15.9	18.8
GAC [2]	30.0	34.4	0.9	15.9	18.8

[1] non-modified film (reference); [2] modified binary (GA); and ternary (GAC) polymer films.

The capsules were prepared using GAC composition (Table 1), by placing 2 pieces of the film (immediately after casting) in a steel form for suppositories. After closing the form, the resulting reservoirs were filled with: (a) MCT oil, (b) PEG 400 or (c) cetearyl alcohol. For a better visual identification of a disintegration test endpoint, the filling material was colored with small amount of a hydrophilic or lipophilic dye. Afterwards, the filling orifice was manually closed with a strip of a film, and to ensure good sealing the capsules were placed for 5 min at 60 °C. Finally, the capsules were stored and dried at ambient temperature and of 15–25% RH for at least 24 h. The measured moisture content in the capsules was around 2.5% (Radwag WPS210S Moisture Analyzer, Radwag, Radom, Poland).

2.3. *Microscopic Imaging*

The imaging of samples was performed with use of a scanning electron microscopy (SEM), confocal laser scanning microscopy (CLSM), confocal Raman microscopy and optical microscopy.

The observation of film samples was performed before and after submersion in 0.1 M HCl at 37 °C, under constant stirring for 2 h (similar to the procedure of swelling test described in our previous work [5]). The films after submersion in acid were frozen in a liquid nitrogen and freeze-dried for 24 h. The investigation was performed with Jeol 7900F SEM (Jeol, Tokyo, Japan), Nikon Ti-E/A1 + CLSM (Nikon, Tokyo, Japan) and WITec Alpha 300 Access Raman microscope equipped with 785 nm laser (WITec, Ulm, Germany).

The imaging of the lab-manufactured capsules was performed using Phenom Pure SEM (Phenom World, Eindhoven, the Netherlands), and Nikon Eclipse 50i optical microscope (Nikon, Tokyo, Japan).

2.4. Gas Permeability

The films GEL, GA and GAC (Table 1) were subjected to oxygen permeability tests, performed with an coulometric detector technique according to method ASTM F 1927-14. The equipment used was OX-TRAN 2-20 (Mocon, Minneapolis, MN, USA). The investigated surface was 50 cm^2.

2.5. Quartz Crystal Microbalance with Dissipation Monitoring (QCM-D)

QCM-D was employed to investigate the affinity of CAP latex particles present in Aquacoat CPD to gelatin. The preparation step comprised coating of the gold-plated quartz crystal sensor with branched polyethyleneimine (PEI), then spin-coating the sensor with 1% gelatin solution (5 s at 2500 rpm and low acceleration, followed by 60 s at 8000 rpm and high acceleration). Afterwards the sensor was dried at 60 °C for 20 min. The gelatin on the sensor was subjected to crosslinking by submersion in 1.5% formaldehyde solution, in order to prevent it from dissolving in aqueous conditions. Finally, the sensor was dried at 60 °C for 60 min.

The sensors were mounted in a Qsense equipment (Qsense, Västra Frölunda, Sweden). A deionized water (at 25 °C) was flushed over the sensors until a stable baseline was obtained. Then the diluted (0.1%) Aquacoat CPD at 25 °C was pumped through the cells, and the changes in fundamental frequency overtones of the crystal were registered. After stabilization of the system, the cells were once again pumped with deionized water to remove all the substances that were not bound to the film.

Additionally, to assess the surface structure and stability of the gelatin films obtained in situ on the sensors, the Atomic Force Microscopy (AFM) was performed with NTEGRA Prima setup (NT-MDT Spectrum Instruments, Moscow, Russia), with a silicon probe (spring constant of 40 N m^{-1} and resonant frequency of 300 kHz) (Tap 300AI-G, Budget Sensors, Sofia, Bulgaria). The images were analyzed using a Gwyddion software (Version 2.55, Free Software Foundation, Boston, MA, USA).

2.6. Disintegration Time

Disintegration time test of the capsules filled with PEG-400, MCT oil or cetearyl alcohol, was performed. The test was performed using: (a) a tablet disintegration tester ED-2SAPO (Electrolab, Mumbai, India); (b) a paddle dissolution apparatus DT800 (Erweka, Langen, Germany), with a capsule placed in a steel sinker (the stirring rate was 50 rpm). The capsules were tested for 120 min in 0.1 M HCl, followed by pH 6.8 phosphate buffer until disintegration.

2.7. Drug Release Test

The study was performed using a vertical diffusion cell (Enhancer cell, Erweka, Langen, Germany) and a paddle dissolution apparatus DT800 (Erweka, Langen, Germany) equipped with a built-in autosampler. The stirring rates of 50, 100 and 150 rpm were used. The enhancer cell with the mounted modified gelatin film is shown in Figure 2.

The film selected for the test was gelatin + Aquacoat + carrageenan (GAC), the same as for disintegration tests. The diffusion cell was filled with 2.5 mL of a 1% diclofenac solution in PEG 400 (the amount of diclofenac sodium was 25 mg). Then the investigated film (cut to a circle of 3 cm in diameter) was carefully placed on the top of the solution and secured with a sealing ring and a screw cap; the active surface was 4.15 cm^2. The test was performed in 900 mL of 0.1 M HCl for 120 min followed by 900 mL phosphate buffer pH 6.8 for 60 min.

Sampling of the acceptor fluid was performed every 15 min in the acid phase, and every 5 min in the buffer phase. Quantification of diclofenac was performed spectrophotometrically at 276 nm wavelength. The study was performed in triplicates.

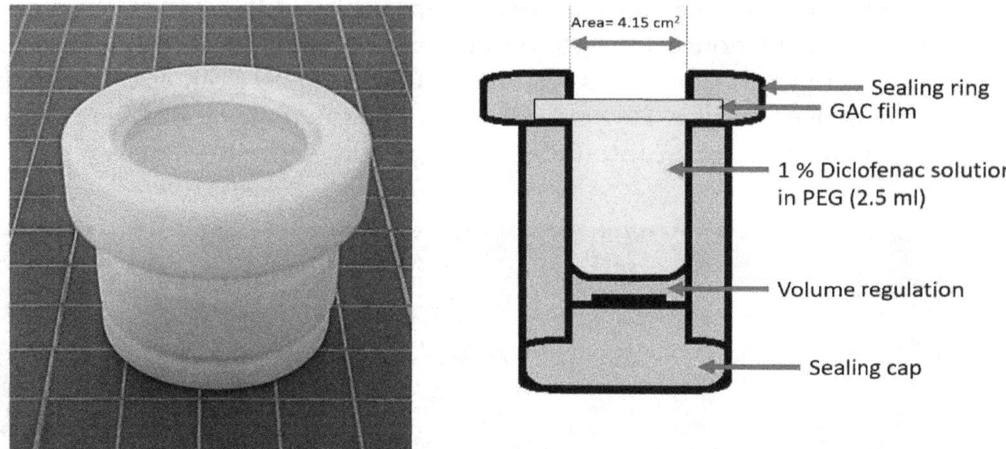

Figure 2. The enhancer cell with gelatin + Aquacoat + carrageenan (GAC) film.

3. Results

3.1. Microscopic Imaging of the Films and Capsules

At the first stage of the study, the prepared GA and GAC films were observed prior to and after submersion in HCl. Macroscopically it was visible that the samples after the acid treatment became opaque and swollen. Under the microscope, the untreated samples had a smooth surface with no structures visible [6]. As presented in Figure 3, the films after submersion in acid revealed a network-like structures, resembling scaffolds.

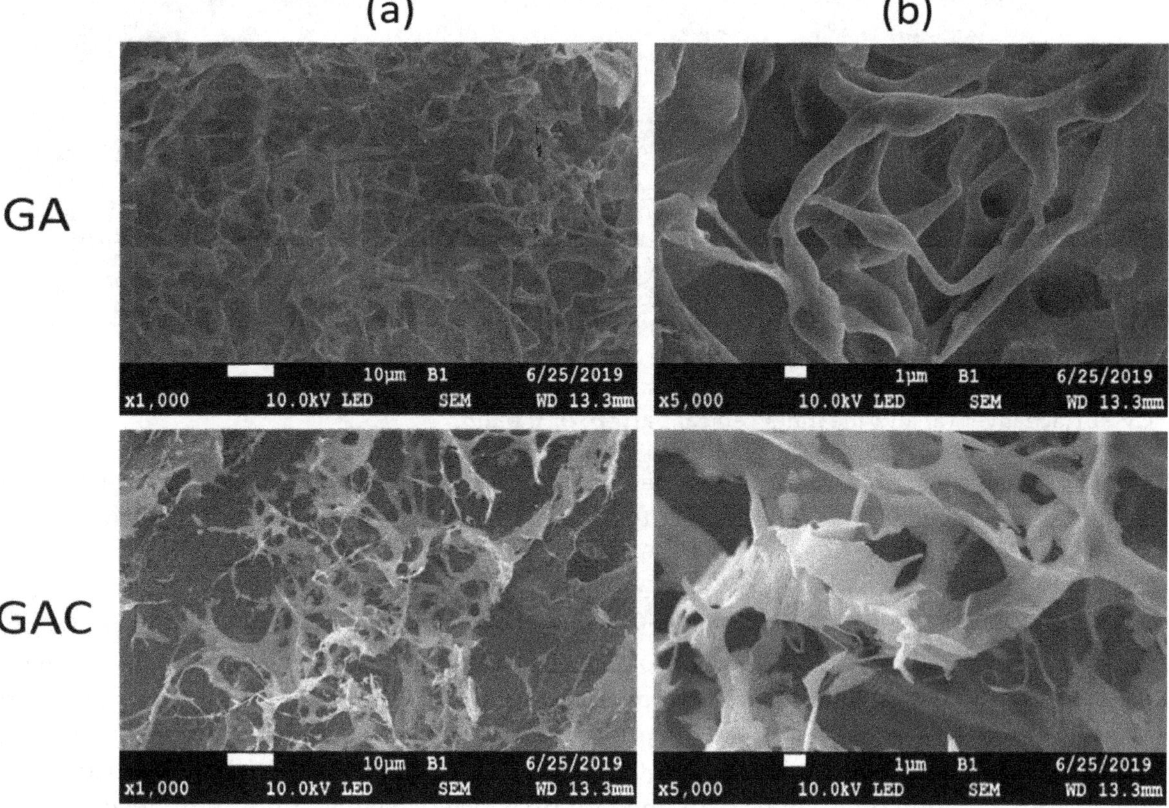

Figure 3. SEM image of GA and GAC films after 2 h in 0.1 M HCl. Scale bar: (**a**) 10 µm, (**b**) 1 µm.

There are clear differences between the images of a top and a middle layer of the sample (Figure 4). It appears that, after 2 h in acid, noticeably less solid material is left on the top of the film, than in the deeper part. The signals registered by CLSM can be potentially both from CAP and gelatin, due to very similar autofluorescence behavior. However, it is suspected that the outer layer consists mostly of CAP, while in the inner layer a swollen and undissolved gelatin can be present as well.

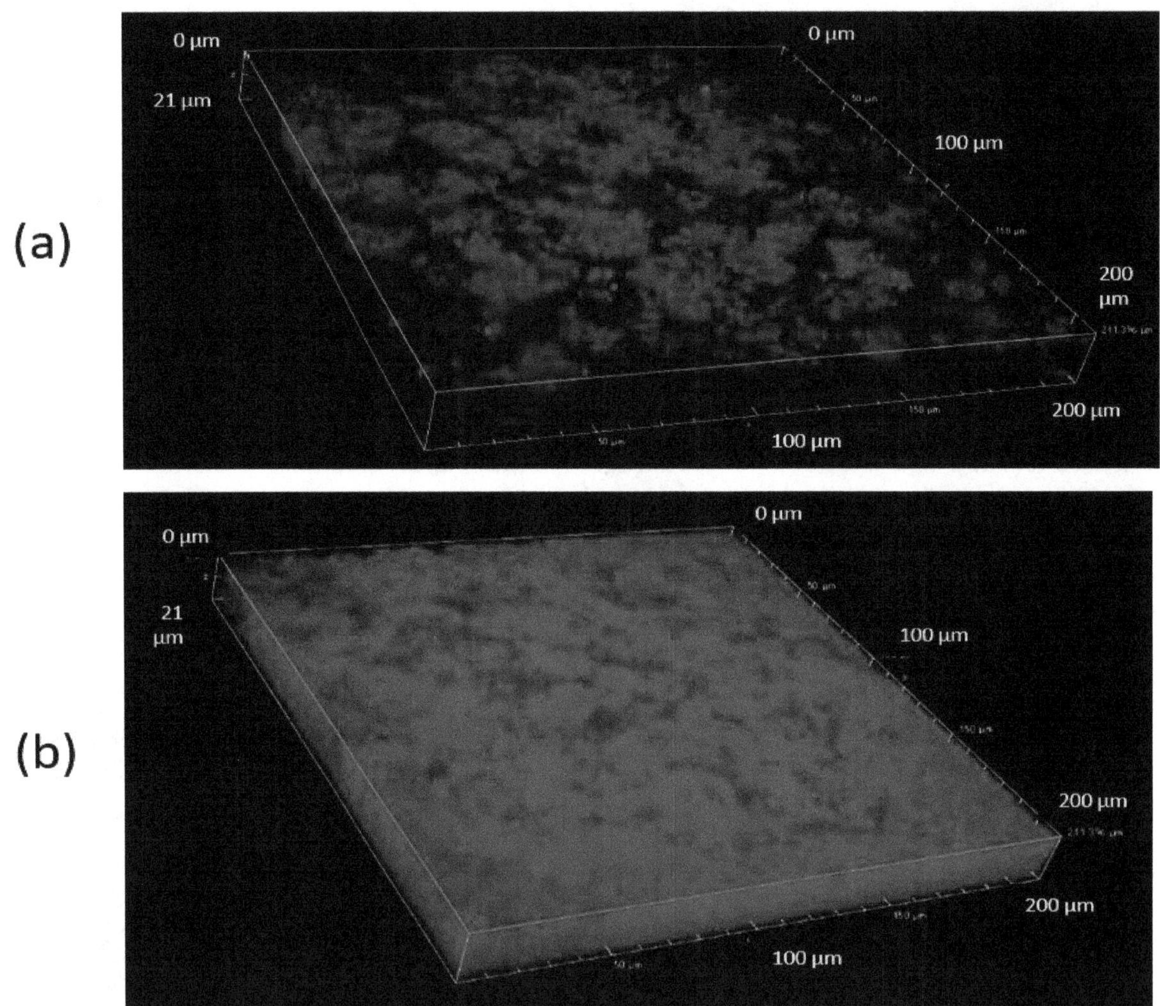

Figure 4. Confocal laser scanning microscopy (CLSM) images of GA film after 2 h immersion in 0.1M HCl: surface layer (**a**) and the inner central part (**b**) of the film.

Raman microscopy investigation was performed on GAC films before and after immersion in 0.1 M HCl. Several points have been scanned to obtain Raman spectra, which have been overlaid and compared. The spectra are shown in Figures 5 and 6.

As it can be seen from the spectra in Figure 5, the surface of the GAC sample is chemically uniform, without any phase separation visible. The acid-treated GAC samples display similar pattern in the spectrum as the untreated GAC. The spectra of the non-modified film (GEL) are not presented in the figure, but they were not different from the spectra of GAC. In Figure 6, different sets of spectra are overlaid. It appears that, in the untreated samples, the gelatin signals are overlapping with the peaks of CAP. After the acid-treatment, the signals from gelatin are weaker, but the signals from CAP are yet undetectable. This outcome can be explained by presence of a small amount of gelatin-rich phase residue undissolved in acid and covering the CAP scaffold. This corresponds well with SEM and CLSM results described above.

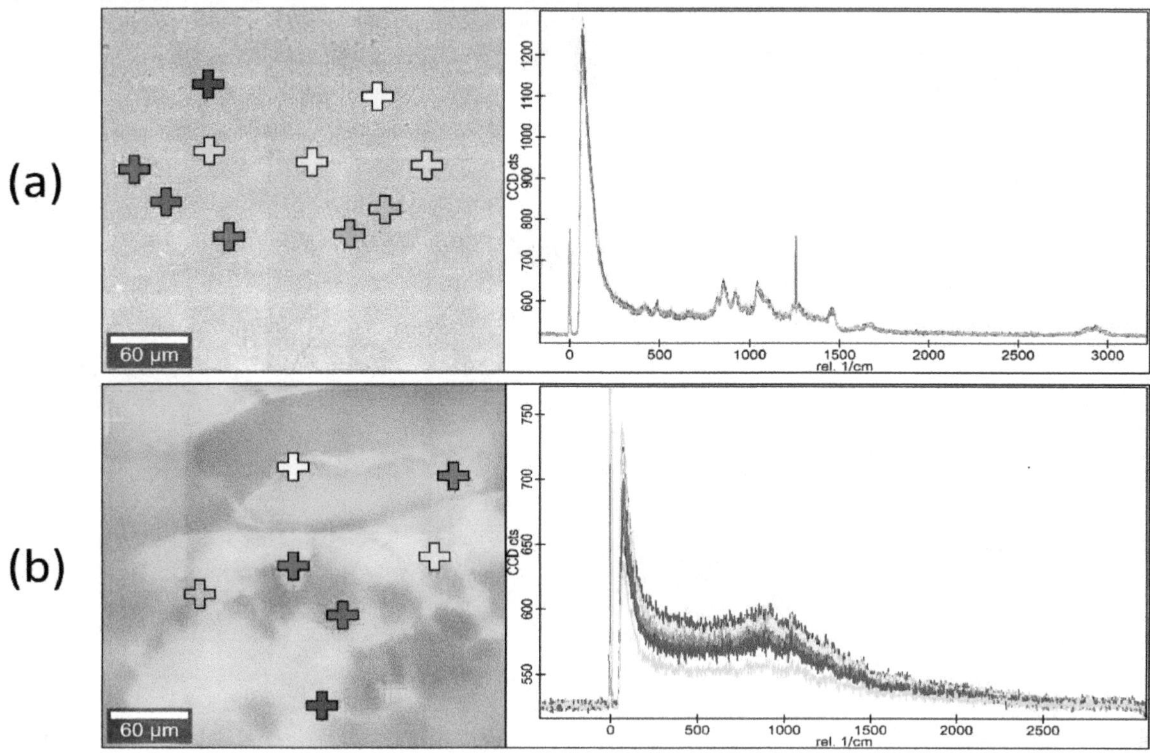

Figure 5. The Raman spectra of several points examined on the surface of GAC film: (**a**) before immersion in acid; (**b**) after immersion for 2 h in 0.1M HCl. Multiple overlaid spectra are presented on each graph.

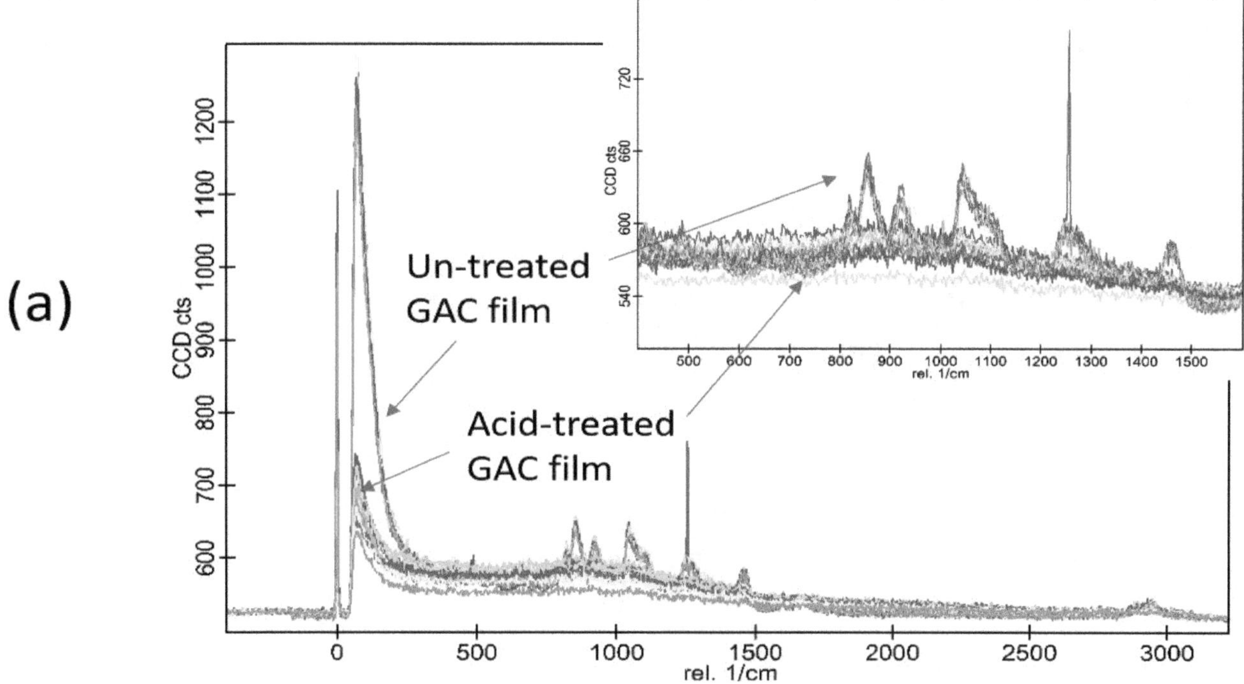

Figure 6. *Cont.*

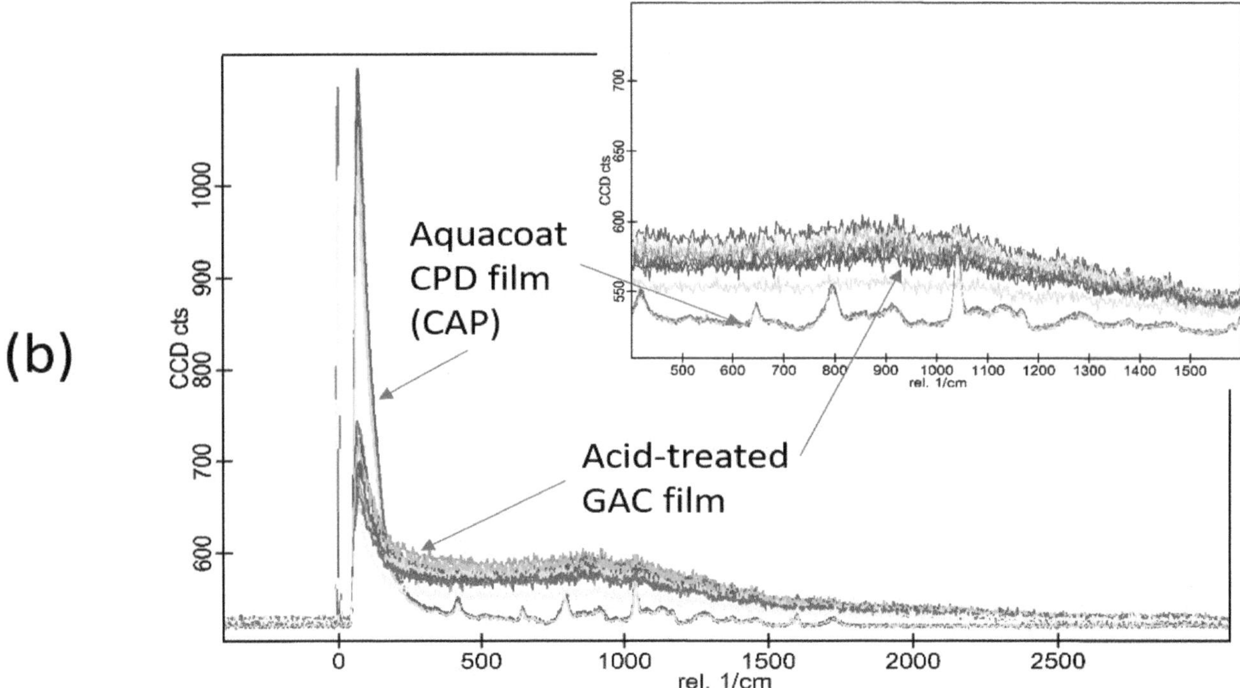

Figure 6. Comparison of the Raman spectra: (**a**) untreated and acid-treated GAC; (**b**) acid-treated GAC and cellulose acetate phthalate (CAP) film (without gelatin). Multiple spectra of each composition are presented.

3.2. QCM-D

A QCM-D study was performed to obtain supporting information on interactions between gelatin and CAP latex particles. Due to the fact that reliable results regarding particle deposition depend on the morphology of the used substrate, the films obtained in situ on the QCM sensors were investigated with AFM. It was confirmed that the films had uniform thickness and smooth surface, as shown in the Figure 7.

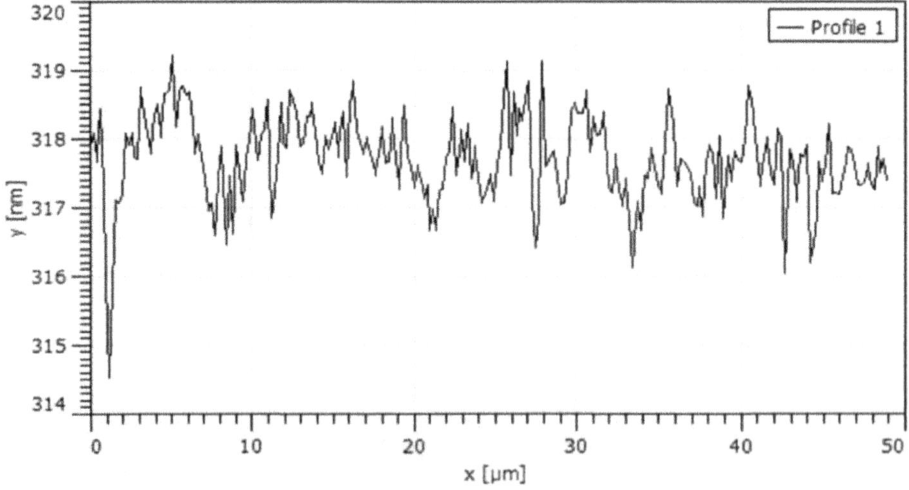

Figure 7. The surface morphology of the gelatin film on the quartz crystal microbalance with dissipation (QCM-D) sensor.

The QCM-D graph is shown in Figure 8. Although a large deposition of CAP particles on the gelatin film was detected, the very high extent of the frequency change (around 550 Hz) of all investigated overtones creates a risk of an error when calculating the mass deposition. Therefore, the obtained results were used only for the qualitative, and not for the quantitative analysis.

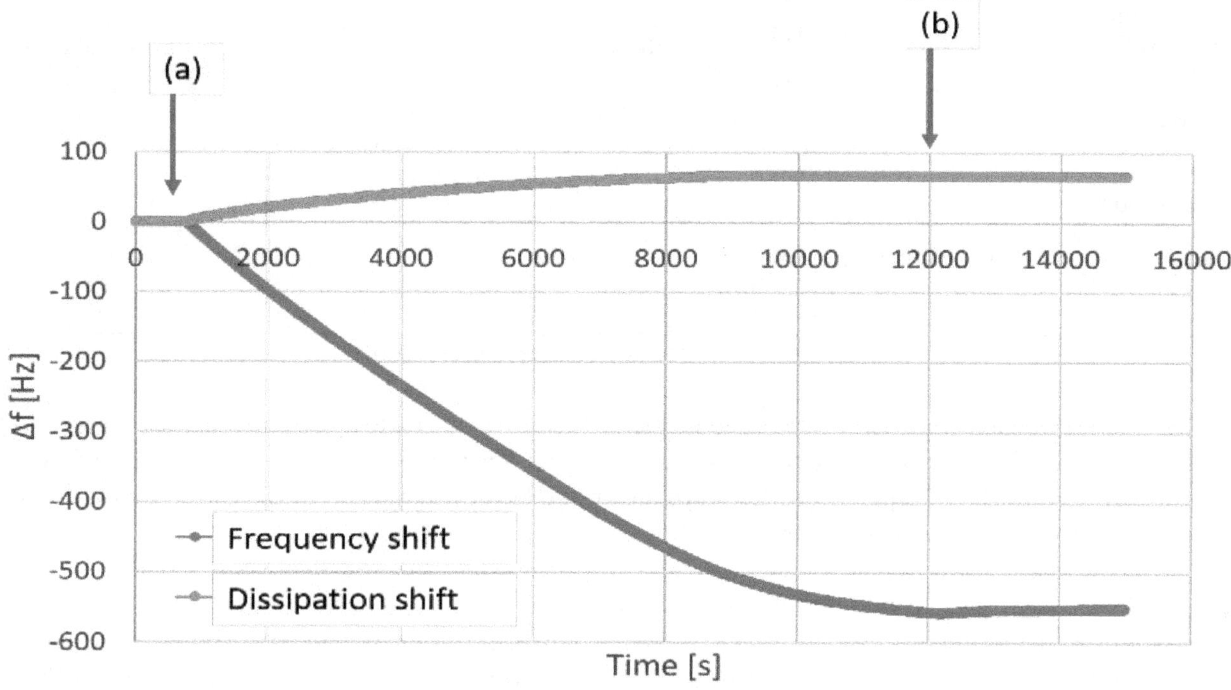

Figure 8. A QCM-D graph obtained at 5th overtone. The approx. 550 Hz drop in frequency carries risk of error on calculating the mass increase: (**a**) start of latex flow; (**b**) start of water flow (to remove particles that are not bound to the film).

The deposition of particles proceeded, until the full coverage of the QCM sensor occurred after approximately 12,000 s, which on the graph in Figure 8 is visible as a plateau in the frequency shift. Afterwards, the system was flushed with deionized water for 50 min, what did not cause any significant decrease in the amount of latex particles adsorbed on the gelatin.

3.3. *Gas Permeability*

Oxygen was a gas used for permeability test. Three compositions were investigated (GEL, GA, GAC). The thickness of investigated films was 650 ± 50 μm. The measured oxygen permeability ($cm^3/(m^2 \times 24\ h \times 0.1\ MPa)$) was 7.58 for GA sample, 3.43 for GAC and 3.43 for GEL samples. The test was performed twice for all the samples, and the same results were obtained.

3.4. *Disintegration Time*

The results of disintegration time measurements are shown in Table 2. The current pharmacopeial standards (European Pharmacopeia 10th) for disintegration time of gastro-resistant capsules state that the investigated sample should not disintegrate in 0.1 M HCl for 2 or 3 h (depending on the composition, however not less than 1 h), which should be followed by disintegration within 1 h at pH 6.8. In the investigated capsules, at the acid stage, no disruption of the capsule shell material was observed. However, the rupture of the capsule sealing was observed in several capsules.

Table 2. Disintegration time of GAC capsules with various fill. Three capsules from each batch were subjected to the test. The results are shown as mean ± standard deviation.

The GAC Capsule Filling Type	Batch No.	Tablet Disintegration Tester		Paddle Apparatus	
		0.1 M HCl	Phosphate Buffer pH 6.8	0.1 M HCl	Phosphate Buffer pH 6.8
MCT oil	1	86 ± 7 min	n/a	>2 h	6 ± 4.6 min
	2	>2 h	3.7 ± 1.5 min	>2 h	10.7 ± 7.4 min
	3	>2 h	2.5 ± 0.7 min	Single capsule leaking [1]	6.5 ± 7.8 min
PEG 400	1	77.7 ± 7.0 min	n/a	Single capsule leaking [1]	12.7 ± 4.2 min
	2	>2 h	7.3 ± 1.5 min	>2 h	39.0 ± 18.5 min
	3	>2 h	4.0 ± 2.0 min	>2 h	43.0 ± 13.2 min
Cetearyl alcohol	1	45.7 ± 7.4 min	n/a	79.3 ± 16.3 min	n/a
	2	48.7 ± 16.0 min	n/a	82.7 ± 23.3 min	n/a
	3	29.0 ± 33.0 min	n/a	81.3 ± 18.5 min	n/a

[1] the leakage was observed on the sealing of capsule.

The results of disintegration time measurements are not significantly different in regard to the method applied. The resistance of capsules to acid was similar when either MCT oil or PEG was used as a filling material. Surprisingly, the capsules filled with cetearyl alcohol disintegrated in acidic conditions within a relatively short time.

A careful observation in acid phase indicated that the shell did not disrupt in any other way but only through the sealing, while the walls of the capsules always retained their integrity. This indicates that the shell material itself is resistant to acid and the filling material does not change this property. The resistance of the capsules to acid, however, lacks reproducibility due to a variability of the seal quality. At pH 6.8, the capsules disintegrated through creation of a breach in the shell, caused by its thinning due to dissolution process. However, similarly to the test in acid, the disintegration always started at the sealing site. It was observed that the disintegration time at pH 6.8 was longer, when the paddle apparatus was used in the test, which can be attributed to different fluid dynamics that had impact on the rate of dissolution of the capsule shell.

The sealing sites of the investigated capsule shells and the reference commercial soft capsules were investigated microscopically. Although with an optical microscopy the image of the seals appeared similar to the commercial capsules, in SEM pictures, in some of the prepared capsules more sharp angle at the contact site of the fused films was observed. Such a defect is likely to induce formation of a rupture when capsules are swollen upon submersion in fluid. An evident difference between "commercial" sealing and the lab-scale sealing of the capsules is presented in Figure 9.

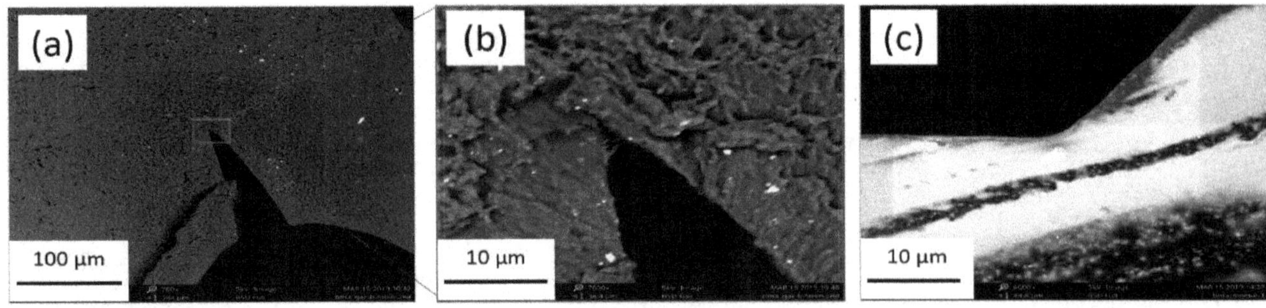

Figure 9. SEM images of the cross-sections of the capsule sealing site: (**a**) an apparently successful sealing; (**b**) close-up of the area; (**c**) a reference commercial soft gelatin capsule.

3.5. *Drug Release Test*

Due to the fact that during disintegration test, the disruption at the sealing zone appeared as a problem, the drug release test was performed in an enhancer cell, described in the Methods section.

Although this system can show potential differences in the kinetics of the drug release in comparison to a filled capsule, still the conclusions about acid-resistance and the rate of drug release can be drawn.

The pharmacopeial standards for drug release test from gastro-resistant forms require the release of less than 10% of the declared drug dose within 2 h in 0.1 M HCl, followed by at least 80% of the dose released at pH 6.8 within a specified time, usually not longer than 45 min.

The drug release test was performed for the diffusion cells filled with 1% m/v solution of diclofenac sodium in PEG (total dose 25 mg of API). The results obtained with different stirring rates are shown in Figure 10.

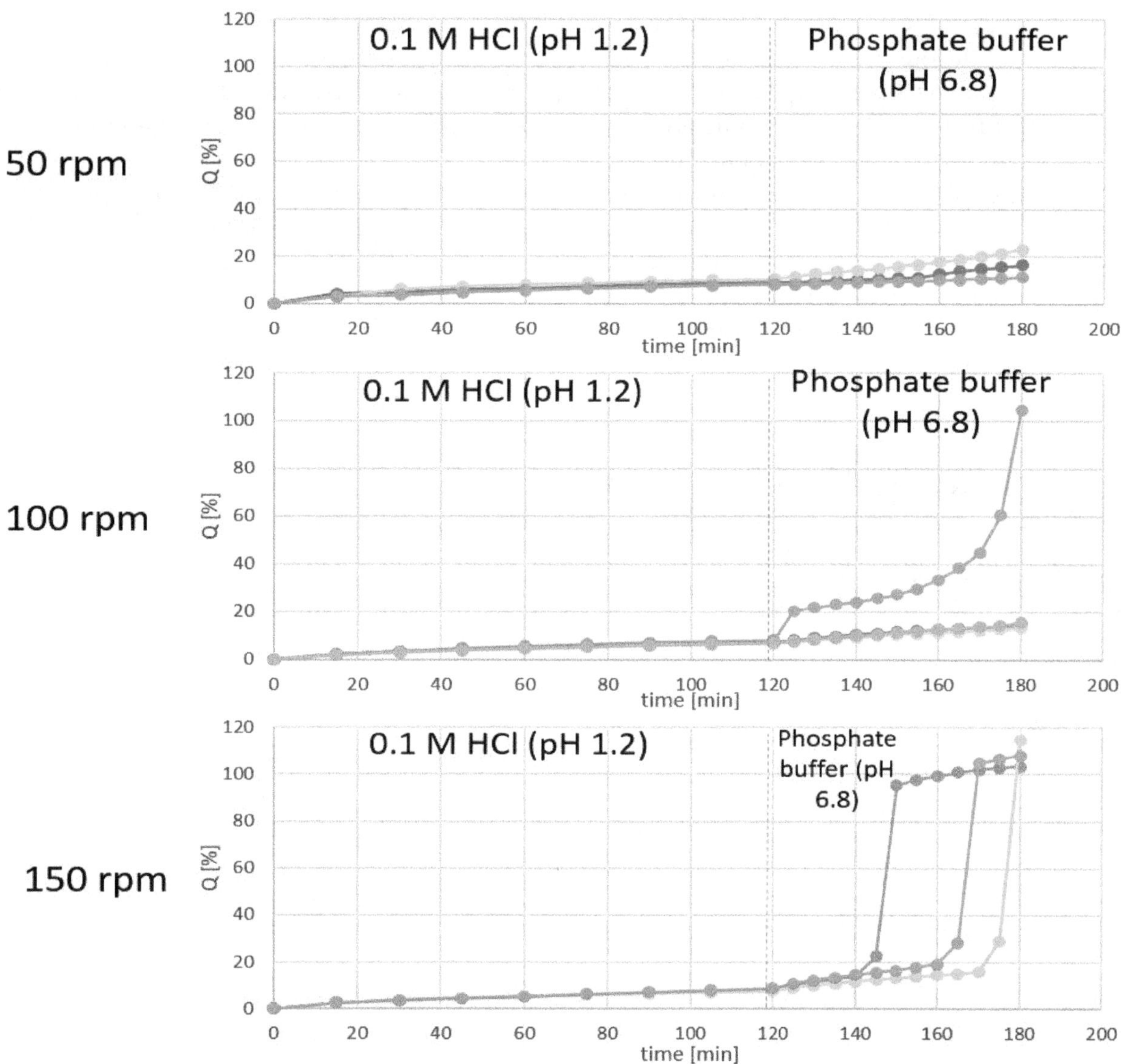

Figure 10. The effect of the stirring rate in a paddle apparatus on the release profiles of diclofenac sodium from the PEG 400 solution in a diffusion cell closed with GAC film.

The results show that at all of the used stirring rates, less than 10% of diclofenac was released during the acid phase of the test, which complies with the pharmacopeial requirements, and confirms the acid-resistance of the investigated films. On the other hand, at the buffer stage of the test, the release occurred in each sample only if they were tested at the high stirring rate, i.e., 150 rpm.

4. Discussion

The structures revealed by SEM in the films after they were treated with an acid (Figure 3) allow for conclusion that the formation of the modified films is based on a phase transformation in a gelatin-CAP mixture at a preparation stage. Due to the fact that pH of the utilized type B gelatin solution was around 4.5, one can expect that CAP should constitute a separate phase as this polymer is insoluble at low pH. The CAP phase can be considered continuous; due to the high temperature at the stage of mixture preparation, which is well above the glass transition temperature (Tg) of CAP, the particles can appear in a rubbery state and coagulate easily. Therefore, the two separate phases: gelatin gel and CAP phase, are physically mixed, forming a bi-continuous network with discreet separate microdomains. The structures revealed with SEM suggest that the phase separation proceeds with a spinodal decomposition mechanism, which is spontaneously initiated, and kinetically limited by increase in the viscosity of gelatin during the gelling process when the temperature drops at the casting stage. Similar "kinetic arrestation" of the phase separation process in the gelatin-containing mixtures was described by Lorén et al. [10] and by Tromp et al. [11].

To better explain the phase separation in the discussed systems, an additional experiment was performed. A premix of GA composition was placed in a glass vial and slowly heated to reach 80 °C. After 5 min at 80°C the temperature was lowered stepwise by 10 °C each 5 min. The appearance of turbidity indicated the phase separation process. After reaching 40 °C the sample was heated again to 80 °C and kept at that temperature for 48 h. The second heating revealed that the temperature-dependent phase separation is reversible (the sample became transparent again). The results are presented in Figure 11.

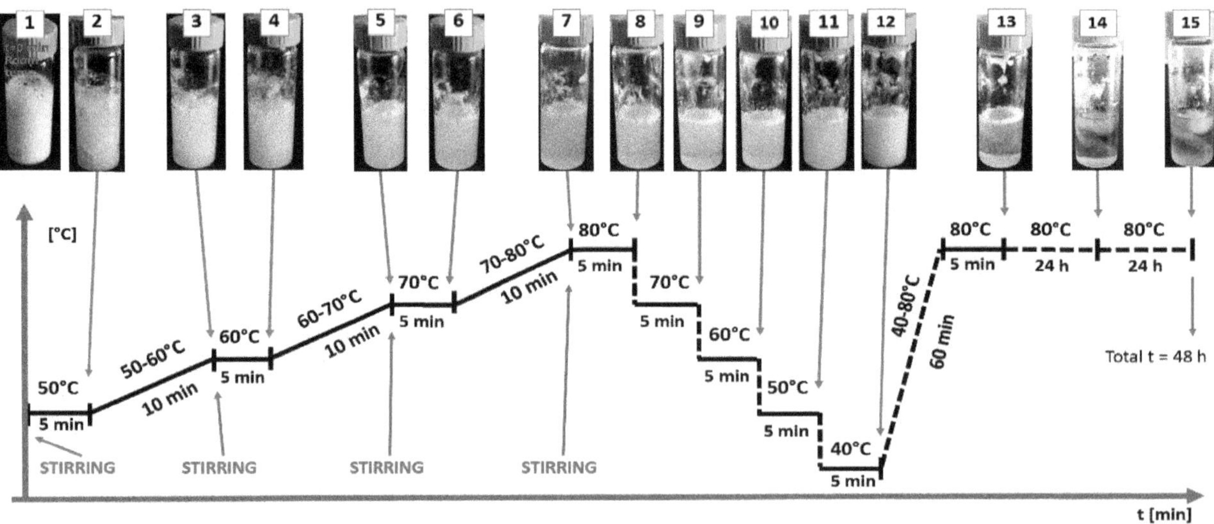

Figure 11. The visible phase-separation on lowering the temperature of the sample, and suspected spinodal decomposition process on storage at 80 °C for a prolonged time.

However, the storage at 80 °C for a prolonged time caused irreversible phase separation, with a fibrillar/sponge-like appearance of the precipitated phase within the liquid continuous phase. Additionally, the alteration of color of the sample and the fact that the gel was partially liquid at room temperature indicated gelatin degradation. The overall results of this experiment confirm that the phase separation process proceeds at high temperature and can be stopped by immobilization of the growing CAP structure in a gelatin gel when the temperature drops below approx. 50 °C. This supports the thesis that the separate phase of CAP acts like a "reinforcement" for the gelatin network, decreasing the rate of penetration of the acidic medium into the water-soluble phase, and explains the structure integrity of the films in acidic media. Furthermore, it appears that the temperature/time balance in the preparation procedure allows to exploit the natural imbalance between phases for the favor of functionality of the films.

The mechanism behind formation and acid-resistance of both binary (GA) and ternary (GAC) polymer systems appears the same. However, in comparison to the GA films, a more significant hindering of disintegration and dissolution can be observed in case of GAC films [5]. This can be explained by a possible interaction between gelatin and carrageenan, which is suspected to be a polyelectrolyte complex formation. This non-covalent interaction has already been reported and is widely described [6,12–16]. Even though carrageenan is present in the film in a small amount, it still can significantly impact the viscosity of the gel phase. Therefore, by increasing the density of the polymer network, it leads to formation of a gel diffusion layer more viscous than the gelatin alone. That causes higher swelling degree and slower dissolution rate of soluble ingredients present in the films, as it was previously described [5]. It appears also possible that the carrageenan in the film-forming mixture accumulates on the CAP-gelatin interface, supporting the CAP scaffold during the immersion in an acid. However, we believe that the more irregular appearance of the CAP scaffolds visible in Figure 4 are actually CAP coated with undissolved gelatin-carrageenan complex. This hypothesis appears to be supported by the results of Raman microscopy (see Figures 6 and 7), in which after immersion in acid, the structure shows a pattern in Raman spectra with the same features as observed in the spectra of the films before the acid treatment (both CAP and GAC), what suggests that during the immersion the gelatin was not fully dissolved and it is still present on the surface of the residual CAP scaffold structure.

The CLSM study (Figure 4) appears to correspond well with the SEM results. Additionally, it was discovered that there are clear differences in the density of the solid material left in structure inside the films and on its surface. Due to the fact that the soluble fraction of the film composition is supposedly gelatin-based gel and plasticizer, the mechanism of erosion of the film when placed in an acid is likely based on the diffusion of the medium through the gel layer. The erosion can be additionally limited by the presence of the insoluble CAP phase, which acts also as a scaffold. Therefore, it can be suspected that the penetration of the acidic medium into the membrane is delayed and can depend on both density of the CAP scaffold and viscosity of the gelatin-based phase.

The higher barrier properties of a ternary system (GAC) than the binary one (GA) also was demonstrated by the oxygen permeability test. However, in the literature the results of oxygen permeability can be found only for very thin gelatin films obtained from dilute gelatin solutions [17], where the values of oxygen permeability can be around 350–600 $cm^3/(m^2 \times 24\ h \times 0.1\ MPa)$. In the present study the permeability was measured for films with thickness around 650 μm, at which the measured values were between 3.5 and 7.5 $cm^3/(m^2 \times 24\ h \times 0.1\ MPa)$. Although, after addition of CAP, the oxygen permeability increased slightly, the differences between formulations were still very low and one can conclude that there is a lack of significant influence of the film ingredients on gas barrier properties.

During the formation of modified GA or GAC films, the CAP spherical particles (average size of 0.43 μm) are being incorporated in the gel structure. QCM-D is a surface sensitive technique which can be applied to analyze the interaction of the particles of CAP with gelatin. Quantitative values can be obtained with well-defined model systems. Saurebrey and Johannsman models [18] are often used to calculate the surface excess after adsorption. In our particular case, those models will not give reliable approximation because of the large size of the CAP particles. However, a qualitative information on interaction between CAP particles and gelatin films can be obtained. The large decrease in frequency of the vibration as soon as the CAP particles were introduced into the flow cell reflects the adsorption of CAP particles on the gelatin films. Due to the fact that the measurements were performed at 25 °C, a coalescence of the CAP is rather negligible, therefore such interaction should be based purely on surface charge of the particles. Although the test could not be performed at high temperature (80 °C), the confirmed high affinity of these two materials at 25 °C may be also relevant at higher temperature.

We assume that such type of interaction can potentially stabilize the CAP inside the gel matrix and allow formation of a network structure during the preparation of the film-forming mass.

Preparation of capsules on a lab scale with the proposed steel mold was a simple process, allowing for application of a liquid fill, and for obtaining visually sealed capsules. However, the results of the disintegration tests show large variability because of the significant tendency of capsules to disrupt at the sealing area. On the other hand, the results prove that formation of the capsules using GAC composition is generally possible, and the capsules can be filled with liquid oil, PEG or melted fatty alcohol. In addition, no case in which a capsule disintegrated in acid at other region than the sealing was observed. This confirms that the films being in contact with a filling, still retain their structural integrity when submersed in acid.

For the purpose of investigation, whether the filling formulation has an impact on acid-resistance of the capsule shell, the capsules were filled with three types of substances: PEG, MCT oil and cetearyl alcohol. The results show that the capsules filled with solid fatty alcohol show lower resistance of the sealing to disintegration in acid. On the other hand, there is no noticeable difference between the capsules filled with MCT oil or PEG. Overall, the mechanism of disintegration of the capsules appears to be related more to the capsule formation process, than to the filling composition. It was observed that the lab-manufactured capsules are prone to leakages on the sealing zone, especially when more intensive mechanical stress was involved, as in the tablet disintegration apparatus. We believe that the imperfect capsule sealing can be corrected when encapsulation process involves the conventional soft capsule manufacturing machines.

The imperfections in the sealing region did not allow to further test the capsules in the drug release test. This is why this study was performed in a vertical diffusion cell placed in a paddle dissolution apparatus. The test was performed to investigate whether the films display barrier properties against diffusion of diclofenac sodium at acidic pH. In addition, it was important that the films allow to release the API after switching the pH to neutral (6.8). In one of our previous articles, the barrier properties of the films towards radio-labeled water were described [5], and preliminary data on the diffusion-hindering by the modified gelatin-CAP compositions was obtained. The present investigation confirms appropriate barrier properties of GAC film, because no diffusion of diclofenac during 2 h in 0.1 M HCl was observed. However, the reproducibility of the diclofenac release at pH 6.8 is not very high. The release was initiated at different time points, what results from the mechanism of film rupture—not dissolving totally in a specified time, but forming a breach. Since at lower stirring rates the release of diclofenac did not occur or was accidental, the proposed model requires higher stirring rates, which shows the significance of the mechanical factor in the dissolution of the GAC film in the pH 6.8 buffer.

Although the performed experiment with diclofenac as a model drug demonstrates lack of the drug diffusion through the modified gelatin film immersed for 2 h in an acid, diffusion of an acid through the membrane was not measured in the course of this stage of the research. Impermeability of the new capsule-forming material to the acid is a condition for using it in the capsules filled with an acid-labile drugs.

5. Conclusions

In this work the discreet kinetically-limited phase separation was identified as the main factor influencing the resistance of the modified gelatin films to disintegration in the acidic environment. The imaging techniques (SEM, CLSM, Raman microscopy) provided the information on the mechanism of film partial dissolution in acid. The QCM-D analysis proved the affinity of the latex particles to the surface-wetted gelatin structures, which may be important in regard to the film formation process. The lab-scale soft capsule formation process was performed, and the tested filling materials were proved to be compatible with the films, however the obtained capsules showed the sealing area as a weak spot, limiting the acid-resistance of the capsules during the disintegration test. On the other hand, a modified dissolution test with a paddle apparatus and diffusion cell allowed to confirm that the films are hampering the drug release in acidic phase, while releasing the drug at pH 6.8. The drug release at pH 6.8 was possible, however, only when higher stirring rates (150 rpm) were applied.

Author Contributions: Conceptualization, B.M. and M.S.; methodology, B.M., M.S. and A.L.; validation, B.M., V.A.; investigation, B.M.; resources, M.S., A.L.; data curation, B.M., V.A.; writing—original draft preparation, B.M.; writing—review and editing, M.S., A.L.; supervision, M.S.; funding acquisition, B.M. All authors have read and agreed to the published version of the manuscript.

Acknowledgments: The oxygen permeability test was performed by COBRO–Packaging Research Institute (Lukasiewicz Research Network, Warsaw, Poland). Katrina Logg and Archana Samanta from Chalmers University of Technology in Gothenburg are acknowledged for the support with the imaging techniques. Authors acknowledge funding from NordForsk for the Nordic University Hub project #85352 (Nordic POP, Patient Oriented Products).

References

1. Soni, H.; Patel, V.A. Gastro retentive drug delivery system. *Int. J. Pharm. Sci. Rev. Res.* **2015**, *31*, 81–85.
2. Benameur, H. Enteric capsule drug delivery technology—Achieving protection without coating. *Drug Dev. Deliv.* **2015**, *15*, 34–37.
3. Felton, L.A.; Haase, M.M.; Shah, N.H.; Zhang, G.; Infeld, M.H.; Malick, A.W.; Mcginity, J.W. Physical and enteric properties of soft gelatin capsules coated with Eutragit L30 D-55. *Int. J. Pharm.* **1995**, *113*, 17–24. [CrossRef]
4. Hassan, E.M.; Fatmi, A.A.; Chidambaram, N. Enteric Composition for the Manufacture of Soft Capsule Wall. U.S. Patent 8,685,445, 1 April 2014.
5. Maciejewski, B.; Ström, A.; Larsson, A.; Sznitowska, M. Soft gelatin films modified with cellulose acetate phthalate pseudolatex dispersion—structure and permeability. *Polymers (Basel)* **2018**, *10*, 981. [CrossRef] [PubMed]
6. Maciejewski, B.; Sznitowska, M. Gelatin films modified with acidic and polyelectrolyte polymers—material selection for soft gastroresistant capsules. *Polymers (Basel)* **2019**, *11*, 338. [CrossRef] [PubMed]
7. Reich, G. Formulation and physical properties of soft capsules. In *Pharmaceutical Capsules*; Podczeck, F., Jones, B., Eds.; Pharmaceutical Press: London, UK, 2004; pp. 201–212.
8. Ulrich, E.; Prosekov, A.; Petrov, A.; Dyshlyuk, L.; Kozlova, O. Properties of plant analogs of pharmaceutical gelatin for shells of soft capsules. *Biol. Med.* **2015**, *7*, 113–115.
9. Kamiya, S.; Nagae, K.; Hayashi, K.; Suzuki, N.; Hayakawa, E.; Kato, K.; Sonobe, T.; Nakashima, K. Development of a new evaluation method for gelatin film sheets. *Int. J. Pharm.* **2014**, *461*, 30–33. [CrossRef] [PubMed]
10. Lorén, N.; Langton, M.; Hermansson, A.-M. Confocal laser scanning microscopy and image analysis of kinetically trapped phase-separated gelatin/maltodextrin gels. *Food Hydrocoll.* **1999**, *13*, 185–198. [CrossRef]
11. Tromp, R.H.; van de Velde, F.; van Riel, J.; Paques, M. Confocal scanning light microscopy (CSLM) on mixtures of gelatine and polysaccharides. *Food Res. Int.* **2001**, *34*, 931–938. [CrossRef]
12. De Kruif, C.G.; Weinbreck, F.; de Vries, R. Complex coacervation of proteins and anionic polysaccharides. *Curr. Opin. Colloid Interface Sci.* **2004**, *9*, 340–349. [CrossRef]
13. McClements, D.J. Non-covalent interactions between proteins and polysaccharides. *Biotechnol. Adv.* **2006**, *24*, 621–625. [CrossRef] [PubMed]
14. De Kruif, C.G.; Tuinier, R. Polysaccharide protein interactions. *Food Hydrocoll.* **2001**, *15*, 555–563. [CrossRef]
15. Michon, C. Gelatin/iota-carrageenan interactions in non-gelling conditions. *Food Hydrocoll.* **2000**, *14*, 203–208. [CrossRef]
16. Derkach, S.R.; Ilyin, S.O.; Maklakova, A.A.; Kulichikhin, V.G.; Malkin, A.Y. The rheology of gelatin hydrogels modified by κ-carrageenan. *Lwt-Food Sci. Technol.* **2015**, *63*, 1–8. [CrossRef]
17. Avena-Bustillos, R.J.; Chiou, B.; Olsen, C.W.; Bechtel, P.J.; Olson, D.; Mchugh, T.H. Gelation, oxygen permeability, and mechanical properties of mammalian and fish gelatin films. *J. Food Sci.* **2011**, *76*, 519–524. [CrossRef] [PubMed]
18. Johannsmann, D.; Mathauer, K.; Wegner, G.; Knoll, W. Visco-elastic properties of thin films probed with a quartz crystal resonator. *Phys. Rev. B* **1991**, *46*, 7809–7815. [CrossRef]

12

Multimodal Decorations of Mesoporous Silica Nanoparticles for Improved Cancer Therapy

Sugata Barui and Valentina Cauda *

Department of Applied Science and Technology, Politecnico di Torino, Corso Duca degli Abruzzi 24, 10129 Turin, Italy; sugata.barui@polito.it
* Correspondence: valentina.cauda@polito.it

Abstract: The presence of leaky vasculature and the lack of lymphatic drainage of small structures by the solid tumors formulate nanoparticles as promising delivery vehicles in cancer therapy. In particular, among various nanoparticles, the mesoporous silica nanoparticles (MSN) exhibit numerous outstanding features, including mechanical thermal and chemical stability, huge surface area and ordered porous interior to store different anti-cancer therapeutics with high loading capacity and tunable release mechanisms. Furthermore, one can easily decorate the surface of MSN by attaching ligands for active targeting specifically to the cancer region exploiting overexpressed receptors. The controlled release of drugs to the disease site without any leakage to healthy tissues can be achieved by employing environment responsive gatekeepers for the end-capping of MSN. To achieve precise cancer chemotherapy, the most desired delivery system should possess high loading efficiency, site-specificity and capacity of controlled release. In this review we will focus on multimodal decorations of MSN, which is the most demanding ongoing approach related to MSN application in cancer therapy. Herein, we will report about the recently tried efforts for multimodal modifications of MSN, exploiting both the active targeting and stimuli responsive behavior simultaneously, along with individual targeted delivery and stimuli responsive cancer therapy using MSN.

Keywords: mesoporous silica nanoparticles; tumor targeting; stimuli responsive; multimodal decorations; targeted and controlled cargo release; cancer therapy and diagnosis

1. Introduction

Cancer is one of the most devastating diseases worldwide, characterized by unregulated cell division and cell growth, a fundamental aberration in cellular behaviors [1]. Consequently, the utmost ongoing challenge for the researchers is to restrain this dreadful disease. Even though, over the past decades, several therapeutic advances have been implemented in cancer treatment, including increases in survival rates [2], the metastasis and invasion associated with the malignant phenotype and heterogenic behavior of this disease still demands new therapeutic strategies [3]. Conventional methods for the treatment of cancer include chemotherapy, surgery and radiation therapy. Unfortunately, surgery and radiation therapy are limited for the treatment of cancers localized to one area of the body (solid cancers) [4]. On the other hand, although chemotherapy is widely used for the systemic treatment of advanced or malignant tumors, most of the chemotherapeutic agents are associated with severe side-effects of destroying the normal healthy cells and limited by cancer cell induced multidrug resistance (MDR) [5,6]. Therefore, developing efficient targeted cancer therapeutic strategies to reduce side-effects and overcome resistances is gaining increasing importance. Herein, researchers start to exploit the enhanced permeability and retention (EPR) effect of solid tumors [7]. Due to the presence of leaky vasculature and the lack of lymphatic drainage of small structures by solid tumors, nanoparticles can easily accrue in the tumor and represent promising delivery vehicles [8–10].

An ideal targeted nanoparticle delivery system should possess (i) the high loading capacity of multiple diverse chemotherapeutics, (ii) efficiency to protect the cargo until reaching the final destination, (iii) circulation stability in blood for prolonged periods without degradation and excretion, (iv) specificity toward target cancer cells to achieve off-target zero-delivery, (v) the ability of intracellular release and to facilitate controlled delivery of the cargo, and (vi) good biocompatibility and low toxicity [11–13]. Over the past decades, various types of organic and inorganic nanoparticles have been proposed as delivery vehicles to address those criteria [14–16]. Among the organic nanoparticles, liposomal-based drug delivery becomes one of the most promising approaches because of its high biocompatibility, flexibility in preparing various formulations, and easy synthesis to incorporate targeting moieties [17–19]. Furthermore, there are some already FDA-approved liposomal formulations; several polymeric and micelle based organic nanoparticles are also in clinical trials for use in cancer therapy [20,21]. However, the liposomal formulations and the polymer-based nanocarriers are limited, due to their invariant size and shape, inadequate loading efficiency, uncontrolled release of the cargo, and change in size and stability by changing loading parameters [22].

There are various inorganic materials developed so far as delivery systems trying to overcome the loading inefficiency, leakage and the uncontrolled release of the cargo, e.g., metal oxide nanoparticles, carbon nanotubes, and mesoporous silica nanoparticles (MSN) [23–27]. Few among the metal oxide nanoparticles are already in process for cancer therapy and diagnosis. A clinical (early phase I) study is also conducted with targeted MSN for image-guided operative sentinel lymph node mapping [28]. Particularly, in comparison to other nanoparticles, the MSN exhibit numerous outstanding features, including good biocompatibility, mechanical thermal and chemical stability, and most importantly, immense loading capacity of various cargos and their possible time-dependent release, thanks to the large surface area, high pore volume and narrow distribution of the tunable pore diameters of MSN [29,30]. For example, because of comprising large surface area one can load nearly a 1000-fold higher amount of doxorubicin in MSN compared to in the FDA-approved liposomal formulation Doxil® [31]. Moreover, silica is recognized by FDA as safe to be used in cosmetics and as a food-additive [32].

A comparative discussion about the pros and cons of MSN with other well-known nanomaterials for bio-applications was excellently provided by Chen et al. [33] and thus is discussed no further here.

In this review, we will discuss the efficacy of mesoporous silica-based systems for cancer therapy, the surface modification of MSN for passive and active targeting cancer therapy, and the modification of MSN for environment-responsive cancer therapy. Importantly, we will focus on multimodal decorations of MSN, which is the most demanding ongoing approach with respect to the present perspectives, and challenges related to MSN application in cancer therapy. Many reviews have summarized the synthesis of MSN, active targeting and environment-responsive drug delivery using MSN, whereas fewer involved in reporting the multimodal decorations of MSN for exploiting both the tumor targeting and stimuli responsive delivery of therapeutics simultaneously. Herein, we will review the multimodal approaches, including both the targeted delivery and stimuli responsive delivery simultaneously, along with individual targeted delivery and stimuli responsive delivery using MSN. As well, we will include the plausible applications of MSN in cancer diagnosis.

2. MSNs as Delivery Vehicles in Cancer Therapy

Despite the increasing numbers of anti-cancer drugs presented in the market and their ability to create potent and lethal interaction with cancer cells, their therapeutic efficacy remains affected by their low aqueous solubility and eventually not reaching a high enough concentration in the site of absorption, i.e., gastrointestinal (GI) lumen [34,35]. As for an example, camptothecin (CPT) is very effective at killing cancer cells in vitro, however, its clinical application has been limited due to poor water solubility. Additionally, researchers have tried to modify CPT as water-soluble salts to make intravenous injection possible, but this modification has altered its physicochemical characteristics and hampered its antitumor activity [36]. Another potent anti-cancer drug, paclitaxel, is also limited in vivo by its insolubility in aqueous systems, although it is very effective against various cancer cell lines [37].

With the aim to improve the drug solubility and oral bioavailability, a growing number of novel drug delivery systems, particularly nanostructures, have been developed [38,39]. The two foremost parameters determining the efficacy of a drug delivery system are the loading capacity and drug release profiles. To this end, with excellent features, including huge surface area and ordered porous interior, MSN can be used as reservoirs to store different anti-cancer drugs with high loading capacity and tunable release mechanisms [40,41]. As a promising drug delivery system, the pore size of MSN can be customized to selectively load either hydrophobic or hydrophilic anticancer agents, and their size and shape can be maintained to have the maximum cellular internalization [41,42]. There are mainly two ways that have been used to load the drug molecules into pores of MSN. One can load either in situ during synthesis or by the adsorption of cargo onto the pores of MSN (by physisorption or chemisorption). The adsorption method is the most widespread approach for the loading of therapeutic molecules, especially for poor water-soluble drugs [31,43]. During soaking of the MSN in a drug solution, the silanol groups present on the surface of MSN play the key role as adsorption sites. As the surface of MSN is negatively charged in the absence of any adsorbent under physiological conditions, the electrostatic adsorption method can be applied for the cargo having positive charge, as well as the lodging of water-soluble therapeutic agents into the pores of MSN. Moreover, the functionalization of MSN will increase the adsorbed amount of this group of cargo having additional interactions between adsorbate and adsorbent [44]. Pore size of MSN is another main controlling parameter to increase the extent of adsorption of hydrophobic molecules from organic solvents, if the molecular size of the cargo is in the range of the pore size of MSN [43,45]. Up until today, there have been various studies reported in favor of using MSN as efficient drug delivery nanosystem in cancer therapy. He et al. have reported the enhanced solubility of paclitaxel after loading into MSN [37]. Lu et al. have performed cytotoxicity assay with camptothecin (CPT)-loaded MSN and showed the clear growth inhibition of pancreatic cancer-cell lines (Capan-1, PANC-1, AsPC-1), stomach cancer-cell line (MKN45) and colon cancer-cell line (SW480) [36]. It was also reported that transplatin, a less potent anticancer drug (an inactive isomer of cisplatin), when loaded in MSN, became effective exhibiting enhanced cytotoxicity compared to that of cisplatin [46].

In this context we should also discuss about the protein adsorption and efficient protein delivery by MSN. The poor solubility and large sizes of the therapeutic proteins and their enzymatic and chemical degradation in the gastrointestinal tract commonly compromise their efficacy in cancer therapy. Additionally, the co-delivery of therapeutic proteins along with other therapeutic molecules is a big challenge for the conventional drug delivery systems, as the physicochemical properties of proteins, such as size, surface charge, stability, and susceptibility are very different than the other therapeutic molecules [47]. Herein, MSN are of special interest for protein delivery due to their possible easily tunable pore sizes, facile surface multi-functionalization, and enormous interior and exterior particle surface [48]. To expand the pore size of MSN depending on the sizes of the protein, generally two ways have been employed, exploiting polymers/surfactants with longer carbon chains/co-surfactants as templates, or the addition of suitable organic swelling agents to enlarge the sizes of surfactant templates [49]. There are variety of reported additives used as pore size expanding agents, such as *N,N*-dimethylhexadecylamine (DMHA), trimethylbenzene (TMB), aromatic hydrocarbons, auxiliary alkyl surfactant, and long-chain alkanes [50]. Moreover, positively charged amino silyl reagents or polymers have been widely used to compensate negative charges of the proteins, such as lysozyme, bovine serum albumin and myoglobin [51]. Protein loading amount in MSN can also be increased utilizing suitable surface functionalization, having strong electrostatic interaction between proteins and the pore channels. In this regards, Slowing et al. have first employed MSN for the intracellular delivery of native cytochrome c, a small protein, into human cervical cancer cells (Hela cells) [52]. There are several other reports about the cytochrome c delivery in cancer cells using MSN [53,54]. Zhang et al. have reported the high protein loading capacity of hollow silica vesicles and demonstrated cancer cell inhibition by the intracellular delivery of RNase A [55]. Besides, Niu et al. have modified MSN by employing hydrophobic C18-functionalization and Yang Y.N. et al. have utilized benzene bridged MSN for the effective intracellular delivery of RNase A [56,57]. Nonetheless, Yang and collaborators have reported multi-shell dendritic mesoporous organosilica nanoparticles to deliver protein antigens for cancer immunotherapy [58].

Along with efficient loading capacity, MSN have been used for controlled release of a variety of pharmaceutical drugs (e.g., DOX, TPT, and CPT) and therapeutic proteins/peptides [59,60]. It can be possible to release the cargo in a controlled manner, without any leakage before reaching the target destination, with the help of "gatekeeper" entities that can seal the pores of MSN. There are infinite gatekeepers reported for the end-capping of MSN to reside the drug molecules in the reservoir of MSNs, e.g., biomolecules, peptides, lipids, polymers, dendrimers, macrocyclic compounds, etc. [61–63] As reported below, we will discuss the gatekeeper systems to be used for controlled drug release.

3. Surface Modification of MSN for Passive and Active Targeting Cancer Therapy

Localizing MSN specifically into the cancer environment is one of the milestones to avoid side effects and damage to healthy cells. Several efforts have been executed to target the MSN to specific tissues, both through passive and/or active targeting [64]. At the beginning, MSN has been developed as anticancer drug delivery systems, mainly based on their efficacy to store high amount of chemotherapeutics into pores and exploit EPR effect for passive targeting to tumor tissues. In this part of the review, we will discuss the EPR effect and passive targeted cancer therapy using MSN. Later on, MSN surface modifications by conjugating targeting ligands have been introduced to enhance the uptake of MSN in targeted cells. Different targeting moieties have been employed to the surface of MSN, e.g., small molecules, aptamers, short peptides, antibodies and antibody fragments, etc. [31,65]. In the following part, we will review the targeted cancer therapy using MSN.

3.1. Passive Targeting

Since the beginning, the foremost important goal in chemotherapy is to achieve the tumor-specific delivery of chemotherapeutics. In this regard, most nanoparticles including MSN can passively target solid tumor tissue due to the EPR effect. In general, the body has its own pre-existing circulation network for the supply of food, nutrients and oxygen to the small primary tumor until the diameter exceeds 1–2 mm. Beyond this size, the tumor growth needs angiogenesis, i.e., the sprouting of new blood vessels from pre-existing vessels around the tumor, in order to supply food, nutrients, oxygen, survival factors etc. [66,67] Angiogenesis generates irregular blood vessels displaying a discontinuous and single thin layer of flattened endothelial cells with an absence of the basal membrane. Hence, nanoparticles having a diameter of at least 10 nm, which is the threshold of renal clearance, can leave the blood vessels and penetrate into the adjacent tumor tissue through the discontinuous leaky membrane. This effect is not applicable in normal tissue [68]. The penetrated nanoparticles remain longer in the tumor tissue without being cleared by the immune system, as the solid tumors commonly lack effective lymphatic drainage [69]. Moreover, particles having a diameter smaller than 4 nm can diffuse through the leaky endothelium back to the blood circulation and be reabsorbed, but the nanomaterials do not naturally return to the blood vessels, accumulating in the perivascular tumoral space [70]. In the nanomedicine field, this phenomenon is popularly known as the enhanced permeability and retention effect, or the "EPR" effect. To avail the efficient passive targeting particle size, the morphology and surface modifications of MSN have been considered. It is observed that the MSN should be at least 10 nm in diameter and have an optimal size of 100–200 nm to avoid the renal clearance of the particles [65]. To this end, Lee and co-workers have shown proficient cell death by the passive targeting of MSN loaded with doxorubicin (DOX) to the tumor site in a melanoma model [71]. Importantly, surface modifications of MSN also have a major influence to achieve efficient passive targeting by prolonging the circulation time of MSN in blood and subsequently reducing the renal clearance [72]. It has been reported by Zhu and colleagues that introducing PEGylation on hollow MSN improves cellular uptake in cervical cancer cells and mouse embryonic fibroblasts, compared to that of naked particles [73]. Huan and colleagues have demonstrated efficient biodistribution, accomplishing an 8% of the EPR effect at the tumor site in vivo of MSN functionalized with polyethyleneimine/polyethylene glycol (PEI/PEG), encapsulating doxorubicin together with P-glycoprotein siRNA [74]. With regard to passive targeting, another important factor is the 10 to 40 fold elevated interstitial fluid pressure (IFP) in solid tumors compared to normal tissue [75]. This pressure gradient may influence reduced nanoparticle distribution in tumor site. Actually, the necrotic tissues that are often present in the larger tumors and metastatic regions are highly hypovascularized, due to slower angiogenesis compared to tumor growth. As a result, the IFP becomes very high and the delivery of nanoparticles to this tumor region by passive targeting is hardly possible. Herein, the active targeting of nanoparticles including MSN is gaining increasing importance and we will discuss the advantage of active targeted drug delivery using MSN in the next part of the review.

3.2. *Active Targeting*

To deliver potent chemotherapeutics selectively to tumor environment, substantial progresses have been made by exploiting tumor cell-specific or tumor-associated cell-specific receptors [76]. A receptor highly expressed on tumor cells or tumor associated cells (compared to the normal cells) is a sensible target receptor for tumor specific drug delivery. If the surfaces of nanoparticles, including MSN, are decorated with ligands able to interact selectively with those overexpressed receptors, the specific retention and uptake of those nanoparticles by tumor cells will be enhanced. To design the targeting ligands grafted to MSN, various receptors over-expressed on the surface of tumor cells or tumor associated cells have been exploited (Figure 1) and we will discuss the decorated MSN mediated active targeted cancer therapy in this part of the review. Usually, the decorated MSN are taken up by the cancer cells via a receptor-mediated endocytosis process. Active targeting allows efficient particle uptake by the tumor cell and tumor microenvironment [77].

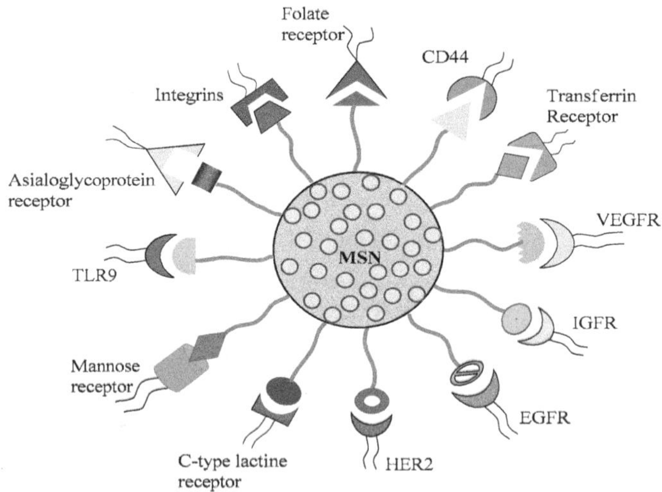

Figure 1. Plausible surface modifications of mesoporous silica nanoparticles (MSN) for active targeting to the over-expressed receptors in cancer microenvironment.

3.2.1. Targeting Folate Receptor

One of the most exploited targeting ligands, folic acid, has been employed to decorate MSN for targeting folate receptor, overexpressed in many tumors compared to healthy tissues [78,79]. The folate receptors are four glycopolypeptide members (FRα, FRβ, FRγ and FRδ), among which the alpha isoform, folate receptor α (FRα) is a glycosylphosphatidylinositol anchored cell surface receptor and has been reported to be overexpressed in solid tumors, such as ovarian, cervical, lung, breast, kidney, colorectal, and brain tumors [80]. In mostly 80–90% of epithelial ovarian cancers, other gynecological cancers, lung cancers and breast cancers, the FRα is highly overexpressed and gaining increasing importance to be exploited for targeted cancer therapy [81]. Considering this fact, several research groups have reported the enhanced specific cellular uptake of MSN in various cancer cells, having overexpressed folate receptors by modifying MSN surface with folic acid [82–86]. Nonetheless, using two different human pancreatic cancer xenografts on different mouse species, Lu et al. have also shown dramatic improvements in tumor-suppression effect by using folic acid functionalized camptothecin-loaded MSN in comparison with unfunctionalized MSN [87]. Moreover, along with using folic acid, López et al. have decorated MSN with triphenylphosphine (TPP), in order to target tumor cells, as well as the mitochondria of the tumor cells [88]. Conversely, instead of using folic acid, Rosenholm et al. have used methotrexate (MTX) as both a targeting ligand and a cytotoxic agent for cancer therapy, due to its high affinity for folate receptors and showed enhanced cancer-cell apoptosis by treating MTX incorporated MSN relative to free MTX [89].

3.2.2. Targeting Transferrin Receptor

There are two subtypes of transferrin receptors (TFRs), TFR1 and TFR2, which complexes with iron to facilitate iron metabolism in cells. Hence, the dysregulated expression of any subtype disorders can impair iron metabolism and eventually induce tumorigenesis and cancer progression [90]. It has been reported that TFR1 is abundantly expressed in many cancer types, e.g., liver, breast, lung, pancreatic, and colon cancer cells [90,91], and thus can be exploited as an important target for drug delivery. In order to improve the tumor specific delivery of MSN carrier, transferrin (Tf) which is a ligand of TFR1, has been widely exploited in surface modification of MSN [92]. As evidenced by the available studies targeting TFR1, Tf-modified MSN exhibit enhancement in nanoparticle uptake by Panc-1 cancer cells [93]. Additionally, Montalvo-Quiros et al. have used MSN as nanovehicles decorated with Tf to provide a nanoplatform for the nucleation and immobilization of silver nanoparticles (AgNPs) and demonstrated that only the nanosystem functionalized with Tf can transport the AgNPs inside the human hepatocarcinoma (HepG2) cells overexpressing Tf receptors [94]. Nevertheless, Tf-decorated MSN have been exploited for sorafenib delivery in thyroid cancer therapy [95]. Importantly, the overexpression of TFRs on the brain capillary endothelial cells (BCECs) of the blood-brain barrier (BBB) and glioblastoma multiforme (GBM) provides a route to allow effective chemotherapeutic penetration to the site of brain tumor [96]. Herein, few research groups have developed Tf-conjugated MSN to deliver the chemotherapeutics to glioma cells across the BBB [97,98].

3.2.3. Targeting Integrin Receptor and Nuclear Targeting

Integrin receptors, the α/β heterodimeric transmembrane glycoproteins, are overexpressed on angiogenetic endothelial cells and certain tumor cells, whereas they are absent (or present in basal levels) in pre-existing endothelial cells and normal tissues [19,99]. This makes integrins, especially $\alpha v\beta 3$ integrin receptors, a promising target in cancer therapy and RGD (arginine-glycine-aspartic acid) based peptides have found widespread exploitations for targeting chemotherapeutics to both tumor and tumor vasculatures via the overexpressed integrin receptors [100]. Therefore, peptides including the RGD motif have been widely used in surface decoration of MSN for targeted cancer therapy [101–106]. Moreover, Pan et al. have shown the in vivo efficacy of doxorubicin-loaded MSN grafted with RGD-motif. The same research group has further determined better tumor accumulation and reduced tumor size by coupling cell-penetrating and nuclear-targeting TAT peptide to the MSN along with RGD. Additionally, side effects of bare MSN to accumulate in liver and spleen have been distinctly minimized by treating RGD/TAT-MSN [107].

3.2.4. Targeting EGF Receptor and HER2 Receptor

Epidermal growth factor receptor (EGFR or ErbB1), a tyrosine kinase receptor, is a key factor in epithelial malignancies, in terms of enhancing tumor growth, invasion, and metastasis [108]. Overexpression of EGFR has been widely observed in many cancers including lung (especially non-small-cell lung carcinoma), colon, ovary, head and neck and breast cancers [109]. As EGFR has emerged as an attractive target for anti-lung cancer drug research, its ligand or antibody has been extensively employed in capping moiety for the active targeting of MSN in lung cancer cells. For example, She et al. have used amine functionalized MSN to conjugate with EGFs (epidermal growth factors) for targeting EGFR positive cells [110]. Sundarraj et al. have shown elevated accumulation of EGFR-MSN-cisplatin drug delivery system in EGFR overexpressed lung adenocarcinoma cells (A549) than that in normal lung cells (L-132). They have also used the non-small cell lung cancer nude mice model to determine the increased and prolonged cisplatin intratumoral distribution and enhanced tumor-cell apoptosis by treating EGFR-MSN-cisplatin [111]. On the other hand, Wang et al. have used cetuximab, a monoclonal antibody of EGFR as a capping agent of MSN loaded with anti-cancer drugs including doxorubicin and gefitinib, to specifically target lung cancer cells exploiting EGFR overexpression [112].

In addition to the EGFR, human epidermal growth factor receptor 2 (HER2)/ErbB2 is another member of the ErbB family of type-1 tyrosine kinases and a proto-oncogene, with a vast role of ErbB receptors in malignant transformation [113]. The overexpression of HER2 receptor in breast cancer alongside lungs, ovary and gastric/gastroesophageal cancers plays a major role in the angiogenic process and makes HER2 an important target in cancer therapy [114]. Furthermore, it has been reported that HER2 specific antibodies or antibody-fragments (e.g., trastuzumab) have been used in the surface modification of MSN for the selective targeting of breast cancer cells [115].

3.2.5. Targeting VEGF Receptor

The vascular endothelial growth factors (VEGFs) and their receptors (VEGFRs) play a critical role in tumor angiogenesis and metastasis. Among the three receptors (VEGFR1, VEGFR2, VEGFR3), VEGFR2 is widely explored as a direct stimulator of angiogenesis [116]. In addition to its constitutive expression on angiogenic endothelial cells, VEGFR2 is found to be overexpressed on several cancer cells such as breast cancer, lung cancer, pancreatic cancer, glioblastoma, gastrointestinal cancer, hepatocellular carcinoma, renal cell carcinoma, ovarian cancer, bladder cancer, and osteosarcoma cells [117]. To target VEGFR2, Weibo and co-workers have used $VEGF_{121}$, a natural VEGFR ligand which has a high binding affinity for VEGFR2 and observed a strong, specific binding of the MSN surface coated with $VEGF_{121}$ in HUVEC (VEGFR+), but not in 4T1 cells (VEGFR−) [118]. The same group has also demonstrated delivery of the MSN encapsulating the anti-cancer drug, sunitinib in a significantly higher amount to the U87MG tumor by targeting VEGFR exploiting $VEGF_{121}$ ligand in comparison with the non-targeted delivery [119]. Moreover, Zhang et al. have shown increased targeting ability and retention time of anti-VEGFR2 targeted MSN in anaplastic thyroid cancer tumor-bearing mouse [120]. Bevacizumab or related antibodies have been also exploited for targeting VEGF receptors.

3.2.6. Targeting Mannose Receptor and C-Type Lectin Receptor

Tumor-associated macrophages (TAMs) that exist in the tumor microenvironment promote tumor immunosuppression, angiogenesis, metastasis, and relapse. TAMs expressing the multi-ligand endocytic receptor mannose receptor (CD206/MRC1) have been suggested as a promising therapeutic target for cancer therapy [121]. It has been reported that MSN coupled with mannosylated polyethylenimine (MP) can target macrophage cells and enhance transfection efficiency through receptor-mediated endocytosis via mannose receptors [122]. Moreover, the C-type lectin receptor is also expressed exclusively by macrophages and exploited for cancer treatment. Lectin-functionalized MSN have recently been experimented in a mouse colon cancer model [123].

3.2.7. Other Active Targeted Delivery

There are several other receptors that have also been exploited for targeted delivery using surface-modified MSN. The overexpression of the insulin-like growth factor (IGF) receptor in ovarian cancer has been employed for the efficient targeted delivery of doxorubicin entrapped in surface modified MSN [124]. Quan et al. have developed lactosaminated MSN (Lac-MSN) for asialoglycoprotein receptor (ASGPR) targeted anticancer drug delivery and showed the effectively inhibited growth of HepG2 and SMMC7721 cells by treatment with docetaxel (DTX) loaded in Lac-MSN [125]. The surface of the MSN has also been functionalized with the ligands of somatostatin receptors [126] and also with hyaluronic acid to target CD44 receptors [127]. Furthermore, Chen et al. have shown the significantly larger tumor uptake of vasculature targeting anti-CD105 antibody (TRC105) conjugated MSN, compared to untargeted nanoparticles in a murine breast cancer model [128]. The same group has employed a TRC105 antibody fragment (Fab) for the surface modification of MSN to target tumor vasculature [129]. Besides, Sweeney et al. have attached a bladder-cancer specific peptide named Cyc6 to MSN for active targeting [130]. Apart from small molecules, peptides and antibodies, the synthetic single-stranded DNA or RNA oligonucleotides (aptamers) have been used to decorate MSN for targeting cancer cells [131,132]. Moreover, Nguyen et al. have shown the Toll-like receptor 9 mediated delivery of mesoporous silica cancer vaccine (antigen) to the dendritic cells (the body's most professional antigen presenting cells) [133].

4. Stimuli-Responsive Drug Delivery Using MSN

Although vast efforts have been devoted to active targeting therapy using MSN, the delivery efficacy still needs to be strengthened. During the blood circulation and penetration into the tumor matrix, anticancer drugs may leak from mesopores of MSN, leading to insufficient drug concentration at the tumor site. To overcome this obstacle, "smart" MSNs-modified with environment-responsive gatekeepers were designed. As the characteristics of tumor microenvironment differ from that of normal tissues (e.g., acidic pH, high concentration of glutathione, etc.), MSN can be modified introducing the moiety sensitive to the tumor microenvironment and release the cargo specifically at the tumor site [134,135]. There are internal and external stimuli that have been exploited for the controlled drug release (Figure 2). In this part of the review, we will discuss the pH, redox and enzyme internal stimuli responsive gatekeepers and also the magnetic, light and ultrasound external stimuli responsive gatekeepers frequently used to prepare stimuli responsive MSN.

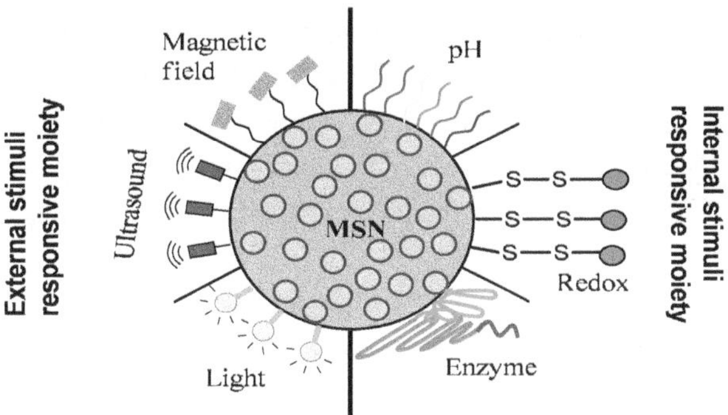

Figure 2. Most relevant stimuli responsive gatekeepers to decorate MSN for controlled cargo release in the cancer site.

4.1. PH-Responsive Gatekeepers

One of the most promising internal stimuli that has been employed for controlled drug release in cancer therapy is to exploit the lower pH values in most of the tumors in comparison with healthy tissues [136]. Actually, in cancer cells, because of high glycolysis rate, the production of lactic acid is high, thus eventually reducing the pH value in the tumor region. There are various reports in the literature regarding the pH-controlled delivery of chemotherapeutics by surface-engineered MSN in cancer therapy. Besides, there are mainly two ways in which they have been used to decorate the MSN for exploiting the pH sensitivity of tumor cells. One approach is to incorporate the pH responsive linkers in between MSN and the capping moiety usually used for blocking the pore entrances of MSN. There are several linkers that have been reported for the intracellular pH-responsive controlled delivery of anti-cancer drugs e.g., acetal linkers [137], boronate ester linkers [138], ferrocenyl linkers [139], aromatic amines [140], imine bonds [141] hydrazine linkers [142], acid labile amide bond [143], etc.

Another widely used approach is to modify the MSN surface with pH sensitive capping moiety, so that the MSN will only open up at acidic pH, release the cargo only in tumor environment and avoid any premature release of drugs on healthy tissues [144,145]. Yang and co-workers have reported that the MSN coated with pH-responsive chitosan/polymethacrylic acid polymer is more efficient to deliver doxorubicin in HeLa cells compared to the uncoated MSN [146]. The modification of the MSN surface using pH-sensitive self-immolative polymers, poly(acrylic acid), nanovalves, such as pseudorotaxane encircled by β-cyclodextrin, tannic acid, lipid coatings and many other nanoparticles have been reported [147–150]. Zhu and coworkers have used a pH-sensitive nanovector for the dissolution of ZnO nanoparticles functionalized onto the surface of MSN for the efficient delivery of doxorubicin in HeLa cells [151]. Moreover, pH degradable calcium phosphate coated MSN and gelatin capped MSN have also been described for intracellular acid-triggered drug delivery [152,153]. In a recent report, the MSN surface was modified with poly (styrene sulfonate) (PSS), which can act as a "nano-gate" for the pH responsive controlled release of curcumin [154].

4.2. *Redox-Responsive Gatekeepers*

Similar to the pH parameter, redox factor can also be exploited to achieve the controlled drug release from MSN specifically to the tumor environment. In general, glutathione (GSH) acts as a biological reducer and can cleave the redox-cleavable groups and trigger the bioactive agents. It has been observed that the GSH concentration in cancer cells is higher than that in normal cells [155]. Moreover, the intracellular concentration of GSH is in the range of 2–10 mM which is quite a bit higher than that in the extracellular part (2–20 nM); this concentration difference can allow the release of cargo from redox-responsive nanocarriers upon entering into the cytoplasm [156,157]. To take advantage of the high GSH concentration in cancer cells, the MSN surface has been decorated either with disulfide linkers or by incorporating any redox-cleavable group in capping moiety for the efficient release of cargo in cancer cells. As for an example, Kim et al. have used disulfide bonds as a linker in between MSN and the surface capping β-cyclodextrin moiety, and reported efficient doxorubicin toxicity in lung adenocarcinoma cells [158]. Moreover, Bräuchle and Bein research groups have reported cystein residues with disulfide linkers to modify the MSN surface [159]. Additionally, Wu et al. have used poly-(β-amino-esters) to seal the MSN pores and reported the intracellular reduction of disulfide linkers present between MSN and poly-(β-amino-esters) capping moiety [160]. The cargo release kinetics upon degradation of MSN can be further controlled by tuning the hindrance of disulfide or tetra-sulfide groups into the silica framework [161–163]. Besides, polymers cross-linked by cystamine, poly (propylene imine) dendrimer and polyethylenimine (PEI) via intermediate disulfide linkers are utilized to close the pores of MSN for a redox-responsive release of the chemotherapeutics by the degradation of polymeric networks in reducing the environment of the tumor site [164,165].

4.3. *Enzyme-Responsive Gatekeepers*

MSN drug release can also be modulated by the enzymatic cleavages of ester, peptide, urea, and oxamide bonds decorated on the MSN surface. Several enzymes such as esterase, protease, galactosidase, amylase, lipase, etc. have been exploited for enzyme responsive controlled drug release [166]. In this regard, Patel et al. have introduced ester bonds between MSN and the adamantine capping moiety, to employ the enzymatic role of porcine liver esterase for the controlled release of cargos [167]. Mondragón et al. have exploited protease cleavable ε-poly-L-lysine moiety to seal the camptothecin encapsulated MSN and reported the reduced viability of human cervix epitheloid carcinoma cells upon treatment of that nanosystem [168]. They have also reported some enzyme-responsive hydrolyzed starch products as saccharides to be used for controlled drug release [169]. There are various other protease-responsive moieties that have been used to cap the MSN pores and improve the drug release, e.g., protease-responsive biotin-avidin [170], arginine-rich protamine proteins [171], matrix metalloproteinase (MMP) degradable gelatin [172], avidin with MMP9-sensitive peptide linker (RSWMGLP) [173], poly (ethylene glycol) diacrylate moiety with protease-sensitive peptide linker (CGPQGIWGQGCR) [174]. Furthermore, cyclodextrin gatekeepers and HRP-polymer nanocapsules have also been employed on the MSN surface for enzyme-responsive drug release [175,176].

4.4. Magnetic Responsive Delivery System

One of the effective ways to exploit external stimuli is to exert the magnetic field on MSN, either to have magnetic guidance by applying the permanent magnetic field, or to increase the temperature by applying an alternating magnetic (AM) field [177,178]. In this regards, iron oxide has been widely exploited as the required magnetic component. There are mainly two ways that have been used to conjugate iron oxide with MSN, either using iron oxide core coated with mesoporous silica or MSN capped with iron oxide nanoparticles [179,180]. The most employed strategy consists on encapsulating superparamagnetic iron oxide nanoparticles (SPIONs) of ca. 5–10 nm within the MSN network during their synthesis [181,182]. These SPIONs are able to convert the magnetic energy into heat and can increase the local temperature of the system upon application of the AM field. If the surface of MSN has already been coated with temperature responsive moieties acting as gatekeepers, e.g., poly (N-isopropylacrylamide), pore opening and drug release from MSN can be triggered by applying an AM field [183]. Taken together, upon application of an AM field, SPIONs encapsulated in MSN can increase the local temperature up to a certain point, to change the conformation of the temperature responsive gatekeepers and open the pore entrances to release the anti-cancer drugs efficiently without having any premature leakage. There are several reports showing the controlled release of anti-cancer therapeutics by applying a magnetic stimulus [180,184,185]. Moreover, there are a few FDA-approved SPIONs for using as imaging agents and EU-approved iron oxide nanoparticles to use in glioblastoma therapy; these can be further exploited in magnetic responsive drug delivery [20].

Another strategy for the design of the magnetic responsive delivery system consists of the functionalization of drug-loaded MSN with a single DNA strand and then mixing this with SPIONs functionalized with the complementary DNA strand, to allow DNA hybridization that can act as a capping agent [186]. The reason behind selecting the DNA sequence is its melting temperature of 47 °C. Thus, upon application of an AM field, SPIONs encapsulated into the MSN network can increase the local temperature that subsequently trigger the double-stranded DNA melting and open the pores of MSN to release the drug. Interestingly, when the magnetic field is switched off, the DNA hybridization occurs again, thus closing the pores and stopping the drug release. This mechanism smartly provides the chance of exploiting the on-off drug release mechanism.

4.5. Light-Responsive Delivery System

The surface of MSN can be decorated introducing photo-cleavable linkers for triggering the cargo release from MSN, by applying lights with different wavelengths (ultraviolet, visible or near-infrared) [187,188]. Among all, as ultraviolet (UV) radiation has the highest power to easily break the bond, it has been the most commonly used light stimulus for the controlled drug release from MSN [187]. It has been reported that MSN coated with photo-responsive azobenzene-modified nucleic acid can trigger the drug release under UV light radiation [189]. However, the biomedical application of the UV light becomes restricted due to its toxicity and low tissue penetrability [190,191]. As an alternate, visible (Vis) light can be employed, as it is less harmful and has a higher tissue penetrability. Few Vis light-triggered MSN drug delivery systems have been reported [192,193]. For example, light responsive porphyrin nanocaps have been used to decorate the MSN. Porphyrin nanocaps are anchored via reactive oxygen species (ROS)-cleavable linkages, so that in response to the Vis light singlet oxygen molecules will be generated to break the sensitive linker and trigger the drug release by opening the pore of MSN [193].

Even though there are several advantages of using light (such as its easy application, non-invasiveness, low toxicity and precise focalization in the desired place), light-responsive delivery is restricted by its low tissue penetration capability (only a few millimeters). It has been observed that the best wavelengths for satisfactory tissue penetration are within the biological spectra, typically 800–1100 nm [134]. Likewise, Guardado-Alvarez et al. have exploited photolabile coumarine-molecules in the capping moiety of MSN surface to control the cargo release upon two-photon excitation at 800 nm [194]. Furthermore, Croissant and colleagues have shown that they can control drug release via a photo-transducer from mesoporous silica nanoimpellers in human cancer cells using two-photon light [195].

4.6. Ultrasound Based Delivery

Ultrasound (US) is an efficient stimulus to be used for controlled drug delivery, because of its advantage of being non-invasive, the absence of ionizing radiations in it and its capability to penetrate deep into living tissues by tuning the parameters, such as frequency, duty cycles and exposure times [171,196]. To exploit the US stimulus, the surface of the MSN has been decorated by employing US sensitive components in capping moiety to prevent the premature release of drugs in healthy tissues, e.g., 2-tetrahydropyranyl methacrylate. A hydrophobic monomer with a US-sensitive group can be transformed to hydrophilic methacrylic acid under US stimulus and this phase change can trigger the drug release from MSN pores [197,198]. Shi and co-workers have reported US responsive perfluorohexane encapsulated MSN to be exploited for drug delivery [199,200]. Moreover, Vallet-Regí and co-workers have decorated the MSN surface by using ultrasound-responsive copolymer (poly (2-(2methoxy-ethoxy) ethylmethacrylate-co-2-tetrahydropyranyl methacrylate) [201]. In fact, certain parts of the copolymer having chemical bonds that are cleavable under US radiation can change the hydrophobicity of the copolymer after their US-triggered cleavage, leading the conformational changes in polymer to open the pores of MSN and release the cargo at the target site [201].

5. Effective Combination of Active Targeting Therapy and Stimuli-Responsive Therapy Using MSN in Cancer Therapy

We have already discussed the various advantages of using MSN for drug delivery. Taken together, MSN exhibit large surface area, porous interior and tunable pore size to act as an excellent reservoir for different drug molecules and other materials of interest. Moreover, the various MSN syntheses approaches, mainly simple and adjustable, offer an ease optimization for sizes and shapes to maximize cellular uptake [202–204]. Importantly, one can easily decorate the surface of MSN by attaching small molecules, antibodies, aptamers, carrier proteins or peptide ligands for active targeting specifically to the cancer region, exploiting overexpressed receptors. Meanwhile, the controlled release of drugs to the disease site without any leakage to healthy tissues can be achieved by employing gatekeepers for the end-capping of MSN, triggered by various internal or external stimuli, such as pH, redox, enzyme activity, heat, light or magnetic field [205,206]. To achieve the precise chemotherapy of cancer, the most desired drug delivery system should possess high drug loading efficiency, site-specificity and the capacity of controlled drug release [207]. Hence, in this part of the review, we will report about the recently tried efforts for surface modification of MSN, exploiting both the active targeting and stimuli responsive behavior simultaneously (Figure 3), to obtain high efficacy with low dosage and minimize the off-target side effects of chemotherapy. Table 1 summarizes these simultaneously employed active targeting and stimuli responsive strategies developed up to date for MSN.

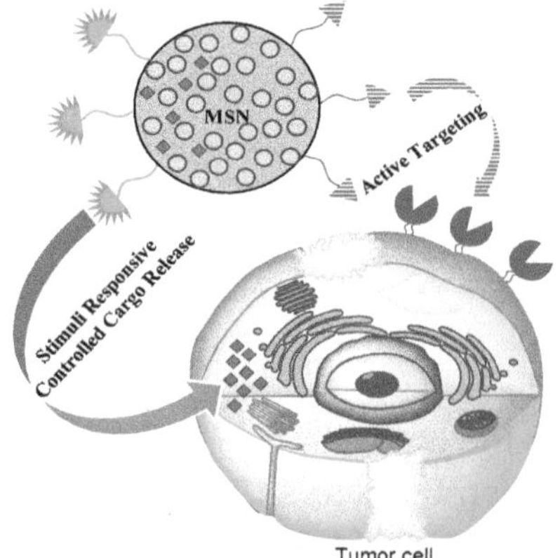

Figure 3. Multimodal decoration of MSN to achieve active targeting and stimuli responsive controlled release simultaneously.

Table 1. Simultaneously employed active targeting and stimuli responsive strategies using MSN in various cancer types.

Active Targeting		Stimuli Responsive Delivery		Cancer Therapeutics	Cancer Type	Outcome	Ref.
Ligand	Receptor	Stimulus	Linker/Moiety				
Folic acid	Folate	pH	poly(ethylene imine) (PEI)	-	cervical cancer	significantly higher number of particle internalization in cancer cells than normal cells	[208]
Folic acid	Folate	pH	poly(ethylene imine) (PEI)	Curcumin	colon cancer	suitable loading of fat-soluble antineoplastic drugs for sustained release	[209]
Folic acid	Folate	pH	polydopamine	Doxorubicin	cervical cancer	higher antitumor efficacy of MSNs@PDA-PEG-FA in vivo	[210]
Folic acid	Folate	Thermo/pH-coupling	poly[(*N*-isopropylacrylamide)-co-(methacrylic acid)]	Cisplatin	laryngeal carcinoma	higher cellular uptake, excellent drug release, greater cytotoxicity	[211],
Folic acid	Folate	Thermo/pH-coupling	poly[(*N*-isopropylacrylamide)-co-(methacrylic acid)]	siRNA against ABCG2 + cisplatin/5-fluorouracil (5-Fu)/paclitaxel	laryngeal carcinoma	down-regulation of ABCG2 significantly enhanced efficacy of chemotherapeutic drug-induced apoptosis of cancer cells	[212]
Folic acid	Folate	Redox	disulfide bonds	Curcumin	breast cancer	good biocompatibility, low toxicity, precise targeting and tumor growth inhibition	[213]
Folic acid	Folate	pH	chitosan-glycine	Colchicine (COL)	colon cancer	enhanced anticancer effects and reduced toxicity of free COL	[214]
Folic acid	Folate	pH	benzimidazole and β-cyclodextrin	valproic acid (VPA)	glioblastoma	enhanced effectiveness of radiotherapy	[215]
Folic acid	Folate	Magnetic field	iron oxide nanoparticles (IONPs)	Doxorubicin	breast cancer	effective active targeting and MRI-guided stimuli-responsive chemotherapy	[216]
Folic acid	Folate	pH and NIR light	polydopamine (PDA)	Doxorubicin	liver cancer	improved antitumor effect combining Dox-loaded MSN and NIR light	[217]
Folic acid	Folate	Enzyme (cathepsin B)	GFLG tetrapeptide linker	organotin-based cytotoxic compound	breast cancer	enhanced tumor growth inhibition with reduced hepatic and renal toxicity	[218]
Folic acid	Folate	Redox (Ascorbic acid)	cisplatin(IV) prodrug	cisplatin(IV) prodrug	cervical cancer	delivering cisplatin into cytosol, inducing DNA adducts and cell death	[219]
Transferrin	Transferrin	pH	chitosan or poly(d,l-lactide-co-glycolide) (PLGA)	Gemcitabine	pancreatic cancer	improved uptake of NPs by cancer cells, inhibition of cancer cell growth	[220]
Transferrin	Transferrin	pH and surface enhanced Raman scattering (SERS)	chitosan/poly(methacrylic acid) (CS-PMAA) and SERS reporter tagged Ag-NPs	Doxorubicin	cervical cancer	pH-responsive drug release, SERS-traceable characteristics and cancer cells targeting	[221]

Table 1. *Cont.*

Active Targeting		Stimuli Responsive Delivery		Cancer Therapeutics	Cancer Type	Outcome	Ref.
Ligand	Receptor	Stimulus	Linker/Moiety				
Transferrin	Transferrin	Redox	disulfide bonds	Doxorubicin	liver cancer	biocompatible system, potential in site-specific and controlled drug release	[222]
Transferrin	Transferrin	UV radiation (366 nm)	avidin, streptavidin and biotinylated photocleavable cross-linker	Doxorubicin	exposed tumors (skin, stomach and oesophagus)	efficient phototriggered drug delivery in accessible tumors and very high tumor cytotoxicity effect	[223]
Cetuximab	EGFR	photo	zinc phthalocyanine	ZnPcOBP	pancreatic Cancer	cell-line dependent photo-killing correlates well with EGFR expression levels	[224]
Trastuzumab	HER2	pH	poly(ethylene imine) (PEI)	siRNA against human HER2 oncogene	breast cancer	high batch-to-batch reproducibility, excellent safety profile, ready for clinical evaluation	[225]
HApt aptamer	HER2	pH	benzimidazole and β-cyclodextrin	Doxorubicin and biotherapeutic agent HApt	breast cancer	synergistic cytotoxic effects of chemotherapeutics in HER2-positive cancer cells	[226]
D-galactose	galactose receptor	pH	chitosan	5-fluorouracil (5-FU)	colon cancer	high drug loading capacity, possessed higher cytotoxicity on cancer cells	[227]
lectin concana-valin A (ConA)	glycans, sialic acids (SA)	pH	polyacrylic acid capping, acetal linker	Doxorubicin	bone cancer	increased antitumor effectiveness and decreased toxicity towards normal cell	[228]
cyclic RGDfC	$\alpha_v\beta_3$ integrin	photons	gold nanorods	-	breast cancer	enhanced radiosensitization of triple-negative breast cancer	[229]
cyclic RGDfC	$\alpha_v\beta_3$ integrin	Glutathione	thiol-functionalization	arsenic trioxide (ATO)	breast cancer	superior therapeutic ability of ATO-MSNs-RGD	[230]
RGD	$\alpha_v\beta_3$ integrin	Glutathione	β-Cyclodextrin, disulfide linker	Doxorubicin	MMP-rich tumor (colorectal and head and neck cancer)	tumor-triggered targeting drug delivery to cancerous cells	[231]
		matrix metallop-roteinase (MMP)	PLGVR peptide				
RGD and Tat_{48-60} peptide	Integrin and nuclear targeting	Glutathione	disulfide linker	Doxorubicin	cervical cancer	facilitated active targeting delivery and enhanced intracellular drug release	[232]
RGD	$\alpha_v\beta_3$ integrin	pH	α-amide-β-carboxyl group	Doxorubicin	glioblastoma	diversified multifunctional nanocomposites	[233]
$(RGDWWW)_2KC$	$\alpha_v\beta_3$ integrin	Glutathione	disulfide linker	Doxorubicin and therapeutic peptide	glioblastoma	tumor targeting and synergism of anticancer drug and therapeutic peptide	[234]

Table 1. *Cont.*

Active Targeting		Stimuli Responsive Delivery		Cancer Therapeutics	Cancer Type	Outcome	Ref.
Ligand	Receptor	Stimulus	Linker/Moiety				
K8(RGD)2	$\alpha_v \beta_3$ integrin	pH	acid-labile amides	Doxorubicin	glioblastoma	electrostatic repulsion induced nanovalve opening and drug release	[235]
RGD	$\alpha_v \beta_3$ integrin	pH	peptide-based amphiphile (P45)	Doxorubicin	Lung and breast cancer	targeted drug delivery and controlled drug release by the nanovalves	[236]
RGD	$\alpha_v \beta_3$ integrin	pH/NIR laser	gold nanostars (Au NSs)	Doxorubicin	glioblastoma	improved therapeutic efficacy combining chemotherapy and photothermal therapy (PTT)	[237]
cRGD and CREKA	$\alpha_v \beta_3$ integrin and fibronectin	radiofrequency (RF)	iron oxide core	Doxorubicin	brain tumor	remarkable increase in intratumoral drug levels	[238]
Asn-Gly-Arg (NGR)	cluster of differen-tiation 13 (CD13)	pH	polydopamine (PDA)	Doxorubicin	neovascular endothelial and glioma	greater BBB permeability, higher accumulation in intracranial tumor region	[239]
EpCAM aptamer	Epithelial cell adhesion molecule (EpCAM)	pH	citrate-capped gold nanoparticles	5-fluorouracil (5-FU)	hepatocellular carcinoma	preferential accumulation in tumor cells in vitro and in vivo	[240]
aptamer (Cy5.5-AS1411)	nucleolin (NCL)	laser irradiation (NIR light)	graphene oxide	Doxorubicin	breast cancer	synergism of chemotherapy and PTT	[241]
galactose (Gal) and TAT peptide	Asialoglycoprotein receptors and nuclear targeting	pH and Redox	poly(allylamine hydrochloride)-citraconic anhydride (PAH-Cit) and cysteine groups	Doxorubicinand VEGF-siRNA	hepato-carcinoma	effective and safe vector, sustained release, synergistic effect of chemodrugs and therapeutic genes	[242]
Phenylboronic acid (PBA)	sialic acid (SA)	MMP-2	PVGLIG peptide	Doxorubicin	liver cancer	tumor growth inhibition, minimal toxic side effects	[243]
YSA-BHQ1 and TAT-FITC	EphA2 receptor and nuclear targeting	pH	citraconic anhydride (Cit)	Doxorubicin	breast cancer	successfully developed anticancer drug delivery and imaging nanosystem	[244]
peptide CSNRDARRC	Targeting bladder cancer	pH	polydopamine (PDA)	Doxorubicin	bladder cancer	significantly superior antitumor effects of loaded nanocarriers than free drug	[245]
galactose (Gal) ligands and TAT peptide	Gal receptors and nuclear targeting	pH	poly(allylamine hydrochloride)-citraconic anhydride	Doxorubicin	hepato-carcinoma	improved tumorous distribution and potent therapeutic efficacy	[246]

Table 1. *Cont.*

Active Targeting		Stimuli Responsive Delivery		Cancer Therapeutics	Cancer Type	Outcome	Ref.
Ligand	Receptor	Stimulus	Linker/Moiety				
oligosaccharide of hyaluronic acid (oHA)	CD44	Glutathione	disulfide linker	6-mercaptopurine (6-MP)	colon cancer	increased stability and biocompatibility, efficient drug release in tumor cell	[247]
hyaluronic acid	CD44	Magnetic field	superparamagnetic Fe_3O_4 nanoparticles	Doxorubicin	breast cancer	active targeting to tumor cells and reduced off-target side effects	[248]
hyaluronic acid	CD44	NIR light	indocyanine green (ICG)	Doxorubicin	breast cancer	synergetic effect of chemotherapy and PTT	[249]
hyaluronic acid	CD44	Enzyme (MMP-2)	gelatin layer	Doxorubicin	breast cancer	successful bienzyme-responsive targeted and optimal drug delivery	[250]
hyaluronic acid	CD44	pH	DMMA (2,3-dimethylmaleic anhydride)	Doxorubicin	lung cancer	synergistic effect of active targeting and charge reversal in drug delivery	[251]

Besides, there are few reports that have used dual or multimodal response systems to improve the controlled release of the cargo. For example, Lu et al. have developed a pH/redox/near infrared (NIR) multi-stimuli responsive MSN to achieve efficient chemo-photothermal synergistic antitumor therapy [252]. Zhou et al. have also reported UV-light cross-linked and pH de-cross-linked coumarin-decorated cationic copolymer functionalized mesoporous silica nanoparticles for the improved co-delivery of anti-cancer drug and gene [253]. Moreover, Xu et al. have prepared a pH and redox dual-responsive (MSN)-sulfur (S)-S- chitosan (CS) controlled release drug delivery system [254]. Besides, a redox- and pH-sensitive dual response MSN system has been developed by Li and colleagues using ammonium salt to seal the pores [255]. Yan et al. have fabricated a pH/redox-triggered MSN nanosystem, for the codelivery of doxorubicin and paclitaxel in cancer cells [256]. Additionally, Anirudhan et al. have exploited both temperature and ultrasound sensitive gatekeepers for the surface modification of MSN [257].

6. MSN as Cancer Theranostics

Possible early detection and diagnosis is one of the most desired objectives to provide appropriate and extra real treatment for cancer. In order to overcome this hurdle along with the targeted and controlled delivery of chemotherapeutics, MSN have also been widely exploited for medical imaging and in situ diagnostics [258,259]. When both functions, i.e., therapy and diagnosis, are combined together, they are referred to as "theranostics" [260]. Herein, in this part of the review, we will discuss about various applications of MSN in cancer diagnosis such as exploiting MSN as imaging contrast agents, and utilizing MSN for proteomic analysis and fluorescent optical imaging.

Among the imaging technologies, magnetic resonance imaging (MRI) and ultrasound (US) have been mostly employed for cancer diagnosis due to their low-cost, low radioactivity and real-time monitoring properties [261]. There are various reports about the application of MSN decorated with specific targeting moiety as hyperpolarized, highly sensitive MRI agents having longer nuclear relaxation time [262,263]. As an example, Matsushita et al. have developed an MRI contrast agent comprising a core micelle with liquid perfluorocarbon inside the MSN for early cancer detection and diagnosis [264]. Additionally, a few research groups have systemically applied functionalized MSN to confer sufficient mean pixel intensity, to generate the higher quality US imaging of tumor bearing mice [265,266]. With imaging guidance from MRI or US, suspected cancerous tissues can be detected through biopsy. Furthermore, mesoporous silica-based chips with specific pore size provide a promising platform for proteomic analysis by mass spectrometry and chromatography, allowing the separation of low molecular weight proteins in serum from the higher weight proteins [267]. An analysis of mass spectrometry can identify unique protein signatures pertaining to various stages of cancer development, demonstrating plausible early cancer detection and therapy [268,269]. In addition, introducing metal ions or other functional groups enhances the selectivity and sensitivity of mesoporous silica chips to concentrate the low molecular weight proteins, analyze post-translational modifications in the human proteome and identify proteomic biomarkers in various cancers [270,271]. Importantly, fluorescent optical imaging exploiting MSN is gaining increasing attention in imaging-based therapy and cancer diagnosis [272,273]. The encapsulation of fluorescent dyes and bioluminescent proteins in MSN can overcome the associated limitations, such as rapid degradation, inadequate photo-stability and unpredictable toxicity of the fluorescent probes [274]. There are mainly two types of fluorescent MSN that have been reported for optical imaging, one is dye-doped MSN, prepared by incorporating fluorescent organic dye into pores of MSN and other one is combining QDs with MSN [275]. Yin et al. have synthesized folic acid-conjugated dye-entrapped MSN for in vivo cancer targeting and imaging [276]. Moreover, in contrast to the conventional organic dye, QDs appear more effective in optical imaging, due to possessing size-tunable wavelength absorption and emission, broad excitation wavelength, narrow emission bandwidth and a long fluorescent lifetime [277]. Functionalized QD-embedded MSN with high quantum yield have been largely exploited for selective tumor imaging in vivo, as well as for cancer cell imaging and detection in vitro by the intracellular internalization of QDs [278,279]. Recently, Zhao et al. have reported the synthesis of fluorescent Carbon Dot-MSN nanohybrids [86]. Nevertheless, Cheng et al. have reported tri-functionalized MSN, effectively decorated to be used in the field of theranostics coordinating the trio of target, imaging, and therapy in a discrete entity [280].

7. Challenges Regarding MSN Application in Cancer Therapy

Despite the recent advances of developing surface decorated MSN as an efficient carrier for the delivery of cancer chemotherapeutics, there are several challenges that need to be addressed for their further development. In particular, the scale up of MSN synthesis is one of the major issues limiting its commercial applications. On a small scale, the reproducibility on the synthesis of MSN can be maintained, but at the large scale, especially at an industrial level, it is very difficult to control batch to batch synthesis, as there are various different factors that need to be taken into account during the synthetic process. Hence, the clinical translation of MSN is taking a longer time than expected, as the therapeutic efficacy is not the only criteria for this [281].

In terms of the biological point of view, the clinical application of MSN is limited, because of the rapid clearance of nanoparticles by immune and excretory systems after administration [282,283]. Recent investigations have shown that MSN may be excreted, either in an intact or a degraded form, through hepatic or renal clearance [72,284]. However, the exact mechanism of the clearance is not known yet. Hence, the detailed in vivo analysis of pharmacokinetic and pharmacodynamic studies, possible immunogenicity and rigorous biodistribution of MSN-based systems should be employed before aiming to translate clinically [285,286]. A few reports highlighting half-life and biodistribution studies have demonstrated that in vivo biodegradation, systematic absorption and excretion, especially liver distribution and urinal excretion, are highly dependent on the physicochemical characteristics of MSN, such as geometries, porosities, surface chemistry, crystallinity, and different bio-nano interface interaction conditions [287–289]. For example, He et al. have evaluated the biodistribution and excretion of spherical MSN having various size ranges (80–360 nm) and pegylation (PEG-MSN) by fluorescence spectroscopy, and revealed accumulation of all the formulations in liver and spleen. They have also determined that, with a decrease in size and the pegylation of MSN, there is a reduction of the excretion rate from 45% to 15%, 30 min after administration [72]. In another study, Dogra et al. have shown that the increasing particle size of MSN from 32 to 142 nm results in a monotonic decrease in systemic bioavailability, along with accumulation in liver and spleen in healthy rats [290]. Furthermore, Sun et al. have completed a pharmacokinetic study of bevacizumab release from MSN-encapsulated bevacizumab nanoparticles in C57B/L mice and determined a significantly greater half-life, along with the sustained and slow release of MSN-encapsulated bevacizumab nanoparticles for a longer period of time than that of bevacizumab alone [291]. Additionally, Kong et al. have performed a biodistribution and pharmacokinetic study of Cy5-loaded hollow MSN in C57BL/6 mice and demonstrated gradual distribution in tumor and highest accumulation of MSN at 36 h after administration using fluorescence imaging. They have used the same MSN to deliver the cancer therapeutics (doxorubicin and interleukin-2) in the tumor microenvironment [292]. Regarding the limitation associated with bio-nano interface interactions, upon administration of MSN in the body and exposure to blood, proteins from blood serum and plasma adsorb onto the MSN surface and form a protein corona, which can eventually block the pores and decrease the release of cargo from the pores of MSN [293]. The protein corona formation is highly dependent upon the geometry of the MSN. Visalakshan et al. have shown a significantly lower amount of protein attaching from both plasma and serum on the spherical MSN, compared to the rod-like particles [294].

To address the biological limitations, a few research groups have started to introduce a lipid bilayer as gatekeeper and platform for surface modifications of MSN [295–298]. The advantages of using a lipid bilayer are its high biocompatibility, low immunogenicity, flexible formulation, and easy to incorporate targeting ligands and stimuli responsive moiety. For example, Brinker and co-workers have demonstrated MSN core for drug loading and a lipid bilayer as a gatekeeper to convey an EGFR-antibody for targeting leukemic cells efficiently in vitro and in vivo [299,300]. Samanta et al. have followed a similar approach of exploiting lipid bilayer around MSN to assist folate receptor targeted drug delivery in ovarian cancer [301]. Several other efforts have also been reported, exploiting organic/inorganic hybrid nanocarriers, L-tartaric acid, mucoadhesive delivery systems, organosilica-based drug delivery systems, to improve the biocompatibility of MSN [302–305]. Besides, cancer cell membranes have been utilized to coat MSN to improve immunocompatibility [306,307]. Moreover, an immunocompatible issue can be further resolved by replacing the commercially available lipids with the lipids derived from autologous extracellular vesicles (EVs) [308].

In conclusion, considering the various advantages of using MSN as a nanocarrier, along with the convincing preclinical results, it can be expected that, with the way out of related issues, MSN-based formulations may make exciting breakthroughs in cancer therapy.

Author Contributions: S.B. and V.C. wrote the paper. All authors have read and agreed to the published version of the manuscript.

References

1. Anand, P.; Kunnumakara, A.B.; Sundaram, C.; Harikumar, K.B.; Tharakan, S.T.; Lai, O.S.; Sung, B.; Aggarwal, B.B. Cancer is a preventable disease that requires major lifestyle changes. *Pharm. Res.* **2008**, *25*, 2097–2116. [CrossRef] [PubMed]
2. Siegel, R.L.; Miller, K.D.; Jemal, A. Cancer statistics, 2020. *CA Cancer J. Clin.* **2020**, *70*, 7–30. [CrossRef]
3. Biankin, A.V.; Piantadosi, S.; Hollingsworth, S.J. Patient-centric trials for therapeutic development in precision oncology. *Nature* **2015**, *526*, 361–370. [CrossRef] [PubMed]
4. Baskar, R.; Itahana, K. Radiation therapy and cancer control in developing countries: Can we save more lives? *Int. J. Med. Sci.* **2017**, *14*, 13–17. [CrossRef]
5. Gillet, J.P.; Gottesman, M.M. Mechanisms of multidrug resistance in cancer. *Methods Mol. Biol.* **2010**, *596*, 47–76. [PubMed]
6. Vasan, N.; Baselga, J.; Hyman, D.M. A view on drug resistance in cancer. *Nature* **2019**, *575*, 299–309. [CrossRef] [PubMed]
7. Greish, K. Enhanced permeability and retention of macromolecular drugs in solid tumors: A royal gate for targeted anticancer nanomedicines. *J. Drug Target.* **2007**, *15*, 457–464. [CrossRef] [PubMed]
8. Davis, M.E.; Chen, Z.G.; Shin, D.M. Nanoparticle therapeutics: An emerging treatment modality for cancer. *Nat. Rev. Drug Discov.* **2008**, *7*, 771–782. [CrossRef]
9. Farokhzad, O.C.; Langer, R. Impact of nanotechnology on drug delivery. *ACS Nano* **2009**, *3*, 16–20. [CrossRef]
10. Maeda, H.; Wu, J.; Sawa, T.; Matsumura, Y.; Hori, K. Tumor vascular permeability and the EPR effect in macromolecular therapeutics: A review. *J. Control. Release* **2000**, *65*, 271–284. [CrossRef]
11. Pérez-Herrero, E.; Fernández-Medarde, A. Advanced targeted therapies in cancer: Drug nanocarriers, the future of chemotherapy. *Eur. J. Pharm. Biopharm.* **2015**, *93*, 52–79. [CrossRef] [PubMed]
12. Stylianopoulos, T.; Jain, R.K. Design considerations for nanotherapeutics in oncology. *Nanomedicine* **2015**, *11*, 1893–1907. [CrossRef]
13. Kydd, J.; Jadia, R.; Velpurisiva, P.; Gad, A.; Paliwal, S.; Rai, P. Targeting Strategies for the Combination Treatment of Cancer Using Drug Delivery Systems. *Pharmaceutics* **2017**, *9*, 46. [CrossRef]
14. Egusquiaguirre, S.P.; Igartua, M.; Hernández, R.M.; Pedraz, J.L. Nanoparticle delivery systems for cancer therapy: Advances in clinical and preclinical research. *Clin. Transl. Oncol.* **2012**, *14*, 83–93. [CrossRef] [PubMed]
15. Bhise, K.; Sau, S.; Alsaab, H.; Kashaw, S.K.; Tekade, R.K.; Iyer, A.K. Nanomedicine for cancer diagnosis and therapy: Advancement, success and structure-activity relationship. *Ther. Deliv.* **2017**, *8*, 1003–1018. [CrossRef] [PubMed]
16. Bayda, S.; Hadla, M.; Palazzolo, S.; Riello, P.; Corona, G.; Toffoli, G.; Rizzolio, F. Inorganic Nanoparticles for Cancer Therapy: A transition from lab to clinic. *Curr. Med. Chem.* **2018**, *25*, 4269–4303. [CrossRef]
17. Torchilin, V.P. Recent advances with liposomes as pharmaceutical carriers. *Nat. Rev. Drug Discov.* **2005**, *4*, 145–160. [CrossRef]
18. Mondal, G.; Barui, S.; Saha, S.; Chaudhuri, A. Tumor growth inhibition through targeting liposomally bound curcumin to tumor vasculature. *J. Control. Release* **2013**, *172*, 832–840. [CrossRef]

19. Barui, S.; Saha, S.; Mondal, G.; Haseena, S.; Chaudhuri, A. simultaneous delivery of doxorubicin and curcumin encapsulated in liposomes of pegylated RGDK-lipopeptide to tumor vasculature. *Biomaterials* **2014**, *35*, 1643–1656. [CrossRef]
20. Bobo, D.; Robinson, K.J.; Islam, J.; Thurecht, K.J.; Corrie, S.R. Nanoparticle-based medicines: A review of FDA-approved materials and clinical trials to date. *Pharm. Res.* **2016**, *33*, 2373–2387. [CrossRef]
21. García-Pinel, B.; Porras-Alcalá, C.; Ortega-Rodríguez, A.; Sarabia, F.; Prados, J.; Melguizo, C.; López-Romero, J.M. Lipid-based nanoparticles: Application and recent advances in cancer treatment. *Nanomaterials (Basel).* **2019**, *9*, 638. [CrossRef]
22. Noble, C.O.; Guo, Z.; Hayes, M.F.; Marks, J.D.; Park, J.W.; Benz, C.C.; Kirpotin, D.B.; Drummond, D.C. Characterization of highly stable liposomal and immunoliposomal formulations of vincristine and vinblastine. *Cancer Chemo. Pharm.* **2009**, *64*, 741–751. [CrossRef]
23. Li, W.; Cao, Z.; Liu, R.; Liu, L.; Li, H.; Li, X.; Chen, Y.; Lu, C.; Liu, Y. AuNPs as an important inorganic nanoparticle applied in drug carrier systems. *Artif. Cells Nanomed. Biotechnol.* **2019**, *47*, 4222–4233. [CrossRef]
24. Pinel, S.; Thomas, N.; Boura, C.; Barberi-Heyob, M. Approaches to physical stimulation of metallic nanoparticles for glioblastoma treatment. *Adv. Drug Deliv. Rev.* **2019**, *138*, 344–357. [CrossRef]
25. Negri, V.; Pacheco-Torres, J.; Calle, D.; López-Larrubia, P. Carbon nanotubes in biomedicine. *Top. Curr. Chem (Cham).* **2020**, *378*, 15. [CrossRef]
26. Li, T.; Shi, S.; Goel, S.; Shen, X.; Xie, X.; Chen, Z.; Zhang, H.; Li, S.; Qin, X.; Yang, H.; et al. Recent advancements in mesoporous silica nanoparticles towards therapeutic applications for cancer. *Acta Biomater.* **2019**, *89*, 1–13. [CrossRef]
27. Wang, Y.; Xie, Y.; Kilchrist, K.V.; Li, J.; Duvall, C.L.; Oupický, D. Endosomolytic and Tumor-Penetrating Mesoporous Silica Nanoparticles for siRNA/miRNA Combination Cancer Therapy. *ACS Appl. Mater. Interfaces* **2020**, *12*, 4308–4322. [CrossRef]
28. Bradbury, M.S.; Pauliah, M.; Zanzonico, P.; Wiesner, U.; Patel, S. Intraoperative mapping of SLN metastases using a clinically-translated ultrasmall silica nanoparticle. *Wiley Interdiscip. Rev. Nanomed. Nanobiotechnol.* **2016**, *8*, 535–553. [CrossRef]
29. Kumar, P.; Tambe, P.; Paknikar, K.M.; Gajbhiye, V. Mesoporous silica nanoparticles as cutting-edge theranostics: Advancement from merely a carrier to tailor-made smart delivery platform. *J. Control. Release* **2018**, *287*, 35–57. [CrossRef]
30. Iturrioz-Rodríguez, N.; Correa-Duarte, M.A.; Fanarraga, M.L. Controlled drug delivery systems for cancer based on mesoporous silica nanoparticles. *Int. J. Nanomed.* **2019**, *14*, 3389–3401. [CrossRef]
31. Watermann, A.; Brieger, J. Mesoporous Silica Nanoparticles as Drug Delivery Vehicles in Cancer. *Nanomaterials* **2017**, *7*, 189. [CrossRef]
32. US Food and Drug Administration GRAS Substances (SCOGS) Database-Select Committee on GRAS Substances (SCOGS) Opinion: Silicates. Available online: https://www.accessdata.fda.gov/scripts/fdcc/?set=SCOGS (accessed on 10 April 2020).
33. Chen, F.; Hableel, G.; Zhao, E.R.; Jokerst, J.V. Multifunctional Nanomedicine with silica: Role of silica in nanoparticles for theranostic, imaging, and drug monitoring. *J. Colloid Interface Sci.* **2018**, *521*, 261–279. [CrossRef]
34. Hauss, D.J. Oral lipid-based formulations. *Adv. Drug Deliv. Rev.* **2007**, *59*, 667–676. [CrossRef] [PubMed]
35. Kawabata, Y.; Wada, K.; Nakatani, M.; Yamada, S.; Onoue, S. Formulation design for poorly water-soluble drugs based on biopharmaceutics classification system: Basic approaches and practical applications. *Int. J. Pharm.* **2011**, *420*, 1–10. [CrossRef] [PubMed]
36. Lu, J.; Liong, M.; Zink, J.I.; Tamanoi, F. Mesoporous silica nanoparticles as a delivery system for hydrophobic anticancer drugs. *Small* **2007**, *3*, 1341–1346. [CrossRef] [PubMed]
37. He, Y.; Liang, S.; Long, M.; Xu, H. Mesoporous silica nanoparticles as potential carriers for enhanced drug solubility of paclitaxel. *Mater. Sci. Eng. C* **2017**, *78*, 12–17. [CrossRef]
38. Badruddoza, A.Z.M.; Gupta, A.; Myerson, A.S.; Trout, B.L.; Doyle, P.S. Low energy nanoemulsions as templates for the formulation of hydrophobic drugs. *Adv. Ther.* **2018**, *1*, 1700020. [CrossRef]
39. Wais, U.; Jackson, A.W.; He, T.; Zhang, H. Formation of hydrophobic drug nanoparticles via ambient solvent evaporation facilitated by branched diblock copolymers. *Int. J. Pharm.* **2017**, *533*, 245–253. [CrossRef]
40. Maleki, A.; Kettiger, H.; Schoubben, A.; Rosenholm, J.M.; Ambrogi, V.; Hamidi, M. Mesoporous silica materials: From physico-chemical properties to enhanced dissolution of poorly water-soluble drugs. *J. Control. Release* **2017**, *262*, 329–347. [CrossRef]

41. Zhou, Y.; Wu, B.; Quan, G.; Huang, Y.; Wu, Q.; Pan, X.; Zhang, X.; Wu, C. Mesoporous silica nanoparticles for drug and gene delivery. *Acta Pharm. Sin. B* **2018**, *8*, 165–177. [CrossRef]
42. Lu, J.; Liong, M.; Li, Z.; Zink, J.I.; Tamanoi, F. Biocompatibility, biodistribution, and drug-delivery efficiency of mesoporous silica nanoparticles for cancer therapy in animals. *Small* **2010**, *6*, 1794–1805. [CrossRef] [PubMed]
43. Jafari, S.; Derakhshankhah, H.; Alaei, L.; Varnamkhasti, B.S.; Saboury, A.A.; Fattahi, A. Mesoporous silica nanoparticles for therapeutic/diagnostic applications. *Biomed. Pharmacother.* **2019**, *109*, 1100–1111. [CrossRef] [PubMed]
44. Barkat, A.; Beg, S.; Panda, S.K.; Alharbi, S.K.; Rahman, M.; Ahmed, F.J. Functionalized mesoporous silica nanoparticles in anticancer therapeutics. *Semin. Cancer Biol.* **2019**, *S1044-579X*, 30104–X. [CrossRef] [PubMed]
45. Narayan, R.; Nayak, U.Y.; Raichur, A.M.; Garg, S. Mesoporous Silica Nanoparticles: A Comprehensive Review on Synthesis and Recent Advances. *Pharmaceutics* **2018**, *10*, 118. [CrossRef]
46. Tao, Z.; Toms, B.; Goodisman, J.; Asefa, T. Mesoporous silica microparticles enhance the cytotoxicity of anticancer platinum drugs. *ACS Nano* **2010**, *4*, 789–794. [CrossRef]
47. Castillo, R.R.; Lozano, D.; Vallet-Regí, M. Mesoporous silica nanoparticles as carriers for therapeutic biomolecules. *Pharmaceutics* **2020**, *12*, 432. [CrossRef]
48. Xu, C.; Lei, C.; Yu, C. Mesoporous silica nanoparticles for protein protection and delivery. *Front. Chem.* **2019**, *7*, 290. [CrossRef]
49. Knezevic, N.Z.; Durand, J.O. Large pore mesoporous silica nanomaterials for application in delivery of biomolecules. *Nanoscale* **2015**, *7*, 2199–2209. [CrossRef]
50. Liu, H.J.; Xu, P. Smart mesoporous silica nanoparticles for protein delivery. *Nanomaterials* **2019**, *9*, 511. [CrossRef]
51. Kim, S.I.; Pham, T.T.; Lee, J.W.; Roh, S.H. Releasing properties of proteins on SBA-15 spherical nanoparticles functionalized with aminosilanes. *J. Nanosci. Nanotechnol.* **2010**, *10*, 3467–3472. [CrossRef]
52. Slowing, I.I.; Trewyn, B.G.; Lin, V.S.Y. Mesoporous silica nanoparticles for intracellular delivery of membrane-impermeable proteins. *J. Am. Chem. Soc.* **2007**, *129*, 8845–8849. [CrossRef]
53. Méndez, J.; Morales Cruz, M.; Delgado, Y.; Figueroa, C.M.; Orellano, E.A.; Morales, M.; Monteagudo, A.; Griebenow, K. Delivery of chemically glycosylated cytochrome c immobilized in mesoporous silica nanoparticles induces apoptosis in HeLa cancer cells. *Mol. Pharm.* **2014**, *11*, 102–111. [CrossRef]
54. Choi, E.; Lim, D.-K.; Kim, S. Hydrolytic surface erosion of mesoporous silica nanoparticles for efficient intracellular delivery of cytochrome c. *J. Colloid Interface Sci.* **2020**, *560*, 416–425. [CrossRef]
55. Zhang, J.; Karmakar, S.; Yu, M.H.; Mitter, N.; Zou, J.; Yu, C.Z. Synthesis of silica vesicles with controlled entrance size for high loading, sustained release, and cellular delivery of therapeutical proteins. *Small* **2014**, *10*, 5068–5076. [CrossRef]
56. Niu, Y.; Yu, M.; Meka, A.; Liu, Y.; Zhang, J.; Yang, Y.; Yu, C. Understanding the contribution of surface roughness and hydrophobic modification of silica nanoparticles to enhanced therapeutic protein delivery. *J. Mater. Chem. B* **2016**, *4*, 212–219. [CrossRef]
57. Yang, Y.; Niu, Y.; Zhang, J.; Meka, A.K.; Zhang, H.; Xu, C.; Xiang, C.; Lin, C.; Yu, M.; Yu, C. Biphasic synthesis of large-pore and well-dispersed benzene bridged mesoporous organosilica nanoparticles for intracellular protein delivery. *Small* **2015**, *11*, 2743–2749. [CrossRef]
58. Yang, Y.; Lu, Y.; Abbaraju, P.L.; Zhang, J.; Zhang, M.; Xiang, G.; Yu, C. Multi-shelled dendritic mesoporous organosilica hollow spheres: Roles of composition and architecture in cancer immunotherapy. *Angew. Chem. Int. Ed.* **2017**, *56*, 8446–8450. [CrossRef]
59. Luo, G.F.; Chen, W.H.; Liu, Y.; Lei, Q.; Zhuo, R.X.; Zhanga, X.Z. Multifunctional enveloped mesoporous silica nanoparticles for subcellular co-delivery of drug and therapeutic peptide. *Sci. Rep.* **2014**, *4*, 6064. [CrossRef]
60. Shao, D.; Li, M.; Wang, Z.; Zheng, X.; Lao, Y.H.; Chang, Z.; Zhang, F.; Lu, M.; Yue, J.; Hu, H.; et al. Bioinspired diselenide-bridged mesoporous silica nanoparticles for dual-responsive protein delivery. *Adv. Mater.* **2018**, *30*, e1801198. [CrossRef]
61. Wen, J.; Yang, K.; Liu, F.; Li, H.; Xu, Y.; Sun, S. Diverse gatekeepers for mesoporous silica nanoparticle based drug delivery systems. *Chem. Soc. Rev.* **2017**, *46*, 6024–6045. [CrossRef]
62. Deodhar, G.V.; Adams, M.L.; Trewyn, B.G. Controlled release and intracellular protein delivery from mesoporous silica nanoparticles. *Biotechnol. J.* **2017**, *12*, 1600408. [CrossRef] [PubMed]

63. Argyo, C.; Weiss, V.; Bräuchle, C.; Bein, T. Multifunctional mesoporous silica nanoparticles as a universal platform for drug delivery. *Chem. Mater.* **2013**, *26*, 435–451. [CrossRef]
64. Vallet-Regí, M.; Colilla, M.; Izquierdo-Barba, I.; Manzano, M. Mesoporous silica nanoparticles for drug delivery: Current insights. *Molecules* **2018**, *23*, 47. [CrossRef] [PubMed]
65. Yang, Y.; Yu, C. Advances in silica based nanoparticles for targeted cancer therapy. *Nanomed. Nanotechnol. Biol. Med.* **2016**, *12*, 317–332. [CrossRef]
66. Folkman, J. Role of angiogenesis in tumor growth and metastasis. *Semin. Oncol.* **2002**, *29*, 15–18. [CrossRef]
67. Carmeliet, P.; Jain, R.K. Angiogenesis in cancer and other diseases. *Nature* **2000**, *407*, 249–257. [CrossRef]
68. Wilhelm, S.; Tavares, A.J.; Dai, Q.; Ohta, S.; Audet, J.; Dvorak, H.F.; Chan, W.C.W. Analysis of nanoparticle delivery to tumours. *Nat. Rev. Mater.* **2016**, *1*, 1–12. [CrossRef]
69. Fang, J.; Nakamura, H.; Maeda, H. The EPR effect: Unique features of tumor blood vessels for drug delivery, factors involved, and limitations and augmentation of the effect. *Adv. Drug Deliv. Rev.* **2011**, *63*, 136–151. [CrossRef]
70. Nakamura, H.; Fang, J.; Maeda, H. Development of next-generation macromolecular drugs based on the EPR effect: Challenges and pitfalls. *Expert Opin. Drug Del.* **2015**, *12*, 53–64. [CrossRef]
71. Lee, J.E.; Lee, N.; Kim, H.; Kim, J.; Choi, S.H.; Kim, J.H.; Kim, T.; Song, I.C.; Park, S.P.; Moon, W.K.; et al. Uniform mesoporous dye-doped silica nanoparticles decorated with multiple magnetite nanocrystals for simultaneous enhanced magnetic resonance imaging, fluorescence imaging, and drug delivery. *J. Am. Chem. Soc.* **2010**, *132*, 552–557. [CrossRef]
72. He, Q.; Zhang, Z.; Gao, F.; Li, Y.; Shi, J. *In vivo* biodistribution and urinary excretion of mesoporous silica nanoparticles: Effects of particle size and PEGylation. *Small* **2011**, *7*, 271–280. [CrossRef]
73. Zhu, Y.; Fang, Y.; Borchardt, L.; Kaskel, S. PEGylated hollow mesoporous silica nanoparticles as potential drug delivery vehicles. *Microporous Mesoporous Mater.* **2011**, *141*, 199–206. [CrossRef]
74. Meng, H.; Mai, W.X.; Zhang, H.; Xue, M.; Xia, T.; Lin, S.; Wang, X.; Zhao, Y.; Ji, Z.; Zink, J.I.; et al. Codelivery of an optimal Drug/siRNA combination using mesoporous silica nanoparticles to overcome drug resistance in breast cancer *in vitro* and *in vivo*. *ACS Nano* **2013**, *7*, 994–1005. [CrossRef]
75. Heldin, C.-H.; Rubin, K.; Pietras, K.; Östman, A. High interstitial fluid pressure-An obstacle in cancer therapy. *Nat. Rev. Cancer* **2004**, *4*, 806–813. [CrossRef]
76. Vyas, S.P.; Singh, A.; Sihorkar, V. Ligand-receptor-mediated drug delivery: An emerging paradigm in cellular drug targeting. *Crit. Rev. Ther. Drug Carrier Syst.* **2001**, *18*, 1–76. [CrossRef]
77. Ruoslahti, E.; Bhatia, S.N.; Sailor, M.J. Targeting of drugs and nanoparticles to tumors. *J. Cell Biol.* **2010**, *188*, 759–768. [CrossRef]
78. Parker, N.; Turk, M.J.; Westrick, E.; Lewis, J.D.; Low, P.S.; Leamon, C.P. Folate receptor expression in carcinomas and normal tissues determined by a quantitative radioligand binding assay. *Anal. Biochem.* **2005**, *338*, 284–293. [CrossRef]
79. Porta, F.; Lamers, G.E.M.; Morrhayim, J.; Chatzopoulou, A.; Schaaf, M.; den Dulk, H.; Backendorf, C.; Zink, J.I.; Kros, A. Folic acid-modified mesoporous silica nanoparticles for cellular and nuclear targeted drug delivery. *Adv. Healthc. Mater.* **2013**, *2*, 281–286. [CrossRef]
80. Zwicke, G.H.; Mansoori, G.A.; Jeffery, C.J. Utilizing the folate receptor for active targeting of cancer nanotherapeutics. *Nano Reviews* **2012**, *3*, 18496. [CrossRef] [PubMed]
81. Cheung, A.; Bax, H.J.; Josephs, D.H.; Ilieva, K.M.; Pellizzari, G.; Opzoomer, J.; Bloomfield, J.; Fittall, M.; Grigoriadis, A.; Figini, M.; et al. Targeting folate receptor alpha for cancer treatment. *Oncotarget* **2016**, *7*, 52553–52574. [CrossRef]
82. Slowing, I.; Trewyn, B.G.; Lin, V.S.Y. Effect of surface functionalization of MCM-41-type mesoporous silica nanoparticles on the endocytosis by human cancer cells. *J. Am. Chem. Soc.* **2006**, *128*, 14792–14793. [CrossRef]
83. Khosravian, P.; Ardestani, M.S.; Mehdi Khoobi, M.; Ostad, S.N.; Dorkoosh, F.A.; Javar, H.A.; Amanlou, M Mesoporous silica nanoparticles functionalized with folic acid/methionine for active targeted delivery of docetaxel. *Onco.Targets Ther.* **2016**, *9*, 7315–7330. [CrossRef]
84. Yinxuea, S.; Binb, Z.; Xiangyang, D.; Yong, W.; Jie, Z.; Yanqiu, A.; Zongjiang, X.; Gaofenge, Z. Folic acid (FA)-conjugated mesoporous silica nanoparticles combined with MRP-1 siRNA improves the suppressive effects of myricetin on non-small cell lung cancer (NSCLC). *Biomed. Pharmacother.* **2020**, *125*, 109561 [CrossRef]

85. Zheng, G.; Shen, Y.; Zhao, R.; Chen, F.; Zhang, F.; Xu, A.; Shao, A. Dual-Targeting Multifuntional Mesoporous Silica Nanocarrier for Codelivery of siRNA and Ursolic Acid to Folate Receptor Overexpressing Cancer Cells. *J. Agric. Food Chem.* **2017**, *65*, 6904–6911. [CrossRef]
86. Zhao, S.; Sun, S.; Jiang, K.; Wang, Y.; Liu, Y.; Wu, S.; Li, Z.; Shu, Q.; Lin, H. In Situ Synthesis of Fluorescent Mesoporous Silica–Carbon Dot Nanohybrids Featuring Folate Receptor Overexpressing Cancer Cell Targeting and Drug Delivery. *Nano-Micro Lett.* **2019**, *11*, 32. [CrossRef]
87. Lu, J.; Li, Z.; Zink, J.I.; Tamanoi, F. *In vivo* tumor suppression efficacy of mesoporous silica nanoparticles-based drug-delivery system: Enhanced efficacy by folate modification. *Nanomedicine* **2012**, *8*, 212–220. [CrossRef]
88. López, V.; Villegas, M.R.; Rodríguez, V.; Villaverde, G.; Lozano, D.; Baeza, A.; Vallet-Regí, M. Janus mesoporous silica nanoparticles for dual targeting of tumor cells and mitochondria. *ACS Appl. Mater. Interfaces.* **2017**, *9*, 26697–26706. [CrossRef]
89. Rosenholm, J.M.; Peuhu, E.; Bate-Eya, L.T.; Eriksson, J.E.; Sahlgren, C.; Linden, M. Cancer-cell-specific induction of apoptosis using mesoporous silica nanoparticles as drug-delivery vectors. *Small* **2010**, *6*, 1234–1241. [CrossRef]
90. Daniels, T.R.; Bernabeu, E.; Rodríguez, J.A.; Patel, S.; Kozman, M.; Chiappetta, D.A.; Holler, E.; Ljubimova, J.Y.; Helguera, G.; Penicheta, M.L. Transferrin receptors and the targeted delivery of therapeutic agents against cancer. *Biochim. Biophys. Acta.* **2012**, *1820*, 291–317. [CrossRef]
91. Shen, Y.; Li, X.; Dong, D.; Zhang, B.; Xue, Y.; Shang, P. The review of TFR1 in cancer. *Am. J. Cancer Res.* **2018**, *8*, 916–931.
92. Jang, M.; Oh, I. Targeted drug delivery of Transferrin-Conjugated Mesoporous Silica Nanoparticles. *Yakhak Hoeji* **2017**, *61*, 241–247. [CrossRef]
93. Ferris, D.P.; Lu, J.; Gothard, C.; Yanes, R.; Thomas, C.R.; Olsen, J.C.; Stoddart, J.F.; Tamanoi, F.; Zink, J.I. Synthesis of Biomolecule-Modified Mesoporous Silica Nanoparticles for Targeted Hydrophobic Drug Delivery to Cancer Cells. *Small* **2011**, *7*, 1816–1826. [CrossRef]
94. Montalvo-Quiros, S.; Aragoneses-Cazorla, G.; Garcia-Alcalde, L.; Vallet-Regí, M.; González, B.; Luque-Garcia, J.L. Cancer cell targeting and therapeutic delivery of silver nanoparticles by mesoporous silica nanocarrirs: Insights into the action mechanisms using quantitative proteomics. *Nanoscale* **2019**, *11*, 4531–4545. [CrossRef]
95. Ke, Y.; Xiang, C. Transferrin receptor-targeted hMsN for sorafenib delivery in refractory differentiated thyroid cancer therapy. *Int. J. Nanomed.* **2018**, *13*, 8339–8354. [CrossRef]
96. Sun, T.; Wu, H.; Li, Y.; Huang, Y.; Yao, L.; Chen, X.; Han, X.; Zhou, Y.; Du, Z. Targeting transferrin receptor delivery of temozolomide for a potential glioma stem cell-mediated therapy. *Oncotarget* **2017**, *8*, 74451–74465. [CrossRef]
97. Luo, M.; Lewik, G.; Ratcliffe, J.C.; Choi, C.H.J.; Mäkilä, E.; Tong, W.Y.; Voelcker, N.H. Systematic evaluation of transferrin-modified porous silicon nanoparticles for targeted delivery of doxorubicin to glioblastoma. *ACS Appl. Mater. Interfaces* **2019**, *11*, 33637–33649. [CrossRef]
98. Sheykhzadeh, S.; Luo, M.; Peng, B.; White, J.; Abdalla, Y.; Tang, T.; Mäkilä, E.; Voelcker, N.H.; Tong, W.Y. Transferrin-targeted porous silicon nanoparticles reduce glioblastoma cell migration across tight extracellular space. *Sci. Rep.* **2020**, *10*, 2320. [CrossRef]
99. Barui, S.; Saha, S.; Yakati, V.; Chaudhuri, A. Systemic co-delivery of a homo-serine derived ceramide analog and curcumin to tumor vasculature inhibits mouse tumor growth. *Mol. Pharm.* **2016**, *13*, 404–419. [CrossRef]
100. Dal Corso, A.; Pignataro, L.; Belvisi, L.; Gennari, C. $\alpha v\beta 3$ Integrin-Targeted Peptide/Peptidomimetic-Drug Conjugates: In-Depth Analysis of the Linker Technology. *Curr. Top. Med. Chem.* **2016**, *16*, 314–329. [CrossRef]
101. Fang, I.J.; Slowing, I.I.; Wu, K.C.; Lin, V.S.; Trewyn, B.G. Ligand conformation dictates membrane and endosomal trafficking of arginine-glycine-aspartate (RGD)-functionalized mesoporous silica nanoparticles. *Chemistry* **2012**, *18*, 7787–7792. [CrossRef]
102. Hu, H.; You, Y.; He, L.; Chen, T. The rational design of NAMI-A-loaded mesoporous silica nanoparticles as antiangiogenic nanosystems. *J. Mater. Chem. B* **2015**, *3*, 6338–6346.
103. Hu, H.; Arena, F.; Gianolio, E.; Boffa, C.; di Gregorio, E.; Stefania, R.; Orio, L.; Baroni, S.; Aime, S. Mesoporous silica nanoparticles functionalized with fluorescent and MRI reporters for the visualization of murine tumors overexpressing $\alpha v\beta 3$ receptors. *Nanoscale* **2016**, *8*, 7094–7104. [CrossRef]

104. Sun, J.; Kim, D.H.; Guo, Y.; Teng, Z.; Li, Y.; Zheng, L.; Zhang, Z.; Larson, A.C.; Lu, G. A c(RGDfE) conjugated multi-functional nanomedicine delivery system for targeted pancreatic cancer therapy. *J. Mater. Chem. B* **2015**, *3*, 1049–1058. [CrossRef]
105. Chakravarty, R.; Goel, S.; Hong, H.; Chen, F.; Valdovinos, H.F.; Hernandez, R.; Barnhart, T.E.; Cai, W. Hollow mesoporous silica nanoparticles for tumor vasculature targeting and PET image-guided drug delivery. *Nanomedicine (Lond).* **2015**, *10*, 1233–1246. [CrossRef]
106. Mo, J.; He, L.; Ma, B.; Chen, T. Tailoring Particle Size of Mesoporous Silica Nanosystem To Antagonize Glioblastoma and Overcome Blood-Brain Barrier. *ACS Appl. Mater. Interfaces* **2016**, *8*, 6811–6825. [CrossRef]
107. Pan, L.; Liu, J.; He, Q.; Shi, J. MSN-mediated sequential vascular-to-cell nuclear-targeted drug delivery for efficient tumor regression. *Adv. Mater.* **2014**, *26*, 6742–6748. [CrossRef]
108. Kari, C.; Chan, T.O.; Rocha de Quadros, M.; Rodeck, U. Targeting the epidermal growth factor receptor in cancer: Apoptosis takes center stage. *Cancer Res.* **2003**, *63*, 1–5.
109. Sharma, S.V.; Bell, D.W.; Settleman, J.; Haber, D.A. Epidermal growth factor receptor mutations in lung cancer. *Nat. Rev. Cancer.* **2007**, *7*, 169–181. [CrossRef]
110. She, X.; Chen, L.; Velleman, L.; Li, C.; He, C.; Denman, J.; Wang, T.; Shigdar, S.; Duanc, W.; Kong, L. The control of epidermal growth factor grafted on mesoporous silica nanoparticles for targeted delivery. *J. Mater. Chem. B* **2015**, *3*, 6094. [CrossRef]
111. Sundarraj, S. Targeting efficiency and biodistribution of EGFR-conjugated mesoporous silica nanoparticles for cisplatin delivery in nude mice with lung cancer. *Ann. Oncol.* **2012**, *23*, ix70–ix71. [CrossRef]
112. Wang, Y.; Huang, H.; Yang, L.; Zhang, Z.; Ji, H. Cetuximab-modified mesoporous silica nano-medicine specifically targets EGFR-mutant lung cancer and overcomes drug resistance. *Sci. Rep.* **2016**, *6*, 25468. [CrossRef]
113. Iqbal, N.; Iqbal, N. Human epidermal growth factor receptor 2 (HER2) in cancers: Overexpression and therapeutic implications. *Mol. Biol. Int.* **2014**, *2014*, 852748. [CrossRef] [PubMed]
114. Orphanos, G.; Kountourakis, P. Targeting the HER2 receptor in metastatic breast cancer. *Hematol. Oncol. Stem Cell Ther.* **2012**, *5*, 127–137. [CrossRef] [PubMed]
115. Tsai, C.; Chen, C.; Hung, Y.; Changb, F.; Mou, C. Monoclonal antibody-functionalized mesoporous silicananoparticles (MSN) for selective targeting breast cancer cells. *J. Mater. Chem.* **2009**, *19*, 5737–5743. [CrossRef]
116. Ellis, L.M.; Hicklin, D.J. VEGF-targeted therapy: Mechanisms of anti-tumour activity. *Nat. Rev. Cancer* **2008**, *8*, 579–591. [CrossRef]
117. Costache, M.I.; Ioana, M.; Iordache, S.; Ene, D.; Costache, C.A.; Săftoiu, A. VEGF Expression in Pancreatic Cancer and Other Malignancies: A Review of the Literature. *Rom. J. Intern. Med.* **2015**, *53*, 199–208. [CrossRef]
118. Goel, S.; Chen, F.; Hong, H.; Valdovinos, H.F.; Barnhart, T.E.; Cai, W. VEGFR-targeted drug delivery in vivo with mesoporous silica nanoparticles. *J. Nucl. Med.* **2014**, *55* (Suppl. 1), 222.
119. Goel, S.; Chen, F.; Hong, H.; Valdovinos, H.F.; Hernandez, R.; Shi, S.; Barnhart, T.E.; Cai, W. $VEGF_{121}$-Conjugated Mesoporous Silica Nanoparticle: A Tumor Targeted Drug Delivery System. *ACS Appl. Mater. Interfaces* **2014**, *6*, 21677–21685. [CrossRef]
120. Zhang, R.; Zhang, Y.; Tan, J.; Wang, H.; Zhang, G.; Li, N.; Meng, Z.; Zhang, F.; Chang, J.; Wang, R. Antitumor effect of 131i-labeled anti-Vegfr2 targeted mesoporous silica nanoparticles in anaplastic thyroid cancer. *Nanoscale Res. Lett.* **2019**, *14*, 96. [CrossRef]
121. Scodeller, P.; Simón-Gracia, L.; Kopanchuk, S.; Tobi, A.; Kilk, K.; Säälik, P.; Kaarel Kurm, K.; Squadrito, M.L.; Kotamraju, V.R.; Rinken, A.; et al. Precision targeting of tumor macrophages with a CD206 binding peptide. *Sci. Rep.* **2017**, *7*, 14655. [CrossRef] [PubMed]
122. Park, I.Y.; Kim, I.Y.; Yoo, M.K.; Choi, Y.J.; Cho, M.H.; Cho, C.S. Mannosylated polyethylenimine coupled mesoporous silica nanoparticles for receptor-mediated gene delivery. *Int. J. Pharm.* **2008**, *359*, 280–287. [CrossRef] [PubMed]
123. Chen, N.-T.; Souris, J.S.; Cheng, S.-H.; Chu, C.-H.; Wang, Y.-C.; Konda, V.; Dougherty, U.; Bissonnette, M.; Mou, C.-Y.; Chen, C.-T.; et al. Lectin-functionalized mesoporous silica nanoparticles for endoscopic detection of premalignant colonic lesions. *Nanomed. Nanotechnol. Biol. Med.* **2017**, *13*, 1941–1952. [CrossRef]
124. Guo, X.; Guo, N.; Zhao, J.; Cai, Y. Active targeting co-delivery system based on hollow mesoporous silica nanoparticles for antitumor therapy in ovarian cancer stem-like cells. *Oncol. Rep.* **2017**, *38*, 1442–1450. [CrossRef] [PubMed]

125. Quan, G.; Pan, X.; Wang, Z.; Wu, Q.; Li, G.; Dian, L.; Chen, B.; Wu, C. Lactosaminated mesoporous silica nanoparticles for asialoglycoprotein receptor targeted anticancer drug delivery. *J. Nanobiotechnol.* **2015**, *13*. [CrossRef] [PubMed]
126. Paramonov, V.M.; Desai, D.; Kettiger, H.; Mamaeva, V.; Rosenholm, J.M.; Sahlgren, C.; Rivero-Müller, A. Targeting somatostatin receptors by functionalized mesoporous silica nanoparticles—are we striking home? *Nanotheranostics* **2018**, *2*, 320–346. [CrossRef] [PubMed]
127. Zhang, M.; Xu, C.; Wen, L.; Han, M.; Xiao, B.; Zhou, J.; Zhang, Y.; Zhang, Z.; Viennois, E.; Merlin, D. A hyaluronidase-responsive nanoparticle-based drug delivery system for targeting colon cancer cells. *Cancer Res.* **2016**, *76*, 7208–7218. [CrossRef] [PubMed]
128. Chen, F.; Hong, H.; Shi, S.; Goel, S.; Valdovinos, H.F.; Hernandez, R.; Theuer, C.P.; Barnhart, T.E.; Cai, W. Engineering of hollow mesoporous silica nanoparticles for remarkably enhanced tumor active targeting efficacy. *Sci. Rep.* **2014**, *4*, 5080. [CrossRef]
129. Chen, F.; Nayak, T.R.; Goel, S.; Valdovinos, H.F.; Hong, H.; Theuer, C.P.; Barnhart, T.E.; Cai, W. *In vivo* tumor vasculature targeted PET/NIRF imaging with TRC105(Fab)-conjugated, dual-labeled mesoporous silica nanoparticles. *Mol. Pharm.* **2014**, *11*, 4007–4014. [CrossRef]
130. Sweeney, S.K.; Luo, Y.; O'Donnell, M.A.; Assouline, J.G. Peptide-Mediated Targeting Mesoporous Silica Nanoparticles: A Novel Tool for Fighting Bladder Cancer. *J. Biomed. Nanotechnol.* **2017**, *13*, 232–242. [CrossRef]
131. Hicke, B.J.; Stephens, A.W.; Gould, T.; Chang, Y.-F.; Lynott, C.K.; Heil, J.; Borkowski, S.; Hilger, C.-S.; Cook, G.; Warren, S.; et al. Tumor targeting by an aptamer. *J. Nucl. Med.* **2006**, *47*, 668–678.
132. Yang, Y.; Zhao, W.; Tan, W.; Lai, Z.; Fang, D.; Jiang, L.; Zuo, C.; Yang, N.; Lai, Y. An efficient cell-targeting drug delivery system based on aptamer-modified mesoporous silica nanoparticles. *Nanoscale Res. Lett.* **2019**, *14*, 390. [CrossRef]
133. Nguyen, T.L.; Cha, B.G.; Choi, Y.; Im, J.; Kim, J. Injectable dual-scale mesoporous silica cancer vaccine enabling efficient delivery of antigen/adjuvant-loaded nanoparticles to dendritic cells recruited in local macroporous scaffold. *Biomaterials* **2020**, *239*, 119859. [CrossRef] [PubMed]
134. Mekaru, H.; Lu, J.; Tamanoi, F. Development of mesoporous silica-based nanoparticles with controlled release capability for cancer therapy. *Adv. Drug Deliv. Rev.* **2015**, *95*, 40–49. [CrossRef] [PubMed]
135. Vivero-Escoto, J.L.; Slowing, I.I.; Trewyn, B.G.; Lin, V.S.Y. Mesoporous silica nanoparticles for intracellular controlled drug delivery. *Small* **2010**, *6*, 1952–1967. [CrossRef] [PubMed]
136. Gatenby, R.A.; Gillies, R.J. Why do cancers have high aerobic glycolysis? *Nat. Rev. Cancer* **2004**, *4*, 891–899. [CrossRef]
137. Liu, R.; Zhang, Y.; Zhao, X.; Agarwal, A.; Mueller, L.J.; Feng, P. pH-responsive nanogated ensemble based on gold-capped mesoporous silica through an acid-labile acetal linker. *J. Am. Chem. Soc.* **2010**, *132*, 1500–1501. [CrossRef]
138. Gan, Q.; Lu, X.; Yuan, Y.; Qian, J.; Zhou, H.; Lu, X.; Shi, J.; Liu, C. A magnetic, reversible pH-responsive nanogated ensemble based on Fe_3O_4 nanoparticles-capped mesoporous silica. *Biomaterials* **2011**, *32*, 1932–1942. [CrossRef]
139. Xu, C.; Lin, Y.; Wang, J.; Wu, L.; Wei, W.; Ren, J.; Qu, X. Nanoceria-triggered synergetic drug release based on CeO_2-capped mesoporous silica host-guest interactions and switchable enzymatic activity and cellular effects of CeO_2. *Adv. Healthc. Mater.* **2013**, *2*, 1591–1599. [CrossRef]
140. Meng, H.; Xue, M.; Xia, T.; Zhao, Y.L.; Tamanoi, F.; Stoddart, J.F.; Zink, J.I.; Nel, A.E. Autonomous *in vitro* anti cancer drug release from mesoporous silica nanoparticles by pH-sensitive nanovalves. *J. Am. Chem. Soc.* **2010**, *132*, 12690–12697. [CrossRef]
141. Gao, Y.; Yang, C.; Liu, X.; Ma, R.; Kong, D.; Shi, L. A multifunctional nanocarrier based on nanogated mesoporous silica for enhanced tumor-specific uptake and intracellular delivery. *Macromol. Biosci.* **2012**, *12*, 251–259. [CrossRef]
142. Lee, C.H.; Cheng, S.H.; Huang, I.P.; Souris, J.S.; Yang, C.S.; Mou, C.Y.; Lo, L.W. Intracellular pH-responsive mesoporous silica nanoparticles for the controlled release of anticancer chemotherapeutics. *Angew. Chem.* **2010**, *122*, 8390–8395. [CrossRef]
143. Li, T.; Chen, X.; Liu, Y.; Fan, L.; Lin, L.; Xu, Y.; Chen, S.; Shao, J. pH-Sensitive mesoporous silica nanoparticles anticancer prodrugs for sustained release of ursolic acid and the enhanced anti-cancer efficacy for hepatocellular carcinoma cancer. *Eur. J. Pharm. Sci.* **2017**, *96*, 456–463. [CrossRef] [PubMed]

144. Feng, W.; Zhou, X.; He, C.; Qiu, K.; Nie, W.; Chen, L.; Wang, H.; Mo, X.; Zhang, Y. Polyelectrolyte multilayer functionalized mesoporous silica nanoparticles for pH-responsive drug delivery: Layer thickness dependent release profiles and biocompatibility. *J. Mater. Chem. B* **2013**, *1*, 5886–5898. [CrossRef] [PubMed]
145. Cauda, V.; Argyo, C.; Schlossbauera, A.; Bein, T. Controlling the delivery kinetics from colloidal mesoporous silicananoparticles with pH-sensitive gates. *J. Mater. Chem.* **2010**, *20*, 4305–4311. [CrossRef]
146. Tang, H.; Guo, J.; Sun, Y.; Chang, B.; Ren, Q.; Yang, W. Facile synthesis of pH sensitive polymer-coated mesoporous silica nanoparticles and their application in drug delivery. *Int. J. Pharm.* **2011**, *421*, 388–396. [CrossRef]
147. Popat, A.; Liu, J.; Lu, G.Q.M.; Qiao, S.Z. A pH-responsive drug delivery system based on chitosan coated mesoporous silica nanoparticles. *J. Mater. Chem.* **2012**, *22*, 11173–11178. [CrossRef]
148. Xiong, L.; Bi, J.; Tang, Y.; Qiao, S.Z. Magnetic Core-Shell Silica Nanoparticles with Large Radial Mesopores for siRNA Delivery. *Small* **2016**, *12*, 4735–4742. [CrossRef]
149. Gisbert-Garzarán, M.; Lozano, D.; Vallet-Regí, M.; Manzano, M. Self-immolative polymers as novel pH-responsive gatekeepers for drug delivery. *RSC Adv.* **2017**, *7*, 132–136. [CrossRef]
150. Yuan, L.; Tang, Q.; Yang, D.; Zhang, J.Z.; Zhang, F.; Hu, J. Preparation of pH-responsive mesoporous silica nanoparticles and their application in controlled drug delivery. *J. Phys. Chem. C* **2011**, *115*, 9926–9932. [CrossRef]
151. Muhammad, F.; Guo, M.; Qi, W.; Sun, F.; Wang, A.; Guo, Y.; Zhu, G. pH-triggered controlled drug release from mesoporous silica nanoparticles via intracelluar dissolution of ZnO nanolids. *J. Am. Chem. Soc.* **2011**, *133*, 8778–8781. [CrossRef]
152. Zou, Z.; He, D.; He, X.; Wang, K.; Yang, X.; Qing, Z.; Zhou, Q. Natural Gelatin Capped Mesoporous Silica Nanoparticles for Intracellular Acid-Triggered Drug Delivery. *Langmuir* **2013**, *29*, 12804–12810. [CrossRef] [PubMed]
153. Rim, H.P.; Min, K.H.; Lee, H.J.; Jeong, S.Y.; Lee, S.C. pH-tunable calcium phosphate covered mesoporous silica nanocontainers for intracellular controlled release of guest drugs. *Angew. Chem. Int. Ed.* **2011**, *50*, 8853–8857. [CrossRef]
154. Wibowo, F.R.; Saputra, O.A.; Lestari, W.W.; Koketsu, M.; Mukti, R.R.; Martien, R. pH-triggered drug release controlled by poly(styrene sulfonate) growth hollow mesoporous silica nanoparticles. *ACS Omega* **2020**, *5*, 4261–4269. [CrossRef]
155. Estrela, J.M.; Ortega, A.; Obrador, E. Glutathione in cancer biology and therapy. *Crit. Rev. Clin. Lab. Sci.* **2006**, *43*, 143–181. [CrossRef]
156. Croissant, J.; Cattoën, X.; Man, M.W.; Gallud, A.; Raehm, L.; Trens, P.; Maynadier, M.; Durand, J.O. Biodegradable ethylene-bis (Propyl) disulfide-based periodic mesoporous organosilica nanorods and nanospheres for efficient *in-vitro* drug delivery. *Adv. Mater.* **2014**, *26*, 6174–6180. [CrossRef]
157. Wang, D.; Xu, Z.; Chen, Z.; Liu, X.; Hou, C.; Zhang, X.; Zhang, H. Fabrication of single-hole glutathione-responsive degradable hollow silica nanoparticles for drug delivery. *ACS Appl. Mater. Interfaces* **2014**, *6*, 12600–12608. [CrossRef]
158. Kim, H.; Kim, S.; Park, C.; Lee, H.; Park, H.J.; Kim, C. Glutathione-induced intracellular release of guests from mesoporous silica nanocontainers with cyclodextrin gatekeepers. *Adv. Mater.* **2010**, *22*, 4280–4283. [CrossRef]
159. Sauer, A.M.; Schlossbauer, A.; Ruthardt, N.; Cauda, V.; Bein, T.; Bräuchle, C. Role of endosomal escape for disulfide-based drug delivery from colloidal mesoporous silica evaluated by live-cell imaging. *Nano Lett.* **2010**, *10*, 3684–3691. [CrossRef]
160. Wu, M.; Meng, Q.; Chen, Y.; Zhang, L.; Li, M.; Cai, X.; Li, Y.; Yu, P.; Zhang, L.; Shi, J. Large pore-sized hollow mesoporous organosilica for redox-responsive gene delivery and synergistic cancer chemotherapy. *Adv. Mater.* **2016**, *28*, 1963–1969. [CrossRef]
161. Nadrah, P.; Maver, U.; Jemec, A.; Tišler, T.; Bele, M.; Dražić, G.; Benčina, M.; Pintar, A.; Planinšek, O.; Gaberšček, M. Hindered disulfide bonds to regulate release rate of model drug from mesoporous silica. *ACS Appl. Mater. Interfaces* **2013**, *5*, 3908–3915. [CrossRef]
162. Prasetyanto, E.A.; Bertucci, A.; Septiadi, D.; Corradini, R.; Castro-Hartmann, P.; de Cola, L. Breakable hybrid organosilica nanocapsules for protein delivery. *Angew. Chem. Int. Ed.* **2016**, *55*, 3323–3327. [CrossRef]
163. Du, X.; Kleitz, F.; Li, X.; Huang, H.; Zhang, X.; Qiao, S.Z. Disulfide-bridged organosilica frameworks: Designed, synthesis, redox-triggered biodegradation, and nanobiomedical applications. *Adv. Funct. Mater.* **2018**, 1707325. [CrossRef]

164. Liu, R.; Zhao, X.; Wu, T.; Feng, P. Tunable Redox-Responsive Hybrid Nanogated Ensembles. *J. Am. Chem. Soc.* **2008**, *130*, 14418–14419. [CrossRef]
165. Sun, L.; Liu, Y.J.; Yang, Z.Z.; Qi, X.R. Tumor specific delivery with redox-triggered mesoporous silica nanoparticles inducing neovascularization suppression and vascular normalization. *RSC Adv.* **2015**, *5*, 55566–55578. [CrossRef]
166. Teng, Z.; Li, W.; Tang, Y.; Elzatahry, A.; Lu, G.; Zhao, D. Mesoporous organosilica hollow nanoparticles: Synthesis and applications. *Adv. Mater.* **2018**, 1707612. [CrossRef]
167. Patel, K.; Angelos, S.; Dichtel, W.R.; Coskun, A.; Yang, Y.-W.; Zink, J.I.; Stoddart, J.F. Enzyme responsive snap-top covered silica nanocontainers. *J. Am. Chem. Soc.* **2008**, *130*, 2382–2383. [CrossRef]
168. Mondragón, L.; Mas, N.; Ferragud, V.; de la Torre, C.; Agostini, A.; Martínez-Máñez, R.; Sancenón, F.; Amorós, P.; Pérez-Payá, E.; Orzáez, M. Enzyme-responsive intracellular-controlled release using silica mesoporous nanoparticles capped with ε-poly-L-lysine. *Chemistry* **2014**, *20*, 5271–5281. [CrossRef]
169. Bernardos, A.; Mondragón, L.; Aznar, E.; Marcos, M.D.; Martínez-Mánez, R.; Sancenón, F.; Soto, J.; Barat, J.M.; Pérez-Payá, E.; Guillem, C.; et al. Enzyme-responsive intracellular controlled release using nanometric silica mesoporous supports capped with "saccharides". *ACS Nano* **2010**, *4*, 6353–6368. [CrossRef]
170. Schlossbauer, A.; Kecht, J.; Bein, T. Biotin-Avidin as a protease-responsive cap system for controlled guest release from colloidal mesoporous silica. *Angew. Chem. Int. Ed.* **2009**, *48*, 3092–3095. [CrossRef]
171. Radhakrishnan, K.; Gupta, S.; Gnanadhas, D.P.; Ramamurthy, P.C.; Chakravortty, D.; Raichur, A.M. Protamine-capped mesoporous silica nanoparticles for biologically triggered drug release. *Part. Part. Syst. Charact.* **2013**, *31*, 449–458. [CrossRef]
172. Xua, J.-H.; Gao, F.-P.; Li, L.-L.; Ma, H.L.; Fan, Y.-S.; Liu, W.; Guo, S.-S.; Zhao, X.-Z.; Wang, H. Gelatin-mesoporous silica nanoparticles as matrix metalloproteinases-degradable drug delivery systems in vivo. *Microporous Mesoporous Mater.* **2015**, *204*, 226–234. [CrossRef]
173. Van Rijt, S.H.; Bölükbas, D.A.; Argyo, C.; Datz, S.; Lindner, M.; Eickelberg, O.; Königshoff, M.; Bein, T.; Meiners, S. Protease-mediated release of chemotherapeutics from mesoporous silica nanoparticles to ex vivo human and mouse lung tumors. *ACS Nano* **2015**, *9*, 2377–2389. [CrossRef]
174. Singh, N.; Karambelkar, A.; Gu, L.; Lin, K.; Miller, J.S.; Chen, C.S.; Sailor, M.J.; Bhatia, S.N. Bioresponsive mesoporous silica nanoparticles for triggered drug release. *J. Am. Chem. Soc.* **2011**, *133*, 19582–19585. [CrossRef]
175. Park, C.; Kim, H.; Kim, S.; Kim, C. Enzyme responsive nanocontainers with cyclodextrin gatekeepers and synergistic effects in release of guests. *J. Am. Chem. Soc.* **2009**, *131*, 16614–16615. [CrossRef]
176. Baeza, A.; Guisasola, E.; Torres-Pardo, A.; González-Calbet, J.M.; Melen, G.J.; Ramirez, M.; Vallet-Regí, M. Hybrid enzyme-polymeric capsules/mesoporous silica nanodevice for in situ cytotoxic agent generation. *Adv. Funct. Mater.* **2014**, *24*, 4625–4633. [CrossRef]
177. Mura, S.; Nicolas, J.; Couvreur, P. Stimuli-responsive nanocarriers for drug delivery. *Nat. Mater.* **2013**, *12*, 991–1003. [CrossRef]
178. Arcos, D.; Fal-Miyar, V.; Ruiz-Hernández, E.; García-Hernández, M.; Ruiz-González, M.L.; González-Calbet, J.; Vallet-Regí, M. Supramolecular mechanisms in the synthesis of mesoporous magnetic nanospheres for hyperthermia. *J. Mater. Chem.* **2012**, *22*, 64–72. [CrossRef]
179. Chen, P.-J.; Hu, S.-H.; Hsiao, C.-S.; Chen, Y.-Y.; Liu, D.-M.; Chen, S.-Y. Multifunctional magnetically removable nanogated lids of Fe3O4–capped mesoporous silica nanoparticles for intracellular controlled release and MR imaging. *J. Mater. Chem.* **2011**, *21*, 2535. [CrossRef]
180. Thomas, C.R.; Ferris, D.P.; Lee, J.H.; Choi, E.; Cho, M.H.; Kim, E.S.; Stoddart, J.F.; Shin, J.S.; Cheon, J.; Zink, J.I. Noninvasive remote-controlled release of drug molecules *in vitro* using magnetic actuation of mechanized nanoparticles. *J. Am. Chem. Soc.* **2010**, *132*, 10623–10625. [CrossRef] [PubMed]
181. Guisasola, E.; Baeza, A.; Talelli, M.; Arcos, D.; Vallet-Regí, M. Design of thermoresponsive polymeric gates with opposite controlled release behaviors. *RSC Adv.* **2016**, *6*, 42510–42516. [CrossRef]
182. Guisasola, E.; Baeza, A.; Talelli, M.; Arcos, D.; Moros, M.; de la Fuente, J.M.; Vallet-Regí, M. Magnetic Responsive Release Controlled by Hot Spot Effect. *Langmuir.* **2015**, *31*, 12777–12782. [CrossRef] [PubMed]
183. Baeza, A.; Guisasola, E.; Ruiz-Hernández, E.; Vallet-Regí, M. Magnetically triggered multidrug release by hybrid mesoporous silica nanoparticles. *Chem. Mater.* **2012**, *24*, 517–524. [CrossRef]

184. Cai, D.; Liu, L.; Han, C.; Ma, X.; Qian, J.; Zhou, J.; Zhu, W. Cancer cell membrane-coated mesoporous silica loaded with superparamagnetic ferroferric oxide and paclitaxel for the combination of chemo/Magnetocaloric therapy on MDA-MB-231 cells. *Sci. Rep.* **2019**, *9*, 14475. [CrossRef]
185. Chen, Y.; Wang, X.; Liu, T.; Zhang, D.S.; Wang, Y.; Gu, H.; Di, W. Highly effective antiangiogenesis via magnetic mesoporous silica-based siRNA vehicle targeting the VEGF gene for orthotopic ovarian cancer therapy. *Int. J. Nanomed.* **2015**, *10*, 2579–2594.
186. Ruiz-Hernández, E.; Baeza, A.; Vallet-Regí, M. Smart drug delivery through DNA/magnetic nanoparticle gates. *ACS Nano* **2011**, *5*, 1259–1266. [CrossRef]
187. Mal, N.K.; Fujiwara, M.; Tanaka, Y. Photocontrolled reversible release of guest molecules from coumarin-modified mesoporous silica. *Nature* **2003**, *421*, 350–353. [CrossRef]
188. Ferris, D.P.; Zhao, Y.-L.; Khashab, N.M.; Khatib, H.A.; Stoddart, J.F.; Zink, J.I. Light-operated mechanized nanoparticles. *J. Am. Chem. Soc.* **2009**, *131*, 1686–1688. [CrossRef]
189. Yuan, Q.; Zhang, Y.; Chen, T.; Lu, D.; Zhao, Z.; Zhang, X.; Li, Z.; Yan, C.-H.; Tan, W. Photon-manipulated drug release from a mesoporous nanocontainer controlled by azobenzene-modified nucleic acid. *ACS Nano* **2012**, *6*, 6337–6344. [CrossRef]
190. Wang, Z.; Boudjelal, M.; Kang, S. Ultraviolet irradiation of human skin causes functional vitamin A deficiency, preventable by all-trans retinoic acid pre-treatment. *Nat. Med.* **1999**, *5*, 418–422. [CrossRef]
191. Shindo, Y.; Witt, E.; Packer, L. Antioxidant defense mechanisms in murine epidermis and dermis and their responses to ultraviolet light. *J. Investig. Dermatol.* **1993**, *100*, 260–265. [CrossRef]
192. Olejniczak, J.; Carling, C.J.; Almutairi, A. Photocontrolled release using one-photon absorption of visible or NIR light. *J. Control. Release* **2015**, *219*, 18–30. [CrossRef]
193. Martínez-Carmona, M.; Lozano, D.; Baeza, A.; Colilla, M.; Vallet-Regí, M. A novel visible light responsive nanosystem for cancer treatment. *Nanoscale* **2017**, *9*, 15967–15973. [CrossRef] [PubMed]
194. Guardado-Alvarez, T.M.; Sudha Devi, L.; Russell, M.M.; Schwartz, B.J.; Zink, J.I. Activation of snap-top capped mesoporous silica nanocontainers using two near-infrared photons. *J. Am. Chem. Soc.* **2013**, *135*, 14000–14003. [CrossRef] [PubMed]
195. Croissant, J.; Maynadier, M.; Gallud, A.; Peindy N'Dongo, H.; Nyalosaso, J.L.; Derrien, G.; Charnay, C.; Durand, J.O.; Raehm, L.; Serein-Spirau, F.; et al. Two-photon-triggered drug delivery in cancer cells using nanoimpellers. *Angew. Chem. Int. Ed.* **2013**, *52*, 13813–13817. [CrossRef] [PubMed]
196. Sirsi, S.R.; Borden, M.A. State-of-the-art materials for ultrasound-triggered drug delivery. *Adv. Drug Deliv. Rev.* **2014**, *72*, 3–14. [CrossRef]
197. Wang, J.; Pelletier, M.; Zhang, H.J.; Xia, H.S.; Zhao, Y. High-frequency ultrasound-responsive block copolymer micelle. *Langmuir* **2009**, *25*, 13201–13205. [CrossRef]
198. Xuan, J.; Boissière, O.; Zhao, Y.; Yan, B.; Tremblay, L.; Lacelle, S.; Xia, H.; Zhao, Y. Ultrasound-responsive block copolymer micelles based on a new amplification mechanism. *Langmuir* **2012**, *28*, 16463–16468. [CrossRef]
199. Wang, X.; Chen, H.; Chen, Y.; Ma, M.; Zhang, K.; Li, F.; Zheng, Y.; Zeng, D.; Wang, Q.; Shi, J. Perfluorohexane-encapsulated mesoporous silica nanocapsules as enhancement agents for highly efficient High Intensity focused Ultrasound (HIFU). *Adv. Mater.* **2012**, *24*, 785–791. [CrossRef]
200. Wang, X.; Chen, H.; Zheng, Y.; Ma, M.; Chen, Y.; Zhang, K.; Zeng, D.; Shi, J. Au-nanoparticle coated mesoporous silica nanocapsule-based multifunctional platform for ultrasound mediated imaging, cytoclasis and tumor ablation. *Biomaterials* **2013**, *34*, 2057–2068. [CrossRef]
201. Paris, J.L.; Cabañas, M.V.; Manzano, M.; Vallet-Regí, M. Polymer-grafted mesoporous silica nanoparticles as ultrasound-responsive drug carriers. *ACS Nano* **2015**, *9*, 11023–11033. [CrossRef]
202. Cauda, V.; Schlossbauer, A.; Kecht, J.; Zürner, A.; Bein, T. Multiple core-shell functionalized colloidal mesoporous silica nanoparticles. *J. Am. Chem. Soc.* **2009**, *131*, 11361–11370. [CrossRef]
203. Cauda, V.; Argyo, C.; Piercey, D.G.; Bein, T. "Liquid-phase calcination" of colloidal mesoporous silica nanoparticles in high-boiling solvents. *J. Am. Chem. Soc.* **2011**, *133*, 6484–6486. [CrossRef]
204. Tang, F.; Li, L.; Chen, D. Mesoporous silica nanoparticles: Synthesis, biocompatibility and drug delivery. *Adv. Mater.* **2012**, *24*, 1504–1534. [CrossRef]
205. Martínez-Carmona, M.; Colilla, M.; Vallet-Regí, M. Smart mesoporous nanomaterials for antitumor therapy. *Nanomaterials* **2015**, *5*, 1906–1937. [CrossRef]
206. Castillo, R.R.; Colilla, M.; Vallet-Regí, M. Advances in mesoporous silica-based nanocarriers for co-delivery and combination therapy against cancer. *Expert Opin. Drug Deliv.* **2017**, *14*, 229–243. [CrossRef]

207. Aquib, M.; Farooq, M.A.; Banerjee, P.; Akhtar, F.; Filli, M.S.; Boakye-Yiadom, K.O.; Kesse, S.; Raza, F.; Maviah, M.B.J.; Mavlyanova, R.; et al. Targeted and stimuli-responsive mesoporous silica nanoparticles for drug delivery and theranostic use. *J. Biomed. Mater. Res.* **2019**, *107A*, 2643–2666. [CrossRef]
208. Rosenholm, J.M.; Meinander, A.; Peuhu, E.; Niemi, R.; Eriksson, J.E.; Sahlgren, C.; Lindén, M. Targeting of Porous Hybrid Silica Nanoparticles to Cancer Cells. *ACS Nano* **2009**, *3*, 197–206. [CrossRef]
209. Sun, X.; Wang, N.; Yang, L.Y.; Ouyang, X.K.; Huang, F. Folic acid and pei modified mesoporous silica for targeted delivery of curcumin. *Pharmaceutics* **2019**, *11*, 430. [CrossRef]
210. Cheng, W.; Nie, J.; Xu, L.; Liang, C.; Peng, Y.; Liu, G.; Wang, T.; Mei, L.; Huang, L.; Zeng, X. A pH-sensitive delivery vehicle based on folic acid-conjugated polydopamine-modified mesoporous silica nanoparticles for targeted cancer therapy. *ACS Appl. Mater. Interfaces* **2017**, *9*, 18462–18473. [CrossRef]
211. Liu, X.; Yu, D.; Jin, C.; Song, X.; Cheng, J.; Zhao, X.; Qi, X.; Zhang, G. A dual responsive targeted drug delivery system based on smart polymer coated mesoporous silica for laryngeal carcinoma treatment. *New J. Chem.* **2014**, *38*, 4830–4836. [CrossRef]
212. Qi, X.; Yu, D.; Jia, B.; Jin, C.; Liu, X.; Zhao, X.; Zhang, G. Targeting CD133+ laryngeal carcinoma cells with chemotherapeutic drugs and siRNA against ABCG2 mediated by thermo/pH-sensitive mesoporous silica nanoparticles. *Tumor Biol.* **2016**, *37*, 2209–2217. [CrossRef]
213. Li, N.; Wang, Z.; Zhang, Y.; Zhang, K.; Xie, J.; Liu, Y.; Li, W.; Feng, N. Curcumin-loaded redox-responsive mesoporous silica nanoparticles for targeted breast cancer therapy. *Artif. Cells Nanomed. Biotechnol.* **2018**, *46*, 921–935. [CrossRef]
214. AbouAitah, K.; Hassan, H.A.; Swiderska-Sroda, A.; Gohar, L.; Shaker, O.G.; Wojnarowicz, J.; Opalinska, A.; Smalc-Koziorowska, J.; Gierlotka, S.; Lojkowski, W. Targeted nano-drug delivery of colchicine against colon cancer cells by means of mesoporous silica nanoparticles. *Cancers* **2020**, *12*, 144. [CrossRef]
215. Zhang, H.; Zhang, W.; Zhou, Y.; Jiang, Y.; Li, S. Dual functional mesoporous silicon nanoparticles enhance the radiosensitivity of VPA in glioblastoma. *Transl. Oncol.* **2017**, *10*, 229–240. [CrossRef]
216. Gao, Q.; Xie, W.; Wang, Y.; Wang, D.; Guo, Z.; Gao, F.; Zhao, L.; Cai, Q. A theranostic nanocomposite system based on radial mesoporous silica hybridized with Fe_3O_4 nanoparticles for targeted magnetic field responsive chemotherapy of breast cancer. *RSC Adv.* **2018**, *8*, 4321. [CrossRef]
217. Cao, Y.; Wu, C.; Liu, Y.; Hu, L.; Shang, W.; Gao, Z.; Xia, N. Folate functionalized pH-sensitive photothermal therapy traceable hollow mesoporous silica nanoparticles as a targeted drug carrier to improve the antitumor effect of doxorubicin in the hepatoma cell line SMMC-7721. *Drug Delivery* **2020**, *27*, 258–268. [CrossRef]
218. Paredes, K.O.; Díaz-García, D.; García-Almodóvar, V.; Chamizo, L.L.; Marciello, M.; Díaz-Sánchez, M.; Prashar, S.; Gómez-Ruiz, S.; Filice, M. Multifunctional silica-based nanoparticles with controlled release of organotin metallodrug for targeted theranosis of breast cancer. *Cancers* **2020**, *12*, 187. [CrossRef]
219. Alvarez-Berríos, M.P.; Vivero-Escoto, J.L. *In vitro* evaluation of folic acid-conjugated redox-responsive mesoporous silica nanoparticles for the delivery of cisplatin. *Int. J. Nanomed.* **2016**, *11*, 6251–6265. [CrossRef]
220. Saini, K.; Bandyopadhyaya, R. Transferrin-Conjugated Polymer-Coated Mesoporous Silica Nanoparticles Loaded with Gemcitabine for Killing Pancreatic Cancer Cells. *ACS Appl. Nano Mater.* **2020**, *3*, 229–240. [CrossRef]
221. Fang, W.; Wang, Z.; Zong, S.; Chen, H.; Zhu, D.; Zhong, Y.; Cui, Y. pH-controllable drug carrier with SERS activity for targeting cancer cells. *Biosens. Bioelectron.* **2014**, *57*, 10–15. [CrossRef]
222. Chen, X.; Sun, H.; Hu, J.; Han, X.; Liu, H.; Hu, Y. Transferrin gated mesoporous silica nanoparticles for redox-responsive and targeted drug delivery. *Colloids Surf. B Biointerfaces* **2017**, *152*, 77–84. [CrossRef]
223. Martínez-Carmona, M.; Baeza, A.; Rodriguez-Milla, M.A.; García-Castro, J.; Vallet-Regí, M. Mesoporous silica nanoparticles grafted with a light-responsive protein shell for highly cytotoxic antitumoral therapy. *J. Mater. Chem. B* **2015**, *3*, 5746–5752. [CrossRef]
224. Er, Ö.; Colak, S.G.; Ocakoglu, K.; Ince, M.; Bresolí-Obach, R.; Mora, M.; Sagristá, M.L.; Yurt, F.; Nonell, S. Selective photokilling of human pancreatic cancer cells using cetuximab-targeted mesoporous silica nanoparticles for delivery of zinc phthalocyanine. *Molecules* **2018**, *23*, 2749. [CrossRef] [PubMed]
225. Ngamcherdtrakul, W.; Morry, J.; Gu, S.; Castro, D.J.; Goodyear, S.M.; Sangvanich, T.; Reda, M.M.; Lee, R.; Mihelic, S.A.; Beckman, B.L.; et al. Cationic polymer modified mesoporous silica nanoparticles for targeted siRNA delivery to HER2 breast cancer. *Adv. Funct. Mater.* **2015**, *25*, 2646–2659. [CrossRef] [PubMed]

226. Shen, Y.; Li, M.; Liu, T.; Liu, J.; Youhua Xie, Y.; Zhang, J.; Xu, S.; Liu, H. A dual-functional HER2 aptamer-conjugated, pH-activated mesoporous silica nanocarrier-based drug delivery system provides *in vitro* synergistic cytotoxicity in HER2-positive breast cancer cells. *Int. J. Nanomed.* **2019**, *14*, 4029–4044. [CrossRef]
227. Liu, W.; Zhu, Y.; Wang, F.; Li, X.; Liu, X.; Pang, J.; Pan, W. Galactosylated chitosan-functionalized mesoporous silica nanoparticles for efficient colon cancer cell-targeted drug delivery. *R. Soc. Open Sci.* **2018**, *5*, 181027. [CrossRef]
228. Martínez-Carmona, M.; Lozano, D.; Colilla, M.; Vallet-Regí, M. Lectin-Conjugated pH-Responsive Mesoporous Silica Nanoparticles for Targeted Bone Cancer Treatment. *Acta Biomater.* **2018**, *65*, 393–404. [CrossRef]
229. Zhao, N.; Yang, Z.; Li, B.; Meng, J.; Shi, Z.; Li, P.; Fu, S. RGD-conjugated mesoporous silica-encapsulated gold nanorods enhance the sensitization of triple-negative breast cancer to megavoltage radiation therapy. *Int. J. Nanomed.* **2016**, *11*, 5595–5610. [CrossRef]
230. Wu, X.; Han, Z.; Schur, R.M.; Lu, Z.R. Targeted mesoporous silica nanoparticles delivering arsenic trioxide with environment sensitive drug release for effective treatment of triple negative breast cancer. *ACS Biomater. Sci. Eng.* **2016**, *2*, 501–507. [CrossRef]
231. Zhang, J.; Yuan, Z.F.; Wang, Y.; Chen, W.H.; Luo, G.F.; Cheng, S.X.; Zhuo, R.X.; Zhang, X.Z. Multifunctional envelope-type mesoporous silica nanoparticles for tumor-triggered targeting drug delivery. *J. Am. Chem. Soc.* **2013**, *135*, 5068–5073. [CrossRef]
232. Cheng, Y.J.; Zhang, A.Q.; Hu, J.J.; He, F.; Zeng, X.; Zhang, X.Z. Multifunctional peptide-amphiphile end-capped mesoporous silica nanoparticles for tumor targeting drug delivery. *ACS Appl. Mater. Interfaces* **2017**, *9*, 2093–2103. [CrossRef]
233. Chen, G.; Xie, Y.; Peltier, R.; Lei, H.; Wang, P.; Chen, J.; Hu, Y.; Wang, F.; Yao, X.; Sun, H. Peptide-decorated gold nanoparticles as functional nano-capping agent of mesoporous silica container for targeting drug delivery. *ACS Appl. Mater. Interfaces* **2016**, *8*, 11204–11209. [CrossRef] [PubMed]
234. Xiao, D.; Hu, J.J.; Zhu, J.Y.; Wang, S.B.; Zhuo, R.X.; Zhang, X.Z. A redox-responsive mesoporous silica nanoparticle with a therapeutic peptide shell for tumor targeting synergistic therapy. *Nanoscale* **2016**, *8*, 16702–16709. [CrossRef] [PubMed]
235. Luo, G.F.; Chen, W.H.; Liu, Y.; Zhang, J.; Cheng, S.X.; Zhuo, R.X.; Zhang, X.Z. Charge-reversal plug gate nanovalves on peptide-functionalized mesoporous silica nanoparticles for targeted drug delivery. *J. Mater. Chem. B* **2013**, *1*, 5723–5732. [CrossRef] [PubMed]
236. Zhao, F.; Zhang, C.; Zhao, C.; Gao, W.; Fan, X.; Wu, G. A facile strategy to fabricate a pH-responsive mesoporous silica nanoparticle end-capped with amphiphilic peptides by self-assembly. *Colloids Surf. B Biointerfaces* **2019**, *179*, 352–362. [CrossRef]
237. Li, X.; Xing, L.; Hu, Y.; Xiong, Z.; Wang, R.; Xu, X.; Du, L.; Shen, M.; Shi, X. An RGD-modified hollow silica@Au core/shell nanoplatform for tumor combination therap. *Acta Biomater.* **2017**, *62*, 273–283. [CrossRef]
238. Turan, O.; Bielecki, P.; Tong, K.; Covarrubias, G.; Moon, T.; Rahmy, A.; Cooley, S.; Park, Y.; Peiris, P.M.; Ghaghada, K.B.; et al. Effect of dose and selection of two different ligands on the deposition and antitumor efficacy of targeted nanoparticles in brain tumors. *Mol. Pharmaceutics* **2019**, *16*, 4352–4360. [CrossRef]
239. Hu, J.; Zhang, X.; Wen, Z.; Tan, Y.; Huang, N.; Cheng, S.; Zheng, H.; Cheng, Y. Asn-Gly-Arg-modified polydopamine-coated nanoparticles for dual-targeting therapy of brain glioma in rats. *Oncotarget* **2016**, *7*, 73681–73696. [CrossRef]
240. Babaei, M.; Abnous, K.; Taghdisi, S.M.; Amel Farzad, S.; Peivandi, M.T.; Ramezani, M.; Alibolandi, M. Synthesis of theranostic epithelial cell adhesion molecule targeted mesoporous silica nanoparticle with gold gatekeeper for hepatocellular carcinoma. *Nanomedicine (Lond).* **2017**, *12*, 1261–1279. [CrossRef]
241. Tang, Y.; Hu, H.; Zhang, M.G.; Song, J.; Nie, L.; Wang, S.; Niu, G.; Huang, P.; Lu, G.; Chen, X. An aptamer-targeting photoresponsive drug delivery system using "off-on" graphene oxide wrapped mesoporous silica nanoparticles. *Nanoscale* **2015**, *7*, 6304–6310. [CrossRef]
242. Han, L.; Tang, C.; Yin, C. Dual-targeting and pH/redox-responsive multi-layered nanocomplexes for smart co-delivery of doxorubicin and siRNA. *Biomaterials* **2015**, *60*, 42–52. [CrossRef]
243. Liu, J.; Zhang, B.; Luo, Z.; Ding, X.; Li, J.; Dai, L.; Zhou, J.; Zhao, X.; Ye, J.; Cai, K. Enzyme responsive mesoporous silica nanoparticles for targeted tumor therapy *in vitro* and *in vivo*. *Nanoscale* **2015**, *7*, 3614–3626. [CrossRef] [PubMed]

244. Zhao, J.; Zhao, F.; Wang, X.; Fan, X.; Wu, G. Secondary nuclear targeting of mesoporous silica nano-particles for cancer-specific drug delivery based on charge inversion. *Oncotarget* **2016**, *7*, 70100–70112. [CrossRef] [PubMed]
245. Wei, Y.; Gao, L.; Wang, L.; Shi, L.; Wei, E.; Zhou, B.; Zhou, L.; Ge, B. Polydopamine and peptide decorated doxorubicinloaded mesoporous silica nanoparticles as a targeted drug delivery system for bladder cancer therapy. *Drug Deliv.* **2017**, *24*, 681–691. [CrossRef] [PubMed]
246. Han, L.; Tang, C.; Yin, C. pH-Responsive Core–Shell Structured Nanoparticles for Triple-Stage Targeted Delivery of Doxorubicin to Tumors. *ACS Appl. Mater. Interfaces* **2016**, *8*, 23498–23508. [CrossRef]
247. Zhao, Q.; Geng, H.; Wang, Y.; Gao, Y.; Huang, J.; Wang, Y.; Zhang, J.; Wang, S. Hyaluronic acid oligosaccharide modified redox-responsive mesoporous silica nanoparticles for targeted drug delivery. *ACS Appl. Mater. Interfaces* **2014**, *6*, 20290–20299. [CrossRef]
248. Fang, Z.; Li, X.; Xu, Z.; Du, F.; Wang, W.; Shi, R.; Gao, D. Hyaluronic acid-modified mesoporous silica-coated superparamagnetic Fe_3O_4 nanoparticles for targeted drug delivery. *Int. J. Nanomed.* **2019**, *14*, 5785–5797. [CrossRef]
249. Li, T.; Geng, Y.; Zhang, H.; Wang, J.; Feng, Y.; Chen, Z.; Xie, X.; Qin, X.; Li, S.; Wu, C.; et al. Versatile nanoplatform for synergistic chemo-photothermal therapy and multimodal imaging against breast cancer. *Expert Opin. Drug Del.* **2020**, *17*, 725–733. [CrossRef]
250. Zhang, Y.; Xu, J. Mesoporous silica nanoparticle-based intelligent drug delivery system for bienzyme-responsive tumour targeting and controlled release. *R. Soc. Open Sci.* **2018**, *5*, 170986. [CrossRef]
251. Liu, Y.; Dai, R.; Wei, Q.; Li, W.; Zhu, G.; Chi, H.; Guo, Z.; Wang, L.; Cui, C.; Xu, J.; et al. Dual-functionalized janus mesoporous silica nanoparticles with active targeting and charge reversal for synergistic tumor-targeting therapy. *ACS Appl. Mater. Interfaces* **2019**, *11*, 44582–44592. [CrossRef]
252. Lu, H.; Zhao, Q.; Wang, X.; Mao, Y.; Chen, C.; Gao, Y.; Sun, C. Siling Wang. Multi-stimuli responsive mesoporous silica-coated carbon nanoparticles for chemo-photothermal therapy of tumor. *Colloids Surf. B* **2020**, *190*, 110941. [CrossRef]
253. Zhou, S.; Ding, C.; Wang, C.; Fu, J. UV-light cross-linked and pH de-cross-linked coumarin-decorated cationic copolymer grafted mesoporous silica nanoparticles for drug and gene co-delivery *in vitro*. *Mater. Sci. Eng. C* **2019**. [CrossRef]
254. Xu, Y.; Xiao, L.; Chang, Y.; Cao, Y.; Chen, C.; Wang, D. pH and redox dual-responsive MSN-S-S-CS as a drug delivery system in cancer therapy. *Materials* **2020**, *13*, 1279. [CrossRef]
255. Li, Y.; Hei, M.; Xu, Y.; Qian, X.; Zhu, W. Ammonium salt modified mesoporous silica nanoparticles for dual intracellular-responsive gene delivery. *Int. J. Pharm.* **2016**, *511*, 689–702. [CrossRef]
256. Yan, J.; Xu, X.; Zhou, J.; Liu, C.; Zhang, L.; Wang, D.; Yang, F.; Zhang, H. Fabrication of a pH/redox-triggered mesoporous silica-based nanoparticle with microfluidics for anticancer drugs doxorubicin and paclitaxel codelivery. *ACS Appl. Bio Mater.* **2020**, *3*, 1216–1225. [CrossRef]
257. Anirudhan, T.S.; Nair, A.S. Temperature and ultrasound sensitive gatekeepers for the controlled release of chemotherapeutic drugs from mesoporous silica nanoparticles. *J. Mater. Chem. B* **2018**, *6*, 428–439. [CrossRef]
258. Lee, J.E.; Lee, N.; Kim, T.; Kim, J.; Hyeon, T. Multifunctional mesoporous silica nanocomposite nanoparticles for theranostic applications. *Acc. Chem. Res.* **2011**, *44*, 893–902. [CrossRef]
259. Nakamura, T.; Sugihara, F.; Matsushita, H.; Yoshioka, Y.; Mizukami, S.; Kikuchi, K. Mesoporous silica nanoparticles for (19)F magnetic resonance imaging, fluorescence imaging, and drug delivery. *Chem. Sci.* **2015**, *6*, 1986–1990. [CrossRef]
260. Chen, N.-T.; Cheng, S.-H.; Souris, J.S.; Chen, C.-T.; Mou, C.-Y.; Lo, L.-W. Theranostic applications of mesoporous silica nanoparticles and their organic/inorganic hybrids. *J. Mater. Chem. B* **2013**, *1*, 3128. [CrossRef]
261. Wu, X.; Wu, M.; Zhao, J.X. Recent development of silica nanoparticles as delivery vectors for cancer imaging and therapy. *Nanomedicine (Lond).* **2014**, *10*, 297–312. [CrossRef]
262. Cassidy, M.C.; Chan, H.R.; Ross, B.D.; Bhattacharya, P.K.; Marcus, C.M. *In vivo* magnetic resonance imaging of hyperpolarized silicon particles. *Nat. Nanotechnol.* **2013**, *8*, 363–368. [CrossRef]
263. Feng, Y.; Panwar, N.; Tng, D.J.H.; Tjin, S.C.; Wang, K.; Yong, K.-T. The application of mesoporous silica nanoparticle family in cancer theranostics. *Coord. Chem. Rev.* **2016**, *319*, 86–109. [CrossRef]
264. Matsushita, H.; Mizukami, S.; Sugihara, F.; Nakanishi, Y.; Yoshioka, Y.; Kikuchi, K. Multifunctional core-shell silica nanoparticles for highly sensitive (19)F magnetic resonance imaging. *Angew. Chem. Int. Ed. Engl.* **2014**, *53*, 1008–1011. [CrossRef] [PubMed]

265. Milgroom, A.; Intrator, M.; Madhavan, K.; Mazzaro, L.; Shandas, R.; Liu, B.L.; Park, D. Mesoporous Silica Nanoparticles as a Breast-Cancer Targeting Ultrasound Contrast Agent. *Colloids Surf. B Biointerfaces* **2014**, *116*, 652–657. [CrossRef] [PubMed]
266. Cha, B.G.; Kim, J. Functional mesoporous silica nanoparticles for bio-imaging applications. *Wiley Interdiscip. Rev. Nanomed. Nanobiotechnol.* **2019**, *11*, e1515. [CrossRef]
267. Bouamrani, A.; Hu, Y.; Tasciotti, E.; Li, L.; Chiappini, C.; Liu, X.; Ferrari, M. Mesoporous silica chips for selective enrichment and stabilization of low molecular weight proteome. *Proteomics* **2010**, *10*, 496–505. [CrossRef]
268. Jäger, T.; Szarvas, T.; Börgermann, C.; Schenck, M.; Schmid, K.; Rübben, H. Use of silicon chip technology to detect protein-based tumor markers in bladder cancer. *Der Urologe. Ausg. A* **2007**, *46*, 1152–1156. [CrossRef]
269. Liang, K.; Wu, H.; Hu, T.Y.; Li, Y. Mesoporous silica chip: Enabled peptide profiling as an effective platform for controlling bio-sample quality and optimizing handling procedure. *Clin. Proteom* **2016**, *13*, 34. [CrossRef]
270. Hu, Y.; Bouamrani, A.; Tasciotti, E.; Li, L.; Liu, X.W.; Ferrari, M. Tailoring of the nanotexture of mesoporous silica films and their functionalized derivatives for selectively harvesting low molecular weight protein. *ACS Nano* **2010**, *4*, 439–451. [CrossRef]
271. Hu, Y.; Peng, Y.; Lin, K.; Shen, H.; Brousseau, L.C., 3rd; Sakamoto, J.; Sun, T.; Ferrari, M. Surface engineering on mesoporous silica chips for enriching low molecular weight phosphorylated proteins. *Nanoscale* **2011**, *3*, 421–428. [CrossRef]
272. Wang, K.; He, X.; Yang, X.; Shi, H. Functionalized silica nanoparticles: A platform for fluorescence imaging at the cell and small animal levels. *Acc. Chem. Res.* **2013**, *46*, 1367–1376. [CrossRef]
273. Shi, S.; Chen, F.; Cai, W. Biomedical applications of functionalized hollow mesoporous silica nanoparticles: Focusing on molecular imaging. *Nanomedicine* **2013**, *8*, 2027–2039. [CrossRef] [PubMed]
274. Alford, R.; Simpson, H.M.; Duberman, J.; Hill, G.C.; Ogawa, M.; Regino, C.; Kobayashi, H.; Choyke, P.L. Toxicity of organic fluorophores used in molecular imaging: Literature review. *Mol. Imaging* **2009**, *8*, 341–354. [CrossRef] [PubMed]
275. Kesse, S.; Boakye-Yiadom, K.O.; Ochete, B.O.; Opoku-Damoah, Y.; Akhtar, F.; Filli, M.S.; Farooq, M.A.; Aquib, M.; Mily, B.J.M.; Murtaza, G.; et al. Mesoporous silica nanomaterials: Versatile nanocarriers for cancer theranostics and drug and gene delivery. *Pharmaceutics* **2019**, *11*, 77. [CrossRef] [PubMed]
276. Yin, F.; Zhang, B.; Zeng, S.; Lin, G.; Tian, J.; Yang, C.; Wang, K.; Xu, G.; Yong, K.-T. Folic acid-conjugated organically modified silica nanoparticles for enhanced targeted delivery in cancer cells and tumor in vivo. *J. Mater. Chem. B* **2015**, *3*, 6081–6093. [CrossRef] [PubMed]
277. Resch-Genger, U.; Grabolle, M.; Cavaliere-Jaricot, S.; Nitschke, R.; Nann, T. Quantum dots versus organic dyes as fluorescent labels. *Nat. Methods* **2008**, *5*, 763–775. [CrossRef]
278. Jun, B.H.; Hwang, D.W.; Jung, H.S.; Jang, J.; Kim, H.; Kang, H.; Kang, T.; Kyeong, S.; Lee, H.; Jeong, D.H.; et al. Ultrasensitive, biocompatible, quantum-dot-embedded silica nanoparticles for bioimaging. *Adv. Funct. Mater.* **2012**, *22*, 1843–1849. [CrossRef]
279. Zhou, S.; Huo, D.; Hou, C.; Yang, M.; Fa, H.; Xia, C.; Chen, M. Mesoporous silica-coated quantum dots functionalized with folic acid for lung cancer cell imaging. *Anal. Methods* **2015**, *7*, 9649–9654. [CrossRef]
280. Cheng, S.-H.; Lee, C.-H.; Chen, M.-C.; Souris, J.S.; Tseng, F.-G.; Yang, C.-S.; Mou, C.-Y.; Chen, C.-T.; Lo, L.-W. Tri-functionalization of mesoporous silica nanoparticles for comprehensive cancer theranostics—The trio of imaging, targeting and therapy. *J. Mater. Chem.* **2010**, *20*, 6149–6157. [CrossRef]
281. Ribeiro, T.; Rodrigues, A.S.; Calderon, S.; Fidalgo, A.; Gonçalves, J.L.M.; André, V.; Teresa Duarte, M.; Ferreira, P.J.; Farinha, J.P.S.; Baleizão, C. Silica nanocarriers with user-defined precise diameters by controlled template self-assembly. *J. Colloid Interface Sci.* **2020**, *561*, 609–619. [CrossRef]
282. He, Q.; Zhang, J.; Shi, J.; Zhu, Z.; Zhang, L.; Bu, W.; Guo, L.; Chen, Y. The effect of PEGylation of mesoporous silica nanoparticles on nonspecific binding of serum proteins and cellular responses. *Biomaterials* **2010**, *31*, 1085–1092. [CrossRef]
283. Manzano, M.; Vallet-Regí, M. Mesoporous silica nanoparticles for drug delivery. *Adv. Funct. Mater.* **2019**, 1902634. [CrossRef]
284. Farjadian, F.; Roointan, A.; Mohammadi-Samani, S.; Hosseini, M. Mesoporous silica nanoparticles: Synthesis, pharmaceutical applications, biodistribution, and biosafety assessment. *Chem. Eng. J.* **2019**, *359*, 684–705. [CrossRef]

285. Li, Z.; Zhang, Y.; Feng, N. Mesoporous silica nanoparticles: Synthesis, classification, drug loading, pharmacokinetics, biocompatibility, and application in drug delivery. *Expert Opin. Drug Deliv.* **2019**, *16*, 219–237. [CrossRef] [PubMed]
286. Rosenholm, J.M.; Mamaeva, V.; Sahlgren, C.; Linden, M. Nanoparticles in targeted cancer therapy: Mesoporous silica nanoparticles entering preclinical development Stage. *Nanomedicine* **2012**, *7*, 111–120. [CrossRef] [PubMed]
287. Huang, X.; Li, L.; Liu, T.; Hao, N.; Liu, H.; Chen, D.; Tang, F. The shape effect of mesoporous silica nanoparticles on biodistribution, clearance, and biocompatibility in vivo. *ACS Nano* **2011**, *5*, 5390–5399. [CrossRef]
288. Yu, T.; Hubbard, D.; Ray, A.; Ghandehari, H. *In vivo* biodistribution and pharmacokinetics of silica nanoparticles as a function of geometry, porosity and surface characteristics. *J. Control. Release* **2012**, *163*, 46–54. [CrossRef]
289. Li, L.; Liu, T.; Fu, C.; Tan, L.; Meng, X.; Liu, H. Biodistribution, excretion, and toxicity of mesoporous silica nanoparticles after oral administration depend on their shape. *Nanomed. Nanotechnol. Biol. Med.* **2015**, *11*, 1915–1924. [CrossRef]
290. Dogra, P.; Adolphi, N.L.; Wang, Z.; Lin, Y.-S.; Butler, K.S.; Durfee, P.N.; Croissant, J.G.; Noureddine, A.; Coker, E.N.; Bearer, E.L.; et al. Establishing the effects of mesoporous silica nanoparticle properties on *in vivo* disposition using imaging-based pharmacokinetics. *Nat. Commun.* **2018**, *9*, 4551. [CrossRef]
291. Sun, J.-G.; Jiang, Q.; Zhang, X.-P.; Shan, K.; Liu, B.-H.; Zhao, C.; Yan, B. Mesoporous silica nanoparticles as a delivery system for improving antiangiogenic therapy. *Int. J. Nanomed.* **2019**, *14*, 1489–1501. [CrossRef]
292. Kong, M.; Tang, J.; Qiao, Q.; Wu, T.; Qi, Y.; Tan, S.; Gao, X.; Zhang, Z. Biodegradable hollow mesoporous silica nanoparticles for regulating tumor microenvironment and enhancing antitumor efficiency. *Theranostics* **2017**, *7*, 3276–3292. [CrossRef]
293. Paula, A.J.; Araujo Júnior, R.T.; Martinez, D.S.T.; Paredes-Gamero, E.J.; Nader, H.B.; Durán, N.; Justo, G.Z.; Alves, O.L. Influence of protein corona on the transport of molecules into cells by mesoporous silica nanoparticles. *ACS Appl. Mater. Interfaces* **2013**, *5*, 8387–8393. [CrossRef] [PubMed]
294. Visalakshan, R.M.; García, L.E.G.; Benzigar, M.R.; Ghazaryan, A.; Simon, J.; Mierczynska-Vasilev, A.; Michl, T.D.; Vinu, A.; Mailänder, V.; Morsbach, S.; et al. The influence of nanoparticle shape on protein corona formation. *Small Nano Micro.* **2020**. [CrossRef]
295. Cauda, V.; Engelke, H.; Sauer, A.; Arcizet, D.; Bräuchle, C.; Rädler, J.; Bein, T. Colchicine-loaded lipid bilayer-coated 50 nm mesoporous nanoparticles efficiently induce microtubule depolymerization upon cell uptake. *Nano Lett.* **2010**, *10*, 2484–2492. [CrossRef]
296. Fei, W.; Zhang, Y.; Han, S.; Tao, J.; Zheng, H.; Wei, Y.; Zhu, J.; Li, F.; Wang, X. RGD conjugated liposome-hollow silica hybrid nanovehicles for targeted and controlled delivery of arsenic trioxide against hepatic carcinoma. *Int. J. Pharm.* **2017**, *519*, 250–262. [CrossRef]
297. Mackowiak, S.A.; Schmidt, A.; Weiss, V.; Argyo, C.; Constantin von Schirnding, C.; Bein, T.; Bräuchle, C. Targeted drug delivery in cancer cells with red-light photoactivated mesoporous silica nanoparticles. *Nano Lett.* **2013**, *13*, 2576–2583. [CrossRef]
298. Li, Y.; Miao, Y.; Chen, M.; Chen, X.; Li, F.; Zhang, X.; Gan, Y. Stepwise targeting and responsive lipid-coated nanoparticles for enhanced tumor cell sensitivity and hepatocellular carcinoma therapy. *Theranostics* **2020**, *10*, 3722–3736. [CrossRef]
299. Durfee, P.N.; Lin, Y.S.; Darren, R.; Dunphy, D.R.; Muñiz, A.J.; Butler, K.S.; Humphrey, K.R.; Lokke, A.J.; Agola, J.O.; Chou, S.S.; et al. Mesoporous silica nanoparticle-supported lipid bilayers (protocells) for active targeting and delivery to individual leukemia cells. *ACS Nano* **2016**, *10*, 8325–8345. [CrossRef]
300. Butler, K.S.; Durfee, P.N.; Theron, C.; Ashley, C.E.; Carnes, E.C.; Brinker, C.J. Protocells: Modular mesoporous silica nanoparticlesupported lipid bilayers for drug delivery. *Small* **2016**, *12*, 2173–2185. [CrossRef] [PubMed]
301. Samanta, S.; Pradhan, L.; Bahadur, D. Mesoporous lipid-silica nanohybrids for folate-targeted drug-resistant ovarian cancer. *New J. Chem.* **2018**, *42*, 2804–2814. [CrossRef]
302. Pan, G.; Jia, T.T.; Huang, Q.X.; Qiu, Y.Y.; Xu, J.; Yin, P.H.; Liu, T. Mesoporous silica nanoparticles (MSNs)-based organic/inorganic hybrid nanocarriers loading 5-Fluorouracil for the treatment of colon cancer with improved anticancer efficacy. *Colloids Surf. B Biointerfaces* **2017**, *159*, 375–385. [CrossRef]

303. Hu, B.; Wang, J.; Li, J.; Li, S.; Li, H. Superiority of L-tartaric acid modified chiral mesoporous silica nanoparticle as a drug carrier: Structure, wettability, degradation, bio-adhesion and biocompatibility. *Int. J. Nanomed.* **2020**, *15*, 601–618. [CrossRef] [PubMed]
304. Wang, B.; Zhang, K.; Wang, J.; Zhao, R.; Zhang, Q.; Kong, X. Poly(amidoamine)-modified mesoporous silica nanoparticles as a mucoadhesive drug delivery system for potential bladder cancer therapy. *Colloids Surf. B Biointerfaces* **2020**, *189*. [CrossRef] [PubMed]
305. Guimarães, R.S.; Rodrigues, C.F.; Moreira, A.F.; Correia, I.J. Overview of stimuli-responsive mesoporous organosilica nanocarriers for drug delivery. *Pharmacol. Res.* **2020**, *155*, 104742. [CrossRef]
306. Liu, C.M.; Chen, G.B.; Chen, H.H.; Zhang, J.B.; Li, H.Z.; Sheng, M.X.; Weng, W.B.; Guo, S.M. Cancer cell membrane-cloaked mesoporous silica nanoparticles with a pH-sensitive gatekeeper for cancer treatment. *Colloids Surf. B Biointerfaces* **2019**, *175*, 477–486. [CrossRef] [PubMed]
307. Yue, J.; Wang, Z.; Shao, D.; Chang, Z.; Hu, R.; Li, L.; Luo, S.; Dong, W. Cancer cell membrane-modified biodegradable mesoporous silica nanocarriers for berberine therapy of liver cancer. *RSC Adv.* **2018**, *8*, 40288–40297. [CrossRef]
308. Cauda, V.; Limongi, T.; Racca, L.; Canta, M.; Susa, F.; Piva, R.; Bergaggio, E.; Vitale, N.; Mereu, E. A biomimetic nanoporous carrier comprising an inhibitor directed towards the native form of IDH2 protein. Patent IB 2020/050401, 23 January 2019.

Permissions

All chapters in this book were first published by MDPI; hereby published with permission under the Creative Commons Attribution License or equivalent. Every chapter published in this book has been scrutinized by our experts. Their significance has been extensively debated. The topics covered herein carry significant findings which will fuel the growth of the discipline. They may even be implemented as practical applications or may be referred to as a beginning point for another development.

The contributors of this book come from diverse backgrounds, making this book a truly international effort. This book will bring forth new frontiers with its revolutionizing research information and detailed analysis of the nascent developments around the world.

We would like to thank all the contributing authors for lending their expertise to make the book truly unique. They have played a crucial role in the development of this book. Without their invaluable contributions this book wouldn't have been possible. They have made vital efforts to compile up to date information on the varied aspects of this subject to make this book a valuable addition to the collection of many professionals and students.

This book was conceptualized with the vision of imparting up-to-date information and advanced data in this field. To ensure the same, a matchless editorial board was set up. Every individual on the board went through rigorous rounds of assessment to prove their worth. After which they invested a large part of their time researching and compiling the most relevant data for our readers.

The editorial board has been involved in producing this book since its inception. They have spent rigorous hours researching and exploring the diverse topics which have resulted in the successful publishing of this book. They have passed on their knowledge of decades through this book. To expedite this challenging task, the publisher supported the team at every step. A small team of assistant editors was also appointed to further simplify the editing procedure and attain best results for the readers.

Apart from the editorial board, the designing team has also invested a significant amount of their time in understanding the subject and creating the most relevant covers. They scrutinized every image to scout for the most suitable representation of the subject and create an appropriate cover for the book.

The publishing team has been an ardent support to the editorial, designing and production team. Their endless efforts to recruit the best for this project, has resulted in the accomplishment of this book. They are a veteran in the field of academics and their pool of knowledge is as vast as their experience in printing. Their expertise and guidance has proved useful at every step. Their uncompromising quality standards have made this book an exceptional effort. Their encouragement from time to time has been an inspiration for everyone.

The publisher and the editorial board hope that this book will prove to be a valuable piece of knowledge for researchers, students, practitioners and scholars across the globe.

List of Contributors

Joanna Goscianska, Aleksander Ejsmont and Anna Olejnik
Department of Chemical Technology, Faculty of Chemistry, Adam Mickiewicz University in Poznań, Uniwersytetu Poznańskiego 8, 61-614 Poznań, Poland

Dominika Ludowicz, Anna Stasiłowicz and Judyta Cielecka-Piontek
Department of Pharmacognosy, Faculty of Pharmacy, Poznań University of Medical Sciences, Święcickiego 4, 61-781 Poznań, Poland

Sumita Swar, Veronika Máková and Ivan Stibor
Department of Nanomaterials in Natural Science, Institute for Nanomaterials, Advanced Technologies and Innovation, Technical University of Liberec, Studentská 1402/2, 46117 Liberec, Czech Republic

Katarzyna Wasilewska and Katarzyna Winnicka
Department of Pharmaceutical Technology, Medical University of Białystok, Mickiewicza 2c, 15-222 Białystok, Poland

Patrycja Ciosek-Skibińska
Chair of Medical Biotechnology, Warsaw University of Technology, Noakowskiego 3, 00 664 Warsaw, Poland

Joanna Lenik
Department of Analytical Chemistry and Instrumental Analysis, Faculty of Chemistry, Maria Curie-Skłodowska University, M. Curie-Skłodowska Sq. 3, 20-031 Lublin, Poland

Stanko Srčič
Department of Pharmaceutical Technology, University of Ljubljana, Aškerčeva c. 7, 1000 Ljubljana, Slovenia

Anna Basa
Department of Physical Chemistry, Faculty of Chemistry, University of Białystok, Ciołkowskiego 1K, 15-245 Białystok, Poland

Muhammad Faizan, Yongxia Hu, Yanyan Wang, Ya Wu, Huaming Sun, Wensheng Dong, Weiqiang Zhang and Ziwei Gao
Key Laboratory of Applied Surface and Colloid Chemistry MOE, School of Chemistry and Chemical Engineering, Shaanxi Normal University, Xi'an 710062, China

Niaz Muhammad
Department of Biochemistry, College of Life Sciences, Shaanxi Normal University, Xi'an 710062, China

Kifayat Ullah Khan Niazi
School of Materials Science and Engineering, Xi'an Jiaotong University, Xi'an 710049, China

Ruixia Liu
Institute of Process Engineering, Chinese Academy of Science, Beijing 100190, China

Xuewu Liu
Department of Nanomedicine, Houston Methodist Research Institute, Houston, TX 77030, USA

Nicola Di Trani
Department of Nanomedicine, Houston Methodist Research Institute, Houston, TX 77030, USA
University of Chinese Academy of Science (UCAS), Shijingshan, 19 Yuquan Road, Beijing 100049, China

Antonia Silvestri
Department of Nanomedicine, Houston Methodist Research Institute, Houston, TX 77030, USA
Department of Electronics and Telecommunications, Polytechnic of Turin, 10129 Turin, Italy

Danilo Demarchi
Department of Electronics and Telecommunications, Polytechnic of Turin, 10129 Turin, Italy

Alessandro Grattoni
Department of Nanomedicine, Houston Methodist Research Institute, Houston, TX 77030, USA
Department of Surgery, Houston Methodist Hospital, Houston, TX 77030, USA
Department of Radiation Oncology, Houston Methodist Hospital, Houston, TX 77030, USA

Kun Nie, Xiang Yu and Yihe Zhang
Beijing Key Laboratory of Materials Utilization of Nonmetallic Minerals and Solid Wastes, National Laboratory of Mineral Materials, School of Materials Science and Technology, China University of Geosciences (Beijing), Beijing 100083, China

Navnita Kumar
Department of Chemistry and Biochemistry, University of California, Los Angeles, CA 90095, USA

Qing Min, Yuchen Zhang and Jiliang Wu
School of Pharmacy, Hubei University of Science and Technology, Xianning 437100, China

Xiaofeng Yu, Jiaoyan Liu and Ying Wan
College of Life Science and Technology, Huazhong University of Science and Technology, Wuhan 430074, China

Witold Jamróz, Jolanta Pyteraf, Mateusz Kurek, Joanna Szafraniec-Szczęsny and Renata Jachowicz
Department of Pharmaceutical Technology and Biopharmaceutics, Jagiellonian University Medical College, Medyczna 9, 30-688 Krakow, Poland

Justyna Knapik-Kowalczuk, Karolina Jurkiewicz and Marian Paluch
Division of Biophysics and Molecular Physics, Institute of Physics, University of Silesia, Uniwersytecka 4, 40-007 Katowice, Poland
Silesian Center for Education and Interdisciplinary Research, University of Silesia, 75 Pulku Piechoty 1a, 41-500 Chorzow, Poland

Bartosz Leszczyński and Andrzej Wróbel
Marian Smoluchowski Institute of Physics, Jagiellonian University, Łojasiewicza 11, 30-348 Krakow, Poland

Tania Limongi, Francesca Susa and Enzo di Fabrizio
Dipartimento di Scienza Applicata e Tecnologia, Politecnico di Torino, Corso Duca Degli Abruzzi 24, 10129 Torino, Italy

Marco Allione
SMILEs Lab, PSE Division, King Abdullah University of Science and Technology, Thuwal 23955-6900, Saudi Arabia

Nan Xu, Dan Wang, Qin Gao, Siyu Xie and Yage Li
State Key Laboratory of New Ceramics and Fine Processing, School of Materials Science and Engineering, Tsinghua University, Beijing 100084, China
Key Laboratory of Advanced Materials of Ministry of Education of China, Tsinghua University, Beijing 100084, China

Yu Wang
State Key Laboratory of New Ceramics and Fine Processing, School of Materials Science and Engineering, Tsinghua University, Beijing 100084, China
Key Laboratory of Advanced Materials of Ministry of Education of China, Tsinghua University, Beijing 100084, China
Department of Nanomedicine, Houston Methodist Research Institute, Houston, TX 77030, USA

Yongkai He and Qiang Cai
State Key Laboratory of New Ceramics and Fine Processing, School of Materials Science and Engineering, Tsinghua University, Beijing 100084, China
Key Laboratory of Advanced Materials of Ministry of Education of China, Tsinghua University, Beijing 100084, China
Tsinghua Shenzhen International Graduate School, Tsinghua University, Shenzhen 518055, China

Ranran Zhang
Tsinghua Shenzhen International Graduate School, Tsinghua University, Shenzhen 518055, China

Jingyun Wang
Shenzhen Geim Graphene Center, Tsinghua-Berkeley Shenzhen Institute, Tsinghua University, Shenzhen 518055, China

Bartosz Maciejewski and Małgorzata Sznitowska
Department of Pharmaceutical Technology, Medical University of Gdansk, 80-416 Gdansk, Poland

Vishnu Arumughan and Anette Larsson
Department of Chemistry and Chemical Engineering, Chalmers University of Technology, 412 96 Gothenburg, Sweden

Sugata Barui and Valentina Cauda
Department of Applied Science and Technology, Politecnico di Torino, Corso Duca degli Abruzzi 24, 10129 Turin, Italy

Index

Printed in the USA
CPSIA information can be obtained
at www.ICGtesting.com
JSHW051625061123
51533JS00005B/109